Nutrition and Health

Series Editors

Adrianne Bendich
Wellington, FL, USA

Connie W. Bales
Durham VA Medical Center
Duke University School of Medicine
Durham, NC, USA

The Nutrition and Health series has an overriding mission in providing health professionals with texts that are considered essential since each is edited by the leading researchers in their respective fields. Each volume includes: 1) a synthesis of the state of the science, 2) timely, in-depth reviews, 3) extensive, up-to-date fully annotated reference lists, 4) a detailed index, 5) relevant tables and figures, 6) identification of paradigm shifts and consequences, 7) virtually no overlap of information between chapters, but targeted, inter-chapter referrals, 8) suggestions of areas for future research and 9) balanced, data driven answers to patient/health professionals questions which are based upon the totality of evidence rather than the findings of a single study.

Nutrition and Health is a major resource of relevant, clinically based nutrition volumes for the professional that serve as a reliable source of data-driven reviews and practice guidelines.

More information about this series at http://www.springer.com/series/7659

Jaime Uribarri • Joseph A. Vassalotti

Editors

Nutrition, Fitness, and Mindfulness

An Evidence-Based Guide for Clinicians

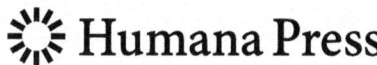 Humana Press

Editors
Jaime Uribarri
Division of Nephrology,
Department of Medicine
Icahn School of Medicine
at Mount Sinai
New York, NY, USA

Joseph A. Vassalotti
Division of Nephrology,
Department of Medicine,
Icahn School of Medicine at Mount Sinai
New York, NY, USA

The National Kidney Foundation, Inc.
New York, NY, USA

Nutrition and Health
ISBN 978-3-030-30894-0   ISBN 978-3-030-30892-6   (eBook)
https://doi.org/10.1007/978-3-030-30892-6

This Humana imprint is published by the registered company Springer Nature Switzerland AG
The registered company address is: Gewerbestrasse 11, 6330 Cham, Switzerland

Preface

Current dietary patterns evolved over millennia as humans transitioned from foraging to farming to fast food. The industrialization of modern society has enabled the distribution of antibiotics, as well as vaccinations, so that premature mortality from acute infection plummeted in the population over the last century, but at the same time it fostered a sedentary lifestyle. Today, the combination of plentiful, inexpensive, and processed food and low physical activity has culminated in an epidemic of obesity and a mosaic of chronic illness, including type-2 diabetes, cardiovascular disease (CVD), and chronic kidney disease (CKD). Morbidity and mortality from these diseases associated with sustained oxidative stress and microinflammation is the greatest challenge facing contemporary medicine. Practitioners have focused on drug therapy and, to a lesser degree, on medicalisation of food with emphasis on the limitation of deleterious elements such as sodium, polyunsaturated fats, and phosphorus. For the patient, navigating multiple chronic conditions, polypharmacy, and a "thou shalt not eat" dietary approach is daunting, discouraging, and difficult to integrate into daily life.

Incorporating healthy and tasty food, active living, and adequate refreshing sleep are all important elements to promote health, to prevent obesity, and to reduce the risk for type-2 diabetes, hypertension, and ultimately CVD and CKD. Large epidemiological studies have shown that the Mediterranean and Dietary Approaches to Stop Hypertension (DASH) diets reduce CVD and incident CKD. There is an existing evidence base in the literature supporting the importance of physical activity to improve cardiovascular health and improve chronic disease management. Like nutrition, physical activity is an essential ingredient of health. Medical literature demonstrates ancient practices of mindfulness have remarkable relevance to health in the twenty-first century for the receptive and motivated individual. Clinicians may know these concepts intuitively, but they need information and tools to help their patients live and schedule their lives accordingly for better health. Hitherto, curricular activities of medical schools emphasize pharmacotherapy rather than lifestyle modification.

The current book presents an approach based on cutting-edge clinical science to the integration of healthy behaviors in clinical practice using three major categories: healthy eating, active living, and mindfulness. A select group of national and international experts in their respective fields develops these concepts for application in routine practice. The editors summarize these approaches in a conclusion.

We are grateful to our collaborators who made this book possible, including the chapter authors, Adrianne Bendich, Samantha Lonuzzi, Kevin Wright, and Springer International Publishing AG.

New York, NY, USA   Jaime Uribarri, MD
                                                                                Joseph A. Vassalotti, MD

Series Editor Page

The great success of the Nutrition and Health Series is the result of the consistent overriding mission of providing health professionals with texts that are essential because each includes (1) a synthesis of the state of the science; (2) timely, in-depth reviews by the leading researchers and clinicians in their respective fields; (3) extensive, up-to-date fully annotated reference lists; (4) a detailed index; (5) relevant tables and figures; (6) identification of paradigm shifts and the consequences; (7) virtually no overlap of information between chapters but targeted, interchapter referrals; (8) suggestions of areas for future research; and (9) balanced, data-driven answers to patient and health professional questions that are based upon the totality of evidence rather than the findings of any single study.

The series volumes are not the outcome of a symposium. Rather, each editor has the potential to examine a chosen area with a broad perspective, both in the subject matter and the choice of chapter authors. The international perspective, especially with regard to public health initiatives, is emphasized where appropriate. The editors, whose trainings are both research and practice oriented, have the opportunity to develop a primary objective for their book, define the scope and focus, and then invite the leading authorities from around the world to be part of their initiative. The authors are encouraged to provide an overview of the field, discuss their own research, and relate the research findings to potential human health consequences. Because each book is developed de novo, the chapters are coordinated so that the resulting volume imparts greater knowledge than the sum of the information contained in the individual chapters.

Nutrition, Fitness, and Mindfulness, edited by Dr. Jaime Uribarri and Dr. Joseph A. Vassalotti, is a very welcome and timely addition to the Nutrition and Health Series and fully exemplifies the series' goals. As clearly stated in the book's title, the editors have identified a major paradigm shift in the management of clinical practice, and the included chapters review the current literature concerning the potential for beneficial consequences when a more holistic approach is taken with patient care. There has been a continuous stream of basic and clinical research over the last decade that has stressed the interactions between exercise, sleep quality, mindfulness programs, and recommended diet patterns. Significant reductions in the ability of patients to cope with serious noncommunicable diseases that are the leading causes of death across economically advantaged countries have been documented. This unique, holistic volume is designed to be an objective resource for clinicians and other health professionals who interact with patients and their families, as well as for graduate and medical students anticipating interactions with patients.

The editors of this volume for health professionals are both clinicians who have extensive experience in patient care, as well as clinical research. Dr. Jaime Uribarri, MD, received his medical degree from the University of Chile School of Medicine and did his postgraduate training in the United States. He has been at the Icahn School of Medicine at Mount Sinai, NYC, since 1990, where he is currently a professor of medicine and director of the Renal Clinic and the Home Dialysis Program at the Mount Sinai Hospital. Dr. Uribarri's main areas of research have been on acid-base, fluid, and electrolyte disorders, as well as nutrition in chronic kidney disease and diabetic patients. He has published over 150 peer-reviewed papers and written many chapters in books. He has lectured extensively on these research topics in New York City, as well as in national and international meetings. Dr. Uribarri has edited a book for health professionals on dietary advanced glycosylated end products (AGEs) and coedited another volume on dietary phosphorus. He serves as a peer reviewer for numerous nutrition, medical, and other scientific journals, and he is an active member of several professional health-related organizations, including the American Society of Nephrology, the American Society for Nutrition, the International Society of Nephrology, The New York Academy of Sciences, and The Maillard Society.

Dr. Joseph A. Vassalotti, MD, is a nephrologist who serves as the chief medical officer of the National Kidney Foundation (NKF) and associate clinical professor of medicine in the Division of Nephrology, at the Icahn School of Medicine at Mount Sinai. He received his medical degree with Distinction in Research from the SUNY Stony Brook School of Medicine and completed an Internal Medicine Residency and Nephrology Fellowship at the Johns Hopkins Hospital. He served on the clinical faculty at George Washington University School of Medicine from 1995 to 2000, where he won the fulltime faculty teaching award in 1998. Since 2000, he has developed an international clinical practice at the Icahn School of Medicine at Mount Sinai and served as Director of Hemodialysis from 2000 to 2005. At the NKF, his major focus is the implementation of evidence-based clinical practice guidelines in chronic kidney disease (CKD), including the NKF's Kidney Disease Outcomes Quality Initiative (KDOQI). He has served as co-PI for the CDC Demonstration Project "CKD Health Evaluation and Risk Information Sharing (CHERISH)," which aimed to identify individuals at high risk for CKD in the USA; he also served as an investigator for the NIH-sponsored clustered practice randomized trial concerning evidenced-based primary care for CKD. Leadership also includes multiple roles over the last decade with the CMS Fistula First national quality improvement initiative for hemodialysis, including as lead physician consultant from 2013 through 2015. He has served in numerous committees that shape innovation and health policy in kidney disease for the CDC, the NIH, and CMS. Currently, he serves as the principal investigator for the Kidney Score Platform, an NKF educational project funded by the Veterans Administration Center for Innovation to improve awareness and education among veterans with and/or at risk for CKD in the primary care setting. Dr. Vassalotti has over 100 publications in peer-reviewed journals and has been featured in Castle Connolly's Top Doctors and Best Doctors in America. Dr. Vassalotti has prioritized patient engagement with their physicians to develop healthier lifestyles, especially for those patients with and/or at risk for kidney disease.

In addition to the exceptional credentials of the editors, the volume includes chapters by the leading authorities in their fields and provides the reader with four parts that examine the areas of nutrition, fitness, mindfulness, and approaches to integrate these into healthful living strategies with emphasis on patients with kidney disease and/or cardiovascular disease. The first part on nutrition, containing seven chapters, includes four chapters that describe the major diets that have been associated with improving markers of heart health and reducing cancer risk. The fifth chapter reviews healthy drinks, and the sixth looks at herbs and spices. The last chapter integrates the findings in the chapters within the part. The part on fitness contains three chapters that examine aerobic, resistive, and less energetic exercises, including yoga and mind-body practices. Five chapters in the mindfulness part include discussions of mindfulness, spirituality, resilience, sleep and a final chapter that integrates the methodologies reviewed. The last part, containing four chapters, looks at the role of electronic devices and software in assisting with the integration of nutrition, fitness, and mindfulness; two chapters delve into the integration of these modalities with regard to reducing the risk of cardiovascular disease and chronic kidney disease. The final chapter summarizes the key learnings from the volume and predicts the potential benefits of adopting the holistic approach to health and its value to patients in an overall treatment strategy.

The volume's objectives are to enhance the clinician's role in providing patients with all avenues available to reduce the stress associated with each major disease and, additionally, disease treatments;

provide guidance in adopting data-driven nutrition strategies; incorporate relevant exercise opportunities into treatment programs; inform patients of the potential benefits of mindfulness training, meditation, spirituality, and other resources that have been shown in clinical settings to be associated with greater peace of mind; and be a comprehensive source of up-to-date electronic and other relevant resources.

Part I – Nutrition

Part 1 begins with its *first chapter*, which provides an in-depth review of the DASH diet. The Dietary Approaches to Stop Hypertension (DASH) diet is an evidence-based dietary pattern that has been proven as an effective strategy for lowering blood pressure (BP), improving lipids, and achieving weight control in several adult patient populations in the USA, and it is also associated with lowering the risk of cardiovascular disease in healthy populations. The chapter includes a comprehensive review of the rationales for the three major DASH intervention studies that confirmed the blood-pressure lowering effectiveness of a diet that contained abundant fruit, vegetables, whole grains, nuts/seeds, and low-fat dairy products; reduced intakes of red meats and sweets; and reduced sodium intake (about 2000 mg/d). In agreement with the holistic approach to reducing the risk of stroke and other serious chronic diseases, the chapter describes the studies where weight loss and/or exercise was added to the DASH diet protocol and resulted in additional benefits. Of great importance is the chapter's evaluation of the difficulties in implementing the DASH diet and the value of behavioral changes. Chapter 2 describes the Mediterranean diet, which is an culturally-based dietary pattern that has been studied by comparing health outcomes seen in Mediterranean countries with those found in Northern European countries. The Mediterranean diet is based on olive oil as the main source of fat, whole grains, legumes, fruits, vegetables, nuts, fish, wine in moderation, and moderate intakes of lean meat and dairy products. The chapter updates the evidence of the benefits of the Mediterranean diet and the Mediterranean lifestyle through its reduction in the risk of developing cardiovascular diseases, metabolic syndrome, type-2 diabetes mellitus, chronic kidney disease, and neurodegenerative diseases. The chapter emphasizes the important role of the cultural, political, religious, agricultural, and economic influences found in the Mediterranean countries that cannot be separated from the diet pattern. There is a review of the impact of this diet on type-2 diabetes, chronic kidney disease, and neurodegenerative diseases and the cellular mechanisms hypothesized to reduce these chronic diseases.

Chapter 3 informs us of the many types of plant-based diets that have been associated with reducing the risk of cardiovascular disease and other chronic age-related diseases by a number of mechanisms. Unlike the first two chapters, this chapter includes specific nutrient/food rather than overall diet plan recommendations. The chapter includes an extensive review of the published literature concerning vegan and other plant-based diets, as well as information concerning certain nutrients that are known to be low in plant-based diets and may require the use of dietary supplements; vitamin B12 is one of the examples discussed. The authors suggest that dieticians and medical staff be trained to help patients adopt plant-based diets. Chapter 4 describes a specific component that may be found in certain diets called advanced glycation end products (AGEs) and their potential effects of increasing the risk of several chronic diseases. Food cooked with high heat is a major source of exogenous AGEs. These food-derived AGEs have been shown to be associated with the development of insulin resistance, type-2 diabetes, kidney disease, and atherosclerosis in mice. Data from several clinical trials show that high dietary intake of exogenous AGEs generates an increase oxidative stress and inflammatory state. Reducing dietary AGE decreases the high oxidative stress characteristic of many chronic diseases. Practical low AGE interventions discussed in the chapter include limiting animal protein and fat intake, cooking slowly without desiccation, marinating food at a lower pH, and use of herbs and spices. The limited number of clinical trials emphasized cooking methods, and no further changes in food constituents were undertaken. This approach to reducing adverse events in patients with diabetes, kidney disease, and other chronic diseases is novel and relatively new.

Chapters 5 and 6 discuss common components of the diet with negligible nutritional value yet significant importance in overall eating habits and caloric intake. Chapter 5 examines the importance of healthy drinks and clearly indicates that water is the primary recommendation. Drinking water is an effective way to promote adequate hydration without calories. Drinking plain water, tap or bottled, rather than high-caloric beverages, reduces dietary calorie consumption and may contribute to maintaining a healthy body weight. There are also certain patient populations that can benefit from increasing water intake. Patients with kidney stones, as well as a subset of patients with CKD, may benefit from increasing water intake above thirst requirements. The chapter reviews sugar sweetened beverages and low calorie, as well as alcoholic drinks, including red wine, green tea, herbal tea, and coffee. Studies suggesting health benefits from moderate intakes of wine and coffee are reviewed. Chapter 6 describes the uses of herbs and spices. We learn that the international committee, CODEX, defines herbs as substances that come from plant leaves or flowering parts, either fresh or dried, and contrasts this with the definition of spices that come from other parts of the plant such as roots, stem, bark, seeds, and bulb. Herbs and spices have been widely used for both food and medicinal purposes over many centuries. In culinary practices, these are used as preservatives, flavor enhancers, and colorants and for ingredient substitution of salt and sugar. Dietary intake levels of spices and herbs are difficult to calculate as these are usually consumed in trace amounts. The chapter includes a review of the regulatory status of herbs and spices in Europe and the USA and also contains detailed tabulations of the clinical data regarding the use of specific herbs and spices for certain medical conditions.

Chapter 7 provides the reader with integrated guidelines for healthy eating and lifestyle modifications that enhance the benefits of recommended food and diet pattern choices. The chapter reviews the educational requirements and the role of the registered dietitian, which is to assist individuals in integrating healthy eating and drinking practices in their lifestyle; reviews strategies for healthy eating, such as volumetrics, mindful eating, and intuitive eating; outlines resources and tools for healthy eating using many resources from the USDA, FDA, and other government functions; and provides guidance in identifying reliable information on the Internet, social media, apps, and blogs about healthy dietary and fitness practices for consumers. The chapter discusses another diet plan, volumetrics. The basic principle of volumetrics is to eat a satisfying volume of food while controlling calories and meeting nutrient requirements. This is a low-calorie, high-volume eating plan that includes food with high water and fiber contents (i.e., fruits and vegetables), since both increase a sense of fullness. The chapter describes relevant apps for dietary intake tracking, watches that are miniature computers, and blogs and provides several web addresses and other useful information, which are presented in seven tables.

Part II – Fitness

Part II contains three chapters that examine the importance of physical fitness to overall health. Chapter 8 describes aerobic physical exercises. Aerobic physical activities are defined as those in which the body's large muscles move in a rhythmic manner for a sustained duration. Examples include walking, jogging, running, bicycling, dancing, swimming and other aquatic activities, and rowing. We are reminded that in the USA, 40% of adults do not meet the minimum recommended amount of physical activity. The chapter focuses on the two most widely practiced modes of aerobic physical activity: walking and cycling. The 2018 guidelines for physical activity levels for adults by age and health conditions are outlined, and the definitions of key exercise-related terms are included. Suggestions for community actions that would support increased walking and cycling are outlined.

Chapter 9 discusses the effect of the aging process on nerves and muscles and the importance of resistance training to help assure a more healthful aging. Reductions in neuromuscular function and skeletal muscle mass (sarcopenia) are experienced during the aging process with exponential declines reported to begin around 60 years of age and can impede functional capabilities, limit activities of daily living, and result in loss of independence. The chapter reviews the types of resistance activities that can overload the neuromuscular system to promote specific neuromuscular responses. Common resistance activities include weight machines, free weights (dumbbells or barbell), resistance tubing/bands, pneumatic machines, aquatic activities, yoga, and body-weight exercises. Participation in resistance activities has a positive effect on enhancing neuromuscular strength, power, and physical function in older adults, and even more benefits are seen in younger, healthy individuals. Methods to maintain exercise routines and assure their safety, especially in patients with certain chronic diseases, such as diabetes and chronic kidney disease, are reviewed. Chapter 10 provides an in-depth examination of the practice of integrated yoga and stresses the need to understand the four principles that are included in this integration. Yoga is defined as an integrated lifestyle consisting of varied practices, including lifestyle and values-related commitments, physical practices, breathing practices, and interior practices (e.g., concentration, meditation), carried out with mindfulness and intention. Integrated yoga is suitable for all persons, regardless of age, physical abilities, gender, or body shape. Yoga is a holistic practice or life philosophy that goes far beyond the posture practice component that is most well known in the USA. The chapter includes advice to clinicians concerning certification of yoga teachers and the differences between the three types of yoga instruction. The chapter includes more than 100 relevant references and four detailed tables.

Part III – Mindfulness

Part III contains five chapters that describe the practices of meditation, spirituality, and resilience; the benefits of sleep; and a final chapter that integrates the methods into daily life. Chapter 11 provides an overview of mindfulness meditation based on mindfulness-based stress reduction (MBSR) and mindfulness-based cognitive therapy (MBCT). The chapter contains discussions of the benefits of practicing mindfulness for physical health, mental health, and cognitive function, along with enhanced performance and wellness promotion. The practice of mindfulness was originally developed for chronic pain patients. The eight-week program taught patients mindfulness meditation and other techniques to increase pain management skills when all else had failed. The philosophy blended eastern practices of yoga and Buddhist teachings with science to assist patients cope with stress, pain, anxiety, and illness. Skills and techniques taught included mindful eating, awareness of the breath, the body scan, various sitting meditations, walking meditation, guided meditations, yoga, and loving kindness meditation. There are about 23,000 certified MBSR instructors who teach mindfulness meditation and techniques with clinics in almost every US state and in over 30 countries. In contrast to MBSR, MBCT is an eight-week group intervention that teaches mindfulness skills and techniques combined with cognitive tools to assist individuals dealing with depression. The chapter reviews the seven core qualities of mindfulness: nonjudging, patience, beginner's mind, trust, nonstriving, acceptance, and letting go. Mindfulness does not eliminate or cure disease states. However, mindfulness has been found to be helpful in the symptom reduction of various diseases. Chapter 12 examines the role of religious and spiritual faith in patient treatment. The chapter reviews the importance of faith as an integral component of the medical field as about 80% of adults in the USA indicate a religious preference. Also, physicians often choose religiously affiliated medical facilities for their patients. For example, in America, there are over 600 Catholic hospitals and more than 1600 Catholic continuing care facilities, and about 1 in 6 patients in the USA is cared for in a Catholic hospital daily. Thus, many Americans' day-to-day healthcare is directly influenced by faith-based facilities' philosophies. Moreover, during illness, many patients rely on their faith to help understand their situation. The chapter reviews the limited number of clinical studies that have shown beneficial effects for patients who practice their religious faith and/or indicate their spirituality. However, in both this chapter and the mindfulness chapter, there are balanced discussions of the potential adverse effects of these faith-based practices on health. The authors recommend that a spiritual history assessment, presented from a neutral perspective, be part of the standard intake procedures and references be cited that suggest standardized questions. Chapter 13 provides a formal definition of resilience and ways to help clinicians help their patients to integrate resilience training into their care program. Resilience is defined as the ability of an individual to bounce back from adversity and move forward with life. The four elements of resilience are reviewed: good emotions, reason and purpose, support from and to others, and wellness flexibility. When patients have high levels of good emotions, a strong sense of reason and purpose, consistent support from and to others, and the ability to be flexible, self-aware, and learn from mistakes, their health outcomes have been shown to improve in certain diseases, including cancer, cardiovascular, metabolic, kidney, and neuropsychiatric illnesses. Methods found to help patients improve their resilience include practicing skills such as gratitude, identifying values and setting goals, yoga, conflict resolution, building and deepening relationships, volunteering and accepting one's faults and failures, and learning from them. The chapter describes three validated published scales of resilience that have been shown to have internal consistency and content validity and are reliably reproducible and discusses the findings using these scales. Optimism has been shown to reduce the risk of developing cardiovascular disease and cancer, as well as reduce the risk of death in both senior men and women. Chapter 14 discusses the functions of sleep and its importance to overall health and maintenance of wellness, especially for patients. The chapter describes what is known about healthy sleep, disrupted sleep, and sleep loss and their general effects on cognitive and physical health. There is also an efficient, practical clinical assessment of sleep quality and quantity that is included in the chapter, and an approach to sleep interventions are overviewed. The stages of sleep are examined and described in detail in the included figures, and their importance is reviewed with the help of clinically relevant sleep deprivation studies. The chapter also includes evaluation of studies on sleep duration. Medicines used to increase sleep duration are reviewed, and benefits/risks are discussed. Sleep apnea causes and consequences, found often in obese and diabetic patients, are examined, and treatment options are also provided. There is an interesting analysis of the value of sleep for memory and the research that links these brain functions to other aspects of sleep benefits. The final chapter in this part is unique in that Chap. 15 provides an early look at the potential to use smartphone apps and web browser studies to enhance the practice of mindfulness. It was thought that mindfulness instruction needed face-to-face experience, but new apps are being developed, and the chapter examines the early data from randomized clinical studies on the usefulness of apps and web-based programs in developing the habits of mindful living. The chapter reviews the potential benefits and risks of both in-person and app-based mindfulness sessions. Some apps are directed to specific clinical conditions, including depression, affect, and stress. There is an example of a large European healthcare company that developed an app that was shown to help patients with general psychiatric conditions.

Part IV – Use of Integrated Approaches in Different Populations

Part IV includes the four final chapters of this highly relevant text for clinicians and other health professionals who interact with healthy individuals, as well as with patients who have to deal with the mental and physical consequences of chronic noninfectious diseases. Chapter 16 is a logical extension of the discussions seen in Chap. 15 dealing with the use of electronic devices to assist in the integration of healthful lifestyles to reduce the risk of chronic diseases, as well as providing new models for patient treatment. Chapter 16 reviews the global benefits of "eHealth," which include the fact that eHealth technologies transcend geographic boundaries to efficiently deliver programs and information to the general population about physical activity, nutrition, and mindfulness. The chapter encourages health providers to increase their awareness of the current state of eHealth literacy in their patients and encourage their patients to enhance their skill set to help reduce the risk of chronic disease. We learn that eHealth technologies include smartphones, tablets, and wearable devices, and eHealth programs include social media, downloadable apps, and electronic health records. eHealth is deeply ingrained in the current healthcare experience. Nearly 90% of the US population has access to the Internet, and nearly 80% have used it for health-related purposes. Of interest, downloading an app is considered an active step toward behavior change. People who are most likely to download an eHealth app are younger and college educated and reside in urban regions and feel motivated to engage in physical activity and healthy eating. Practitioners must we aware that patients are using eHealth before a healthcare appointment to learn about their symptoms and prepare questions in order to make the best of their brief time with the clinician. Nearly 80% of patients refer to the Internet following a healthcare appointment to seek clarification and second opinion from users on online discussion forums. The Internet is also a temporal healthcare substitute when patients, especially those who are uninsured or have low income, cannot obtain immediate access to a clinician.

Chapter 17 reviews the real potential to reduce the risk of cardiovascular disease (CVD) by implementing the scientifically based modalities of fitness, nutrition, and mindfulness. In addition, the usefulness of these lifestyle factors as part of CVD therapy is addressed. Physical inactivity is widely recognized as an independent risk factor for CVD, whereas physical activity and fitness are associated with a 25% reduction in all-cause mortality in coronary artery disease patients and 20–30% in the general population. Despite the well-known cardiovascular benefits of exercise, 50% of men and 53% of women in the USA fail to meet general aerobic physical activity guidelines for adults of about 30 minutes of moderate intensity physical activity on most days of the week. Of great importance is the exercise-based cardiac rehabilitation that is prescribed to patients following their first cardiovascular event, such as a heart attack. This structured exercise program is the cornerstone for the prevention of a second cardiac event. The chapter reviews the types of physical activity that clinicians need to encourage in patients with CVD. Mindfulness training has been shown to reduce all-cause mortality and CVD morbidity in two preliminary studies. Stress, anxiety, and depression have been recognized as nontraditional risk factors for CVD that can benefit from mindfulness training. Additionally, smoking cessation programs in CVD patients that include mindfulness training have more success than those without this intervention. More data in larger patient populations are needed to increase the implementation by clinicians treating CVD patients. With regard to nutritional recommendations, we learn that dietary patterns influence cardiometabolic risk factors, including adiposity, blood pressure, glucose-insulin homeostasis, lipids, endothelial function, inflammation, cardiac function, thrombosis, and vascular adhesion. The chapter recommends the DASH and Mediterranean diets reviewed in Chaps. 1 and 2 for patients with CVD and those who are at risk as well. Also recommended is the selection of a nutrient-dense dietary pattern that leads to the maintenance of a healthy body weight; this is crucial for maintaining cardiometabolic health. Chapter 18 reviews the serious adverse effects of chronic kidney disease (CKD) and end-stage renal disease, kidney transplant, dialysis effects, and overall burden of this disease on the nutritional status and needs, as well as the physical and mental health, of the CKD patient. CKD has many causes, but the leading causes are diabetes and obesity. Moreover, the functions of the kidney, including filtering the blood and reducing the risk of anemia, keeping protein and other large molecules in the blood and not lost in the urine, maintaining the acid-base balance of the body, and synthesizing the active form of vitamin D, are critical to the functioning of all the cells of the body. Thus, the multiple functions of kidney are examined in this chapter with an emphasis on a holistic and integrative approach to the management of CKD patients who are given different and complex drugs, have specific nutritional requirements, need fitness training, and often have an overall depressed sense of well-being. There is a detailed discussion of the importance of certain sources of protein, sodium, phosphorus, and potassium and the central role of the Renal Registered Dietitian Nutritionist, who is trained in the treatment of kidney disease patients. Low to moderate exercise programs are recommended based upon the results from published studies that are cited. The chapter, containing five helpful tables, outlines the multidisciplinary approach, including physicians, dietitians, nurses, healthcare technicians, and renal social workers, that is required to facilitate patients' transition to the optimum renal replacement therapy (dialysis or transplant) and to help them deal with the strain that this endeavor places on their schedules, employment, personal relations, finances, and appearances. There are recommendations for the use of trained renal social workers that have a pivotal role to play in the care of patients with CKD. The chapter also reviews the importance of the use of the Internet, video conferencing, media streaming, text messaging, and wireless communications, which can be used by providers to help improve CKD-related care and education, especially for patients in remote areas who do not have access to clinicians. Online healthcare system portals have drastically improved physician–patient communication, with expedited refill requests for medications and access to their test results electronically at home or on the go. The final chapter in this clinically informative volume, Chap. 19, strongly suggests that the medical school curriculum be redeveloped as a holistic approach to patient health, including healthy patient education concerning critical nutrition information and encouragement to maintain a fitness program and be open to mindfulness training. With regard to the patients with chronic diseases, emphasis should be placed on clinician understanding and the communication of relevant drug-nutrient interactions and specific dietary recommendations that are based upon the published literature. Clinicians in practice should widen their referral lists to include trained dieticians, physical activity and sleep experts, and psychologist/social workers, who can help patients to better cope with their illnesses. By highlighting the information in each chapter, the editors of this volume, who are also the authors of this chapter, provide a path for clinicians to follow to better integrate the critical patient needs of better nutrition, physical activity, sleep, and mental health.

Conclusions

The above description of the volume's 19 chapter contents attests to the depth of information provided by the 41 highly respected chapter authors and volume editors. Each chapter includes complete definitions of terms with the abbreviations fully defined and the consistent use of terms between chapters. Key features of the comprehensive volume include 55 detailed tables and informative figures; an extensive, detailed index; and more than 1100 up-to-date references that provide the reader with excellent sources of worthwhile practice-oriented information that will be of great value to cardiologists, nephrologists, and related health providers, as well as graduate and medical students.

In conclusion, *Nutrition, Fitness, and Mindfulness*, edited by Dr. Jaime Uribarri and Dr. Joseph A. Vassalotti, provides health professionals in many areas of chronic disease practice, with particular emphasis on cardiovascular and kidney disease research, with the most current and well-referenced volume on the integration of nutrition, fitness, mindfulness, and other important lifestyle areas into the care of the overall health of their patients. The in-depth guidance provided by each chapter includes methods to integrate these factors into their medical treatment strategies. Special attention is given to reducing the risk of adverse effects in patients with kidney disease and cardiovascular disease. This volume serves the reader as the benchmark for integrating the complex interrelationships between nutritionally related risk factors, such as obesity, aging, CKD, and CVD with the potential benefits of exercise programs, sleep, and mindfulness training. Practice-oriented chapters examine the medical diagnosis, management, and prevention of these two major chronic diseases with emphasis on holistic medical practice. Many of the chapters of this valuable volume provide unique and relevant data on the most relevant Internet resources, national initiatives, and well-recognized diet, including the DASH and Mediterranean diets. The recommended resources are from national research centers, academic departments, and related organizations that provide reliable, up-to-date information based upon the totality of the research on integrated patient care. The broad scope, as well as in-depth reviews, of each chapter's topic makes this excellent volume a very welcome addition to the Nutrition and Health Series.

Adrianne Bendich, PhD, FACN, FASN
Series Editor

About the Series Editors

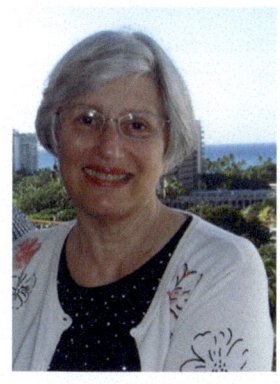

Adrianne Bendich, PhD, FASN, FACN has served as the *Nutrition and Health* Series Editor for more than 20 years and has provided leadership and guidance to more than 200 editors who have developed the 80+ well-respected and highly recommended volumes in the Series.

In addition to *Nutrition, Fitness, and Mindfulness*, edited by Dr. Jaime Uribarri and Dr. Joseph A. Vassalotti, 2020, major new editions published from 2012 to 2020 include the following:

1. *Vitamin E in Human Health* 2019 edited by Peter Weber, Marc Birringer, Jeffrey B. Blumberg, Manfred Eggersdorfer, Jan Frank
2. *Handbook of Nutrition and Pregnancy, Second Edition*, edited by Carol J. Lammi-Keefe, Sarah C. Couch and John P. Kirwan, 2019
3. *Dietary Patterns and Whole Plant Foods in Aging and Disease*, edited as well as written by Mark L. Dreher, Ph.D, 2018
4. *Dietary Fiber in Health and Disease*, edited as well as written by Mark L. Dreher, Ph.D., 2017
5. *Clinical Aspects of Natural and Added Phosphorus in Foods*, edited by Orlando M. Gutierrez, Kamyar Kalantar-Zaden\h and Rajnish Mehrotra, 2017
6. *Nutrition and Fetal Programming"* edited by Rajendram Rajkumar, Victor R. Preedy and Vinood B. Patel, 2017
7. *Nutrition and Diet in Maternal Diabetes"*, edited by Rajendram Rajkumar, Victor R. Preedy and Vinood B. Patel, 2017
8. *Nitrite and Nitrate in Human Health and Disease, Second Edition*, edited by Nathan S. Bryan and Joseph Loscalzo, 2017
9. *Nutrition in Lifestyle Medicine*, edited by James M. Rippe, 2017
10. *Nutrition Guide for Physicians and Related Healthcare Professionals 2nd Edition* edited by Norman J. Temple, Ted Wilson and George A. Bray, 2016
11. *Clinical Aspects of Natural and Added Phosphorus in Foods*, edited by Orlando M. Gutiérrez, Kamyar Kalantar-Zadeh and Rajnish Mehrotra, 2016
12. *L-Arginine in Clinical Nutrition*, edited by Vinood B. Patel, Victor R. Preedy, and Rajkumar Rajendram, 2016
13. *Mediterranean Diet: Impact on Health and Disease* edited by Donato F. Romagnolo, Ph.D. and Ornella Selmin, Ph.D, 2016

14. *Nutrition Support for the Critically Ill* edited by David S. Seres, MD and Charles W. Van Way, III, MD, 2016
15. *Nutrition in Cystic Fibrosis: A Guide for Clinicians*, edited by Elizabeth H. Yen, M.D. and Amanda R. Leonard, MPH, RD, CDE, 2016
16. *Preventive Nutrition: The Comprehensive Guide For Health Professionals, Fifth Edition*, edited by Adrianne Bendich, Ph.D. and Richard J. Deckelbaum, M.D., 2016
17. *Glutamine in Clinical Nutrition*, edited by Rajkumar Rajendram, Victor R. Preedy and Vinood B. Patel, 2015
18. *Nutrition and Bone Health, Second Edition*, edited by Michael F. Holick and Jeri W. Nieves, 2015
19. *Branched Chain Amino Acids in Clinical Nutrition, Volume 2*, edited by Rajkumar Rajendram, Victor R. Preedy and Vinood B. Patel, 2015
20. *Branched Chain Amino Acids in Clinical Nutrition, Volume 1*, edited by Rajkumar Rajendram, Victor R. Preedy and Vinood B. Patel, 2015
21. *Fructose, High Fructose Corn Syrup, Sucrose and Health*, edited by James M. Rippe, 2014
22. *Handbook of Clinical Nutrition and Aging, Third Edition*, edited by Connie Watkins Bales, Julie L. Locher and Edward Saltzman, 2014
23. *Nutrition and Pediatric Pulmonary Disease*, edited by Dr. Youngran Chung and Dr. Robert Dumont, 2014
24. *Integrative Weight Management"* edited by Dr. Gerald E. Mullin, Dr. Lawrence J. Cheskin and Dr. Laura E. Matarese, 2014
25. *Nutrition in Kidney Disease, Second Edition* edited by Dr. Laura D. Byham-Gray, Dr. Jerrilynn D. Burrowes and Dr. Glenn M. Chertow, 2014
26. *Handbook of Food Fortification and Health, volume I* edited by Dr. Victor R. Preedy, Dr. Rajaventhan Srirajaskanthan, Dr. Vinood B. Patel, 2013
27. *Handbook of Food Fortification and Health, volume II* edited by Dr. Victor R. Preedy, Dr. Rajaventhan Srirajaskanthan, Dr. Vinood B. Patel, 2013
28. *Diet Quality: An Evidence-Based Approach, volume I* edited by Dr. Victor R. Preedy, Dr. Lan-Ahn Hunter and Dr. Vinood B. Patel, 2013
29. *Diet Quality: An Evidence-Based Approach, volume II* edited by Dr. Victor R. Preedy, Dr. Lan-Ahn Hunter and Dr. Vinood B. Patel, 2013
30. *The Handbook of Clinical Nutrition and Stroke*, edited by Mandy L. Corrigan, MPH, RD Arlene A. Escuro, MS, RD, and Donald F. Kirby, MD, FACP, FACN, FACG, 2013
31. *Nutrition in Infancy, volume I* edited by Dr. Ronald Ross Watson, Dr. George Grimble, Dr. Victor Preedy and Dr. Sherma Zibadi, 2013
32. *Nutrition in Infancy, volume II* edited by Dr. Ronald Ross Watson, Dr. George Grimble, Dr. Victor Preedy and Dr. Sherma Zibadi, 2013
33. *Carotenoids and Human Health*, edited by Dr. Sherry A. Tanumihardjo, 2013
34. *Bioactive Dietary Factors and Plant Extracts in Dermatology*, edited by Dr. Ronald Ross Watson and Dr. Sherma Zibadi, 2013
35. *Omega 6/3 Fatty Acids*, edited by Dr. Fabien De Meester, Dr. Ronald Ross Watson and Dr. Sherma Zibadi, 2013
36. *Nutrition in Pediatric Pulmonary Disease*, edited by Dr. Robert Dumont and Dr. Youngran Chung, 2013
37. *Nutrition and Diet in Menopause*, edited by Dr. Caroline J. Hollins Martin, Dr. Ronald Ross Watson and Dr. Victor R. Preedy, 2013.
38. *Magnesium and Health*, edited by Dr. Ronald Ross Watson and Dr. Victor R. Preedy, 2012.

39. *Alcohol, Nutrition and Health Consequences*, edited by Dr. Ronald Ross Watson, Dr. Victor R. Preedy, and Dr. Sherma Zibadi, 2012
40. *Nutritional Health, Strategies for Disease Prevention, Third Edition*, edited by Norman J. Temple, Ted Wilson, and David R. Jacobs, Jr., 2012
41. *Chocolate in Health and Nutrition*, edited by Dr. Ronald Ross Watson, Dr. Victor R. Preedy, and Dr. Sherma Zibadi, 2012
42. *Iron Physiology and Pathophysiology in Humans*, edited by Dr. Gregory J. Anderson and Dr. Gordon D. McLaren, 2012

Earlier books included *Vitamin D*, Second Edition, edited by Dr. Michael Holick; *Dietary Components and Immune Function*, edited by Dr. Ronald Ross Watson, Dr. Sherma Zibadi, and Dr. Victor R. Preedy; *Bioactive Compounds and Cancer*, edited by Dr. John A. Milner and Dr. Donato F. Romagnolo; *Modern Dietary Fat Intakes in Disease Promotion*, edited by Dr. Fabien De Meester, Dr. Sherma Zibadi, and Dr. Ronald Ross Watson; *Iron Deficiency and Overload*, edited by Dr. Shlomo Yehuda and Dr. David Mostofsky; *Nutrition Guide for Physicians*, edited by Dr. Edward Wilson, Dr. George A. Bray, Dr. Norman Temple, and Dr. Mary Struble; *Nutrition and Metabolism*, edited by Dr. Christos Mantzoros; and *Fluid and Electrolytes in Pediatrics*, edited by Leonard Feld and Dr. Frederick Kaskel. Recent volumes include *Handbook of Drug-Nutrient Interactions*, edited by Dr. Joseph Boullata and Dr. Vincent Armenti; *Probiotics in Pediatric Medicine*, edited by Dr. Sonia Michail and Dr. Philip Sherman; *Handbook of Nutrition and Pregnancy*, edited by Dr. Carol Lammi-Keefe, Dr. Sarah Couch, and Dr. Elliot Philipson; *Nutrition and Rheumatic Disease*, edited by Dr. Laura Coleman; *Nutrition and Kidney Disease*, edited by Dr. Laura Byham-Grey, Dr. Jerrilynn Burrowes, and Dr. Glenn Chertow; *Nutrition and Health in Developing Countries*, edited by Dr. Richard Semba and Dr. Martin Bloem; *Calcium in Human Health*, edited by Dr. Robert Heaney and Dr. Connie Weaver; and *Nutrition and Bone Health*, edited by Dr. Michael Holick and Dr. Bess Dawson-Hughes.

Dr. Bendich is past President of Consultants in Consumer Healthcare LLC and is the editor of ten books, including *Preventive Nutrition: The Comprehensive Guide for Health Professionals, Fifth Edition*, coedited with Dr. Richard Deckelbaum (www.springer.com/series/7659). Dr. Bendich serves on the Editorial Boards of the *Journal of Nutrition in Gerontology and Geriatrics*, and *Antioxidants*, and has served as Associate Editor for *Nutrition: The International Journal of Applied and Basic Nutritional Sciences*; served on the Editorial Board of the *Journal of Women's Health and Gender-Based Medicine*; and served on the Board of Directors of the American College of Nutrition.

Dr. Bendich was Director of Medical Affairs at GlaxoSmithKline (GSK) Consumer Healthcare and provided medical leadership for many well-known brands, including TUMS and Os-Cal. Dr. Bendich had primary responsibility for GSK's support for the Women's Health Initiative (WHI) intervention study. Prior to joining GSK, Dr. Bendich was at Roche Vitamins Inc. and was involved in groundbreaking clinical studies showing that folic-acid-containing multivitamins significantly reduced major classes of birth defects. Dr. Bendich has coauthored over 100 major clinical research studies in the area of preventive nutrition. She is recognized as a leading authority on antioxidants, nutrition and immunity and pregnancy outcomes, vitamin safety, and the cost-effectiveness of vitamin/mineral supplementation.

Dr. Bendich received the Roche Research Award, is a *Tribute to Women and Industry* Awardee, and was a recipient of the Burroughs Wellcome Visiting Professorship in Basic Medical Sciences. Dr. Bendich was given the Council for Responsible Nutrition (CRN) Apple Award in recognition of her many contributions to the scientific understanding of dietary supplements. In 2012, she was recognized for her contributions to the field of clinical nutrition by the American Society for Nutrition and was elected a *Fellow of ASN* (FASN). Dr. Bendich served as an Adjunct Professor at Rutgers University. She is listed in Who's Who in American Women.

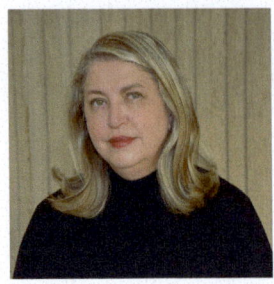 **Connie W. Bales, PhD, RD** is a Professor of Medicine in the Division of Geriatrics, Department of Medicine, at the Duke School of Medicine and Senior Fellow in the Center for the Study of Aging and Human Development at Duke University Medical Center. She is also Associate Director for Education/Evaluation of the Geriatrics Research, Education, and Clinical Center at the Durham VA Medical Center. Dr. Bales is a well-recognized expert in the field of nutrition, chronic disease, function, and aging. Over the past two decades, her laboratory at Duke has explored many different aspects of diet and activity as determinants of health during the latter half of the adult life course. Her current research focuses primarily on enhanced protein as a means of benefiting muscle quality, function, and other health indicators during geriatric obesity reduction and for improving perioperative outcomes in older patients. Dr. Bales has served on NIH and USDA grant review panels and is Past-Chair of the Medical Nutrition Council of the American Society for Nutrition. She has edited three editions of the *Handbook of Clinical Nutrition and Aging*, is Editor-in-Chief of the *Journal of Nutrition in Gerontology and Geriatrics* and is a Deputy Editor of *Current Developments in Nutrition*.

About the Volume Editors

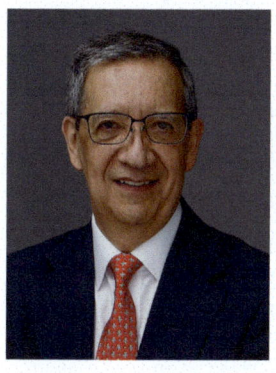

Jaime Uribarri, MD is a physician and clinical investigator. He was born in Chile and received his medical degree from the University of Chile School of Medicine. He did all his postgraduate training in the United States. He has been in The Icahn School of Medicine at Mount Sinai, NYC, since 1990, where he is currently Professor of Medicine and Director of the Renal Clinic and the Home Dialysis Program at the Mount Sinai Hospital.

In parallel with his clinical activities, Dr. Uribarri has been very active in clinical investigation for the past 30 years. His main areas of research have been on acid-base and fluid and electrolyte disorders, as well as nutrition in chronic kidney disease and diabetic patients. He has published over 150 peer-reviewed papers and written many chapters in books. He has lectured extensively on these research topics in New York City, as well as in national and international meetings.

He has edited a book on dietary AGEs and coedited a book on dietary phosphorus published by the CRC Press. He serves as an ad hoc referee for numerous nutrition, medical, and other scientific journals, and he is an active member of several health organizations and professional associations, including the American Society of Nephrology, the American Society of Nutrition, the International Society of Nephrology, The New York Academy of Sciences, and The Maillard Society.

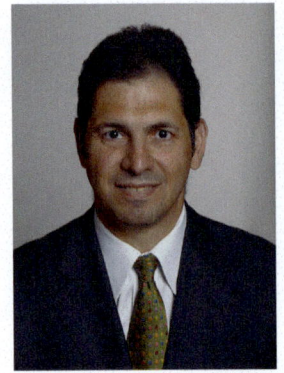

Joseph A. Vassalotti, MD is a nephrologist who serves as the Chief Medical Officer of the National Kidney Foundation (NKF) and Associate Clinical Professor of Medicine in the Division of Nephrology, at Icahn School of Medicine at Mount Sinai. He received his medical degree with Distinction in Research from the SUNY Stony Brook School of Medicine and completed an Internal Medicine Residency and Nephrology Fellowship at the Johns Hopkins Hospital. Next, he served in the clinical faculty at George Washington University School of Medicine from 1995 to 2000, where he won the full-time faculty teaching award in 1998. Since 2000, he has developed a busy regional and international clinical practice at Icahn School of Medicine at Mount Sinai, including as Director of Hemodialysis from 2000 to 2005.

At NKF, his major focus is the implementation of evidence-based clinical practice guidelines in chronic kidney disease (CKD), including the NKF's Kidney Disease Outcomes Quality Initiative (KDOQI), particularly through the guidance of the NKF's primary care initiative, called CKD intercept. He has served as co-PI for the CDC Demonstration Project "CKD Health Evaluation and Risk Information Sharing (CHERISH)," which aimed to identify individuals at high risk for CKD in the USA, and as an investigator for the NIH-sponsored clustered practice randomized trial entitled, evidenced-based primary care for CKD. Leadership also includes multiple roles over the last decade with the CMS Fistula First national quality improvement initiative for hemodialysis, including as Lead Physician Consultant from 2013 through 2015. He has served on numerous committees that shape innovation and health policy in kidney disease for the CDC, the NIH, and CMS. Currently, he serves as Principal Investigator for the Kidney Score Platform an NKF educational project funded by the Veterans Administration Center for Innovation to improve awareness and education among veterans with and at risk for CKD in the primary care setting. Dr. Vassalotti has over 100 publications in peer-reviewed journals and has been featured in Castle Connolly's Top Doctors and Best Doctors in America. He has developed respect and passion for the import of patient engagement for those with and at risk for kidney disease to lead a healthy lifestyle through partnerships with clinicians.

Contents

Contributors

Edlyn Bustamante Alghafir, PhD, MPH, RD, LD Department of Clinical Nutrition, Ben Taub Hospital (Harris Health System), Houston, TX, USA

Samaya Javed Anumudu, MD Department of Nephrology, Baylor College of Medicine, Houston, TX, USA

Ahmed Arslan Yousuf Awan, MD Department of Medicine, Division of Nephrology, Baylor College of Medicine, Houston, TX, USA

Christiane Brems, PhD, ABPP, RYT500, C-IAYT Department of Psychiatry and Behavioral Sciences, Stanford University School of Medicine, Stanford, CA, USA

Jerrilynn D. Burrowes, PhD, RD, CDN, FNKF Department of Nutrition, School of Health Professions and Nursing, Brookeville, NY, USA

Martha R. Crowther, PhD The University of Alabama, Tuscaloosa, AL, USA

María Dolores del Castillo Department of Bioactivity and Food Analysis, Instituto de Investigación en Ciencias de la Alimentación (CIAL) (CSIC-UAM), Madrid, Spain

Devinder Singh Dhindsa, MD Division of Cardiology, Department of Medicine, Emory University School of Medicine, Emory Clinical Cardiovascular Research Institute, Atlanta, GA, USA

Deanna Dragan, MA Department of Psychology, The University of Alabama, Tuscaloosa, AL, USA

Jared M. Gollie, PhD Muscle Morphology, Mechanics and Performance Laboratory, Human Performance Research Unit, Clinical Research Center, Veterans Affairs Medical Center, Washington, DC, USA

Department of Health, Human Function, and Rehabilitation Sciences, School of Medicine & Health Sciences, The George Washington University, Washington, DC, USA

Francisco M. Gutierrez-Mariscal, PhD Department of Lipids and Atherosclerosis Unit, Maimonides Institute for Biomedical Research in Cordoba, Reina Sofia University Hospital, University of Córdoba, Córdoba, Spain

CIBER Physiopathology of Obesity and Nutrition (CIBEROBN), Institute of Health Carlos III, Madrid, Spain

Michael O. Harris-Love, Dsc, MPT Director, Physical Therapy Program, University of Colorado Anschutz Medical Campus, Aurora, CO, USA

Eastern Colorado Geriatric Research Education and Clinical Center, Rocky Mountain Regional VA Medical Center, Aurora, CO, USA

Teresa Herrera, PhD Department of Bioactivity and Food Analysis, Instituto de Investigación en Ciencias de la Alimentación (CIAL) (CSIC-UAM), Madrid, Spain

Amaia Iriondo-DeHond, Msc Department of Bioactivity and Food Analysis, Instituto de Investigación en Ciencias de la Alimentación (CIAL) (CSIC-UAM), Madrid, Spain

Robin Keijzer, BSc Department of Clinical Psychology, University of Amsterdam, Amsterdam, The Netherlands

Pao-Hwa Lin, PhD Department of Medicine, Nephrology Division, Sarah W. Stedman Nutrition and Metabolism Center, Duke University Medical Center, Durham, NC, USA

Lia S. Logio, MD, MACP Department of Medicine, Drexel University College of Medicine, Philadelphia, PA, USA

Jose Lopez-Miranda, PhD, MD Department of Lipids and Atherosclerosis Unit, Maimonides Institute for Biomedical Research in Cordoba, Reina Sofia University Hospital, University of Córdoba, Córdoba, Spain

CIBER Physiopathology of Obesity and Nutrition (CIBEROBN), Institute of Health Carlos III, Madrid, Spain

Danielle McDuffie, MA Department of Psychology, The University of Alabama, Tuscaloosa, AL, USA

Darshan H. Mehta, MD, MPH Department of Medicine, Benson-Henry Institute for Mind Body Medicine at Massachusetts General Hospital|Osher Center for Integrative Medicine at Brigham & Women's Hospital and Harvard Medical School, Boston, MA, USA

Sankar Dass Navaneethan, MD, MS, MPH Department of Medicine, Section of Nephrology, Baylor College of Medicine, Houston, TX, USA

Samantha R. Paige, PhD, MPH Department of STEM Translational Communication Center, University of Florida, Gainesville, FL, USA

Hena N. Patel, MD Department of Cardiology, Rush University Medical Center, Chicago, IL, USA

Lauren A. Peccoralo, MD, MPH Department of Medicine, Department of Medical Education, Icahn School of Medicine at Mount Sinai, New York, NY, USA

Pablo Perez-Martinez, PhD, MD Department of Lipids and Atherosclerosis Unit, Maimonides Institute for Biomedical Research in Cordoba, Reina Sofia University Hospital, University of Córdoba, Córdoba, Spain

CIBER Physiopathology of Obesity and Nutrition (CIBEROBN), Institute of Health Carlos III, Madrid, Spain

Ingrid M. Provident, EdD Department of Occupational Therapy, Chatham University, Pittsburgh, PA, USA

Pratik B. Sandesara, MD Division of Cardiology, Department of Medicine, Emory University School of Medicine, Emory Clinical Cardiovascular Research Institute, Atlanta, GA, USA

Gabrielle Schiller Department of Geriatric and Palliative Medicine, Icahn School of Medicine at Mount Sinai, New York, NY, USA

Tim M. Schoenmakers, PhD Department of Clinical Psychology, University of Amsterdam, Amsterdam, The Netherlands

Jia Shen, MD Division of Cardiology, University of California San Diego, San Diego, CA, USA

Kathleen C. Spadaro, PhD, PMHCNS, RN Department of Nursing, Chatham University, Pittsburgh, PA, USA

Laurence S. Sperling, MD, FACC, FAHA, FACP, FASPC Division of Cardiology, Department of Medicine, Emory University School of Medicine, Emory Clinical Cardiovascular Research Institute, Atlanta, GA, USA

Laura P. Svetkey, MD, MHS Department of Medicine, Nephrology Division, Sarah W. Stedman Nutrition and Metabolism Center, Duke University Medical Center, Durham, NC, USA

Matthew A. Tucker, PhD Department of Biomedical Sciences, University of South Carolina School of Medicine, Greenville, Greenville, SC, USA

Crystal C. Tyson, MD Department of Medicine, Nephrology Division, Sarah W. Stedman Nutrition and Metabolism Center, Duke University Medical Center, Durham, NC, USA

Jaime Uribarri, MD Division of Nephrology, Department of Medicine, Icahn School of Medicine at Mount Sinai, New York, NY, USA

Arnold A. P. van Emmerik, PhD Department of Clinical Psychology, University of Amsterdam, Amsterdam, The Netherlands

Joseph A. Vassalotti, MD Division of Nephrology, Department of Medicine, Icahn School of Medicine at Mount Sinai, New York, NY, USA

The National Kidney Foundation, Inc., New York, NY, USA

Ilkka M. Vuori, MD, PhD The UKK Institute for Health Promotion Research, Tampere, Finland

Kim Allan Williams Sr., MD, MACC, FAHA, MASNC, FESC Department of Cardiology, Rush University Medical Center, Chicago, IL, USA

Josephine Wright, PhD, RD, CDN Department of Nutrition, School of Health Professions and Nursing, Brookeville, NY, USA

Elena M. Yubero-Serrano, PhD Department of Lipids and Atherosclerosis Unit, Maimonides Institute for Biomedical Research in Cordoba, Reina Sofia University Hospital, University of Córdoba, Córdoba, Spain

CIBER Physiopathology of Obesity and Nutrition (CIBEROBN), Institute of Health Carlos III, Madrid, Spain

Part I
Nutrition

Chapter 1
The DASH Dietary Pattern

Pao-Hwa Lin, Crystal C. Tyson, and Laura P. Svetkey

Keywords DASH dietary pattern · Hypertension · Diet · Blood pressure

Key Points
- Dietary Approaches to Stop Hypertension (DASH) diet is an evidence-based dietary pattern that is effective in lowering blood pressure, improving lipids, and achieving weight control, and it is associated with lower risk of cardiovascular diseases and other adverse health conditions.
- DASH dietary pattern is rich in fiber, potassium, magnesium, protein and calcium and lower in total and saturated fats and cholesterol and emphasizes fruits, vegetables, whole grains, nuts/seeds, and low-fat dairy products and reduces red meats and sweets.
- Adherence to DASH remains suboptimal at a national level in the United States across race/ethnicity, education, and income level.
- Clinicians play a critical role in endorsing and promoting the implementation of DASH.
- Efforts are needed to understand the minimum effective "dose" of DASH, identify effective strategies for implementation, establish safety and efficacy of DASH in a wide range of clinical conditions and across the life span, and engage/empower healthcare system, providers, and food industry in promoting DASH.

Introduction

The Dietary Approaches to Stop Hypertension (DASH) diet is an evidence-based dietary pattern that is effective in lowering blood pressure (BP), improving lipids, and achieving weight control, and it is associated with lower risk of cardiovascular diseases and other adverse health conditions. In this chapter, we outline the background of how DASH was developed and tested, its application in hypertensive and non-hypertensive populations, and challenges and potential strategies for implementation.

P.-H. Lin (✉) · C. C. Tyson · L. P. Svetkey
Department of Medicine, Nephrology Division, Sarah W. Stedman Nutrition and Metabolism Center, Duke University Medical Center, Durham, NC, USA
e-mail: pao.hwa.lin@dm.duke.edu; cs206@duke.edu; svetk001@mc.duke.edu

© Springer Nature Switzerland AG 2020
J. Uribarri, J. A. Vassalotti (eds.), *Nutrition, Fitness, and Mindfulness*, Nutrition and Health, https://doi.org/10.1007/978-3-030-30892-6_1

What Is the DASH Dietary Pattern?

Rationale, Design, and Results of DASH Feeding Trials

The DASH feeding trial was conducted from 1993 to 1997 to identify a whole dietary pattern that included several dietary elements that were associated with lower BP. Prior to the conduct of this trial, dietary approaches to control BP relied mainly on caloric restriction for weight loss and sodium reduction; however, there was strong epidemiologic evidence that other dietary factors were relevant to BP control. Thus, the DASH trial was intentionally designed to test the effect of dietary factors independent of the effect of sodium and weight reduction on BP. The original DASH trial [5] was a multicenter randomized controlled feeding trial (RCFT) of 459 individuals, with systolic blood pressure (SBP) of less than 160 mm Hg and diastolic blood pressure (DBP) between 80 and 95 mm Hg (corresponding to prehypertension and stage 1 hypertension at the time), testing three dietary patterns varying in amounts of macro- and micronutrients (Table 1.1). In brief, the dietary patterns were (1) the control diet, which mimicked what most Americans were consuming at the time the trial was conducted; (2) a fruits and vegetables diet, which contained a nutrient profile similar to that of the control diet except with higher content of potassium, magnesium, and fiber; and (3) the DASH dietary pattern, which contained a nutrient profile similar to that of the fruits and vegetables diet but was higher in protein and calcium and lower in total and saturated fats and cholesterol. To achieve this nutrient profile, the DASH diet emphasizes fruits, vegetables, whole grains, nuts/seeds, and low-fat dairy products and reduces red meats and sweets. Sodium and energy intake (3000 mg/2100 kcal/day), body weight, and alcohol consumption were kept constant throughout the intervention.

Table 1.1 DASH trial nutrient and food group targets for each study diet based on 2100 kcal/day

	Control diet	Fruits and vegetables diet	DASH diet
Food group, daily servings			
Fruit	1.6	5.2	5.2
Vegetable	2.0	3.3	4.4
Grains	8.2	6.9	7.5
Dairy	0.5	0.3	2.7
Meat/seafood	2.5	2.5	1.6
Nuts/seeds/legumes	0	0.6	0.7
Fats	5.8	5.3	2.5
Sweets	4.1	1.4	0.7
Macronutrients			
Carbohydrate (% of kcal)	48	48	55
Total fat (%)	37	37	27
Saturated fat (%)	16	16	6
Monounsaturated fat (%)	13	13	13
Polyunsaturated fat (%)	8	8	8
Protein (%)	15	15	18
Cholesterol (mg/day)	300	300	150
Fiber (g/day)	9	31	31
Micronutrients			
Potassium (mg/2100 kcal)	1700	4700	4700
Magnesium (mg)	165	500	500
Calcium (mg)	450	450	1240
Sodium (mg)	3000	3000	3000

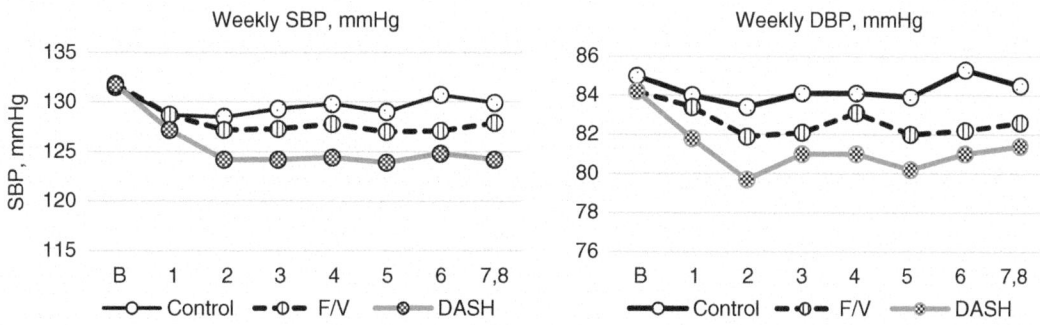

Fig. 1.1 Systolic (left panel) and diastolic (right) blood pressure responses in the 379 participants in the DASH trial. The DASH diet group is identified here as "Combination Diet" [5]

After 8 weeks of feeding, the DASH diet reduced BP by 5.5/3.0 mm Hg more than the control diet ($p < 0.001$ for both SBP and DBP). The reductions in BP were significant after participants consumed the diets for 2 weeks and were sustained for the following 6 weeks (Fig. 1.1). BP lowering was similarly effective in men and women and in younger and older persons, and it was twice as effective among African Americans compared to non-African Americans and three times more effective in those who had higher compared to lower baseline BP. Among the 133 participants with hypertension (baseline SBP $\geq$140 mm Hg and/or DBP $\geq$90 mm Hg), the DASH diet lowered BP by 11.4/5.5 mm Hg. These effects in hypertensives are similar to reductions seen with single drug therapy [37]. These reductions occurred, while body weight, sodium intake, alcohol consumption, and exercise patterns remained stable.

The fruits and vegetables diet had an intermediate effect, reducing BP by 2.8/1.1 mm Hg relative to control diet ($p < 0.001$ for SBP and $p = 0.07$ for DBP), indicating that only half of the BP reduction by DASH could be attributed to fruit and vegetables (i.e., potassium, magnesium, and fiber). Because whole foods rather than individual nutrients were manipulated in the DASH trial, other nutrients or dietary factors that were not controlled for in the study may also have contributed to the BP lowering. Further details on DASH can be found in the following website: http://www.nhlbi.nih.gov/health/resources/heart/hbp-dash-index.

Since the DASH trial was conducted independent of testing the effect of sodium reduction, a subsequent RCFT was conducted (DASH-sodium) to specifically examine the effect on BP of consuming the DASH diet at three sodium levels (high, 3500 mg/day, comparable to typical American intake; intermediate, 2400 mg/day, the recommended limit; and low, 1500 mg/day) [49]. The results of the DASH-sodium feeding trial demonstrate that the combination of DASH and reduced sodium (either 2400 or 1500 mg/day) had a larger BP-lowering effect than either dietary change alone (Fig. 1.2) [49], leading to current recommendations to implement both changes [21]. Similar to the DASH study, the effect of the DASH diet with reduced sodium intake was significant in all subgroups defined by age, sex, and race [49, 64].

The BP-lowering effect of the DASH diet has been replicated several times, indicating a robust and consistent finding. In fact, the effect estimate in a meta-analysis of 20 studies involving 1900 participants was 5.2/2.6 mm Hg [53], remarkably similar to the finding of 5.5/3.0 mm Hg reduction in the original DASH trial [5]. In addition, BP lowering with the DASH dietary pattern has been demonstrated in the context of treatment with antihypertensive medication. The combination of the angiotensin receptor antagonist losartan and the DASH diet lowered BP more than either losartan or DASH alone [17].

It is noteworthy that the effect of the DASH dietary pattern cannot be achieved using dietary supplements. Trials of calcium, magnesium, potassium, and fiber supplements do not demonstrate a consistent BP effect [2, 66]. Therefore, it is likely that the effect of DASH on BP requires consumption of key DASH nutrients from food sources in the context of an overall dietary pattern.

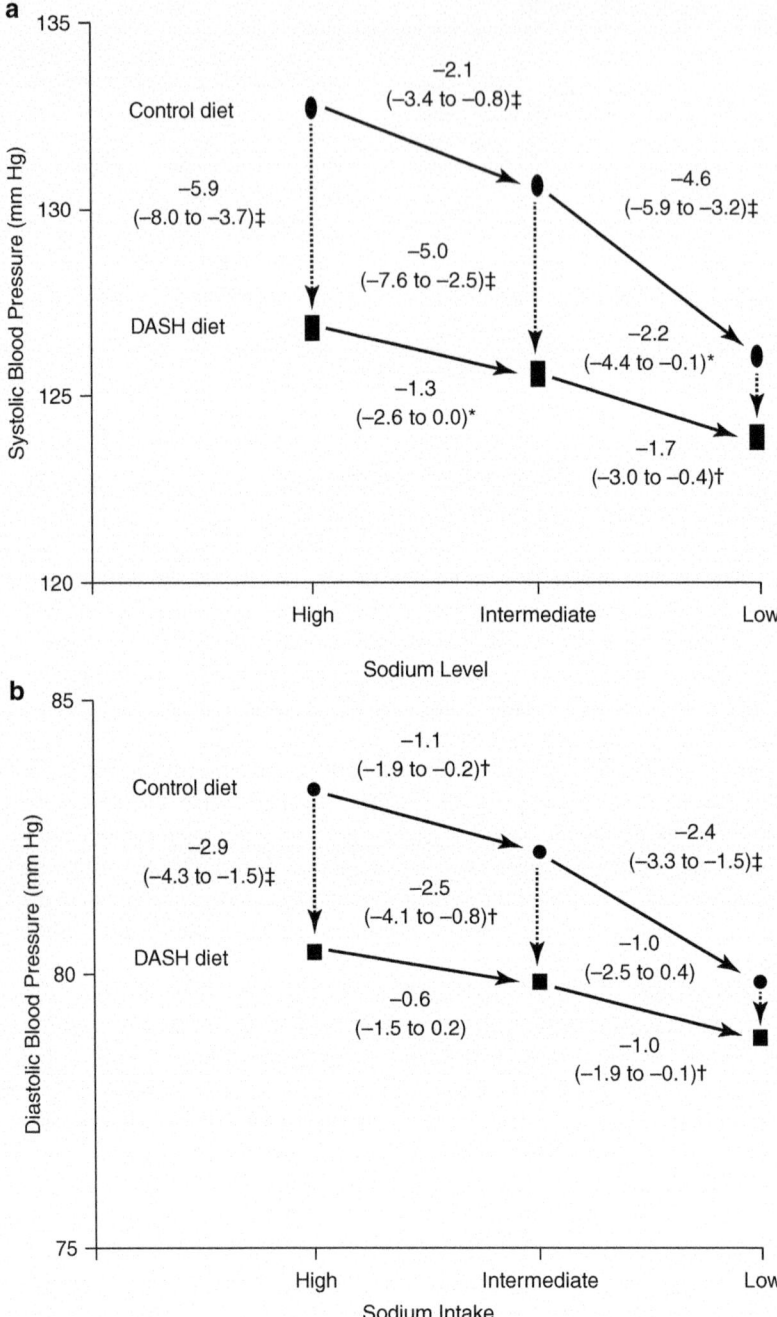

Fig. 1.2 The effect on systolic blood pressure (Panel **a**) and diastolic blood pressure (Panel **b**) of reduced sodium intake and the DASH diet [49]. $^*p < 0.05$, $\dagger p < 0.01$, $\ddagger p < 0.001$

DASH in Racial and Ethnic Subgroups

Although elevated BP (previously referred to as prehypertension) and hypertension are ubiquitous [67], affecting more than half of the adult U.S. population, certain racial and ethnic groups carry a disproportionate burden and may have both a unique need for and response to DASH.

Among African Americans, hypertension is more common, more severe, more resistant to treatment, and more likely to lead to adverse cardiovascular, cerebrovascular, and kidney complications [11, 29, 59]. However, there is also evidence that both DASH [58] and reduced sodium intake [27] are particularly effective in this subgroup.

Among Hispanic adults in the USA, the prevalence of hypertension was similar to that of the non-Hispanic white (27.8%) but is less likely to be controlled [25]. Unfortunately, to date, most DASH trials have not included sufficient numbers of Hispanics for subgroup analysis, markedly limiting generalizability to this group. Although there is no expectation that biologic response to DASH would differ, implementation will no doubt need to be informed by cultural norms.

Among Asian Americans, prevalence of hypertension is lower than among Whites, but the control rate is the lowest of subgroups reported [25]. Although there is no Asian subgroup analysis in any randomized trial, a prospective observational study of Chinese adults showed that adherence to DASH was associated with lower BP and stroke risk [36]. Therefore, it is likely that cultural adaptation to promote DASH adherence among various Asian American groups can improve BP control in these groups.

Mechanisms of Action

BP-lowering mechanisms of DASH are unclear. Some studies suggest a natriuretic effect: DASH shifts the pressure-natriuresis curve [1], and potassium intake itself promotes natriuresis [54]. In addition, a small feeding study demonstrated that DASH increases plasma nitrite after hyperemia, suggesting BP-lowering effects that are mediated through upregulation of nitric oxide bioavailability [35]. Other data suggest genetic regulation: BP response to DASH is associated with polymorphisms both in renin-angiotensin-aldosterone and in adrenergic system genes [56]. In addition, our preliminary data suggest that the high fiber in DASH affects the gut microbiome to promote the mucosal barrier, potentially improving intestinal tight junction and thus reducing absorption of inflammatory toxins that may elevate BP (unpublished data).

Other DASH Effects

Lipids

As noted above, the DASH diet is reduced in total and saturated fat. Thus, as expected, it lowered total and LDL-cholesterol [42]. However, it also lowered HDL-cholesterol slightly and had no effect on triglycerides. Therefore, a subsequent RCFT replaced 10% of carbohydrate in DASH with mono- and polyunsaturated fat while holding other DASH nutrients constant. With this modification, the OmniHeart study demonstrated similar BP and LDL-cholesterol lowering, increased HDL-cholesterol, and reduced triglycerides [6]. Although OmniHeart was a small trial ($N = 161$), and a subsequent smaller trial ($N = 36$) demonstrates similar effects with substituting saturated fat for some carbohydrate [14], the OmniHeart results suggest that a "Mediterraneanized"[24] version of DASH could lower BP with additional benefits to lipid profile.

Other Outcomes

Although there is no other direct evidence of DASH effects on disease outcomes, there is a large body of observational data linking DASH to important public health priorities. A report analyzing 68 studies with a total of 1,670,179 participants and multiple other epidemiologic studies show that concordance with the DASH dietary pattern is associated with lower risk for all-cause mortality, cardiovascular disease in general, coronary artery disease, stroke [20, 33, 36, 50], cancer [19, 26, 30, 34, 51, 63], diabetes [13, 18, 31, 52], chronic kidney disease [47], and neurodegenerative diseases [52]. Associations between DASH and health have also been observed in populations of children and adolescents [16]. Future research will determine whether these associations are causal and thus potential outcomes of successful DASH implementation.

Implementing DASH

Effectiveness Trials

While feeding trials established the efficacy of DASH, its ultimate implementation requires evidence of effectiveness in individuals selecting and preparing their own meals. Several studies provide evidence of effectiveness. In the PREMIER clinical trial [4], the effects on BP of two 18-month multicomponent lifestyle behavioral interventions compared to an advice-only control group were tested in 810 adults with above-optimal BP (>120/80 mm Hg). The two behavioral interventions were designed to stimulate adoption of what were at the time the well-established lifestyle guidelines for BP control (EST) or the well-established guidelines plus the DASH dietary pattern (EST + DASH). The well-established guidelines included weight loss if overweight (95% of participants), reducing sodium intake to 2300 mg or less per day, increasing physical activity to at least 180 minutes of moderate activity/week, and no more than moderate alcohol consumption. Participants in both intervention groups significantly reduced weight, improved physical activity, and lowered sodium intake, and the EST + DASH group also increased intake of DASH food groups (fruit, vegetable, and dairy). Mean reduction in SBP, net of the control group, was 3.7 mm Hg (p < 0.001) in EST group and 4.3 mm Hg (p < 0.001) in EST + DASH group [4]. Each individual lifestyle modification was independently and significantly associated with SBP reduction at 6 and 18 months [22].

Since PREMIER tested the effects of DASH within a combined lifestyle intervention program which included weight loss, sodium reduction, and increased physical activity, it did not determine the effectiveness of the DASH dietary pattern alone. In contrast, the ENCORE behavioral intervention trial compared DASH alone, DASH combined with a weight management program, and usual diet in 144 adults with prehypertension or stage 1 hypertension (>130/80 mm Hg), according to the classification at the time of the trial [9]. Both clinic and ambulatory BP fell by 11.2/7.5 mm Hg with DASH alone and by 16.1/9.9 mm Hg in the DASH plus weight management group. Thus, this study confirms that adoption of DASH in free-living individuals lowers BP, with greater effects when combined with a weight loss intervention. Incidentally, ENCORE demonstrated favorable effects of DASH on pulse wave velocity, baroreflex sensitivity, and left ventricular mass, all of which suggest improvement in vascular and autonomic function and cardiac morphology that could lead to reduced cardiovascular disease risk.

Both PREMIER and ENCORE trials involved extremely intense behavioral intervention and were provided in an academic medical center without engagement of a health system. In order to move closer to implementation in the real world, we conducted a DASH effectiveness trial in community-based primary care clinics. In the Hypertension Improvement Project (HIP), we compared BP effects of a physician intervention, patient intervention, both, or neither. The physician intervention included Internet-based training, self-monitoring, and quarterly feedback reports related to management of hypertension and counseling on nonpharmacologic interventions, including DASH. The patient intervention included 20 weekly group sessions in the clinic, followed by 12 monthly telephone counseling contacts to promote behavior change leading to adoption of the DASH dietary pattern, reduced sodium intake, weight loss (if overweight), and increased physical activity. Among 32 physicians in 8 primary care practices, 574 patients (mean age 60 years, 61% women, 37% self-identified Black) were randomized to 1 of the 4 groups. The physician intervention itself did not significantly impact BP. At 6 months, the patient intervention reduced SBP by 2.6 mm Hg (95% CI: 4.4–0.7; p = 0.01). The combination of physician and patient intervention had an interactive impact on SBP (p-value for interaction = 0.03; mean SBP effect −9.7 +/− 12.7 mm Hg). Although differences between treatment groups did not persist at 18 months, highlighting the need for research on sustained impact, HIP suggests that physicians play an important role in promoting DASH and other nonpharmacologic interventions for BP control [57].

Implementation Challenges

The Joint National Committee on Prevention, Detection, Evaluation, and Treatment of High BP (JNC) adopted the DASH diet as a dietary pattern for hypertension prevention and nonpharmacologic treatment from 1997 [32] until the final iteration in 2017 [15, 67]. DASH has also been consistently endorsed by the American Dietetic Association [3] and the NHLBI Lifestyle Guidelines [21], and it was adopted in 2005 as the dietary guideline for all Americans 2 years and older [61]. Inclusion of the DASH dietary pattern in national policy and clinical guidelines sets the stage for large-scale implementation of this dietary pattern. However, the challenges in implementation remain strong as indicated by the low levels of DASH adherence noted in national survey data [55].

For example, in 1999–2000 [12, 68], Americans were consuming far less than the nationally recommended amounts of fruit, vegetables, fiber, calcium, magnesium, and potassium—all of which are key components of the DASH dietary pattern. More than 10 years after DASH results were published, half of the total US population consumed <1 cup of fruit and <1.5 cups of vegetables daily, and three quarters did not meet fruit and vegetable intake recommendations [40].

Nonetheless, from 1999 to 2012, US dietary intake improved somewhat, including more whole grains and less fruit juice and sugar-sweetened beverages, but there was no significant improvement in intake of total fruit and vegetables, processed meats, saturated fat, and sodium. In fact, overall adherence to DASH decreased in this time period so that only about 11% of the population was categorized in the highest quartile of DASH adherence score [10]. In addition, in a survey (1999–2004) among 4386 participants with hypertension, only 19.4% were classified as DASH accordant after adjustment for age and energy intake [38]. Thus, adherence to DASH remains suboptimal at a national level in the USA [55], and this is true across race/ethnicity, education, and income level.

Despite the disappointing adherence data, there is evidence that even half accordance with DASH may convey meaningful BP and health benefits. In the ENCORE study [9], DASH accordance was found to be associated with BP change in a dose-response fashion, with significant BP lowering in the top two quartiles of intake, corresponding roughly to "half DASH" [23]. Future study is needed to verify the dose-response relationship between DASH accordance and BP effect. If this relationship is confirmed, strategies may be developed to encourage at least partial DASH adherence.

Many challenges contribute to low DASH adherence. At the individual level, factors such as emotional eating, family and social support, social significance of food, knowledge, and even health insurance coverage for dietary coaching serve as barriers [62]. At the environmental level, studies have shown that close proximity to convenience and fast-food outlets and a high density of fast-food outlets and the lack of access to a sufficient quantity of affordable, nutritious food in the community are associated with low dietary quality [28, 43]. Another major challenge is the lack of training, time, and resources for clinicians to provide dietary coaching to patients. Thus, a multi-approach strategy is needed to overcome challenges and improve DASH adherence rates.

Potential Strategies to Improve DASH Adherence

As noted above, intensive behavioral intervention trials lead to improvements in dietary pattern, and yet adoption of DASH is low. Individual, health-system, and environmental level barriers contribute to poor implementation. What is badly needed are evidence-based strategies for implementing what we know to be effective. Lessons learned from past research indicate that behavioral intervention programs that result in successful behavior change are generally rooted in social cognitive theory [7] and techniques of behavioral self-management [65]. They are ideally constructed using the transtheoretical or stages-of-change model [45, 46] and use motivational enhancement approaches [39, 48]. These approaches emphasize the importance of the individual's ability to regulate behavior by setting goals, developing specific behavior change plans, monitoring progress toward the goals, and attaining skills necessary to reach the goals. Self-efficacy (one's confidence in performing a given behavior) and outcome expectancies (one's expectations concerning the outcome of that behavior) are critical mediators of behavior change [8, 48]. The transtheoretical model recognizes that behavior change is a dynamic process of moving through different motivational stages of readiness for change. Different behavioral strategies may need to be emphasized at different times, depending on the individual's life circumstances and stage of change.

In addition, behavioral interventions conducted with small groups can take advantage of the economy of scale and the social support provided by a group of peers. For example, in the PREMIER trial of lifestyle intervention for lowering BP [4], the behavioral strategies discussed earlier were incorporated into an intervention consisting of frequent group sessions conducted by a trained interventionist in which participants provided extensive peer support. It is also important to design culturally appropriate intervention program. Examples of cultural appropriateness may include but are not limited to (1) having intervention encounters take place at a location in the community familiar to the participants; (2) employing staff from the same cultural background as participants; (3) selecting foods, activities, or examples from within the culture; and (4) involving staff and/or community stakeholders of diverse cultural backgrounds in program design.

Despite considerable understanding of the theory and practice of behavior change, additional research is needed to develop effective strategies for sustaining long-term dietary and lifestyle change. In addition, strategies are needed for scalability. With over 50% of the US population needing BP-lowering strategies [41, 67], a model that requires intensive on-site individual or small-group coaching cannot hope to adequately disseminate intervention. Early efforts at implementing DASH through mobile technology appear promising [60].

Tips for Clinicians

Previous research has shown that including clinicians in the care of hypertensive patients is more effective for BP control than lifestyle intervention by a coach alone [57]. Table 1.2 shows a simple tool utilizing the evidence-based 5 As approach (ask, advise, assess, assist, and arrange) [44] in assisting patients in following the DASH dietary pattern. This tool allows clinicians or other healthcare professionals to (1) ask the patient to recall his/her own eating pattern, (2) advise the patient what DASH is, (3) assess the patient's readiness to change his/her eating pattern, (4) assist the patient in identifying a goal toward better DASH adherence and setting an action plan, and (5) arrange a follow-up visit to provide accountability. Table 1.3 includes a list of tips that may help clinicians assist patients in achieving a DASH-adherent dietary pattern.

Available Resources

There are many resources available to help patients follow the DASH dietary pattern. Table 1.4 contains a list of examples.

Even though these tools are very helpful to set the foundation for how one may start to change dietary pattern toward DASH, the motivation to change usually comes from within the individual and may be "discovered" through an interactive coaching process led by a trained professional. Thus, clinicians are strongly encouraged to collaborate with dietitians to help their patients make dietary changes toward DASH. Resources of local dietitians can be found in the American dietetic association website (https://www.eatright.org/find-an-expert).

Future Needs and Directions

In order for DASH to reach its full potential to improve the public health, steps are needed to (1) deepen the understanding of the minimum effective "dose" of DASH and its mechanisms of action; (2) develop and test strategies for implementation and dissemination; (3) establish safety and efficacy of DASH in a wide range of clinical conditions and across the life span; (4) determine ways for a health system and healthcare policy to support DASH adherence, for example,

Table 1.2   "Follow the DASH dietary pattern" Guide sheet

Food group serving sizes	1. *Ask*: How many servings do you usually eat in a day?	2. *Advise*: DASH guidelines (per 2000 kcal per day)	3. *Assess*: How likely will you make changes in your eating in the next month? 4. *Assist*: Identify one goal to work on before next visit
Vegetables (1/2 cup cooked, 1 cup raw leafy greens)		4–5 per day	Goal: Action plan:
Fruit (1/2 cup, 1 medium-sized fruit)		4–5 per day	Goal: Action plan:
Dairy (1 cup milk/yogurt, 1 oz cheese)		2–3 per day	Goal: Action plan:
Whole grains (1/2 cup cooked, 1 slice bread)		3–4 per day	Goal: Action plan:
Meat/seafood (3 oz cooked)		2 or fewer per day	Goal: Action plan:
Nuts/seeds/legumes (1/4 cup nuts/seeds, ½ cup legumes)		4–5 per week	Goal: Action plan:
Sweets (1 serving of dessert, 8 oz sweet drink)		5 or fewer per week	Goal: Action plan:
5. *Arrange*. Next visit date/time: _____			

Table 1.3 Tips for clinicians

No	Tips	Rationale
1	Make diet a visit priority	Discussing diet at beginning of visit conveys the message that diet is important for BP management. If necessary, schedule visit to discuss diet specifically
2	Prescribe DASH	Prescribing DASH rather than just recommending it conveys the message that following DASH is a critical component of BP treatment
3	Identify gap, set goal and action plan	Use "Follow the DASH dietary pattern" guide sheet (Table 1.2) to help patients identify areas that need improvement. Assist patients in setting goals and developing action plans
4	Use familiar terms	Use common food terms and examples that patients can understand when discussing how to follow the DASH diet
5	Seek resources	Engage dietitians or lifestyle counselors to help patients make long-term changes
6	Schedule follow-up visits	Accountability is critical in making and maintaining lifestyle changes. Scheduling follow-up visits may motivate patients to initiate and maintain changes
7	Model for the patients	Set a good model for the patients about following the DASH diet. Design the clinic to be DASH friendly by serving healthy food, snacks, and drinks

Table 1.4 Resources for patients

Tool	Source	Notes
Websites	1. http://www.nhlbi.nih.gov/health/resources/heart/hbp-dash-index 2. https://www.dashforhealth.com	Helpful overview and pamphlets about DASH
Phone apps	There are more than 20 smartphone apps designed to help users follow the DASH diet; most provide recipes, meal plans, and shopping list concordant with DASH	Apps that provide recipes and menu ideas but rarely with self-monitoring tool
Pamphlet	*Your Guide to Lowering Your Blood Pressure with DASH* published by the NIH/NHLBI (NIH Publication No. 06-5834)	A brief summary of what DASH is and how to follow it
Books	*The DASH Diet for Hypertension* by T. Moore *The DASH diet for weight loss* by T, Moore	Complete guide for following DASH for BP control and for weight loss

through increased access to and insurance coverage for nutritional coaching; (5) empower providers to participate in the delivery of behavioral intervention for promoting DASH adherence; and (6) engage the food and restaurant industry in promoting more healthful dietary patterns across the nation.

Conclusion

Strong evidence supports the benefit of the DASH dietary pattern for BP and lipids. Further, following DASH is also associated with overall health and health benefits including reduced risk for cardiovascular disease, coronary heart disease, diabetes, and chronic kidney disease. There is some evidence suggesting that the greater the adherence to DASH, the greater the benefit and that partial adherence still conveys significant health benefit. Effective strategies are urgently needed to improve the implementation of this dietary pattern at both the individual and public health levels, and clinicians play a critical role in endorsing and promoting its implementation.

References

1. Akita S, Sacks FM, Svetkey LP, Conlin PR, Kimura G, DASH-Sodium Trial Collaborative Research Group. Effects of the Dietary Approaches to Stop Hypertension (DASH) diet on the pressure-natriuresis relationship. Hypertension. 2003;42:8–13.

2. Al-Solaiman Y, Jesri A, Mountford WK, Lackland DT, Zhao Y, Egan BM. DASH lowers blood pressure in obese hypertensives beyond potassium, magnesium and fibre. J Hum Hypertens. 2010;24:237–46.

3. Andf. DASH diet: reducing hypertension through diet and lifestyle [Online]. Academy of Nutrition and Dietetics Foundation. 2019. Available: https://www.eatright.org/health/wellness/heart-and-cardiovascular-health/dash-diet-reducing-hypertension-through-diet-and-lifestyle. Accessed 6 Jan 2019.

4. Appel LJ, Champagne CM, Harsha DW, Cooper LS, Obarzanek E, Elmer PJ, Stevens VJ, Vollmer WM, Lin PH, Svetkey LP, Stedman SW, Young DR, Writing Group of the PREMIER Collaborative Research Group. Effects of comprehensive lifestyle modification on blood pressure control: main results of the PREMIER clinical trial. JAMA. 2003;289:2083–93.

5. Appel LJ, Moore TJ, Obarzanek E, Vollmer WM, Svetkey LP, Sacks FM, Bray GA, Vogt TM, Cutler JA, Windhauser MM, Lin PH, Karanja N. A clinical trial of the effects of dietary patterns on blood pressure. DASH Collaborative Research Group. N Engl J Med. 1997;336:1117–24.

6. Appel LJ, Sacks FM, Carey VJ, Obarzanek E, Swain JF, Miller ER 3rd, Conlin PR, Erlinger TP, Rosner BA, Laranjo NM, Charleston J, Mccarron P, Bishop LM. Effects of protein, monounsaturated fat, and carbohydrate intake on blood pressure and serum lipids: results of the OmniHeart randomized trial. J Am Med Assoc. 2005;294:2455–64.

7. Bandura A. Social foundations of thought and action: a social cognitive theory. Englewood Cliffs: Prentice-Hall; 1986.

8. Bandura A. The anatomy of stages of change. Am J Health Promot. 1997;12:8–10.

9. Blumenthal JA, Babyak MA, Hinderliter A, Watkins LL, Craighead L, Lin PH, Caccia C, Johnson J, Waugh R, Sherwood A. Effects of the DASH diet alone and in combination with exercise and weight loss on blood pressure and cardiovascular biomarkers in men and women with high blood pressure: the ENCORE study. Arch Intern Med. 2010;170:126–35.

10. Booth JN 3rd, Li J, Zhang L, Chen L, Muntner P, Egan B. Trends in prehypertension and hypertension risk factors in US adults: 1999–2012. Hypertension. 2017;70:275–84.

11. Broderick J, Brott T, Kothari R, Miller R, Khoury J, Pancioli A, Gebel J, Mills D, Minneci L, Shukla R. The greater Cincinnati/Northern Kentucky Stroke Study: preliminary first-ever and total incidence rates of stroke among blacks. Stroke. 1998;29:415–21.

12. Casagrande SS, Wang Y, Anderson C, Gary TL. Have Americans increased their fruit and vegetable intake? The trends between 1988 and 2002. Am J Prev Med. 2007;32:257–63.

13. Chen GC, Koh WP, Neelakantan N, Yuan JM, Qin LQ, Van Dam RM. Diet quality indices and risk of type 2 diabetes mellitus: the Singapore Chinese health study. Am J Epidemiol. 2018;187:2651–61.

14. Chiu S, Bergeron N, Williams PT, Bray GA, Sutherland B, Krauss RM. Comparison of the DASH (Dietary Approaches to Stop Hypertension) diet and a higher-fat DASH diet on blood pressure and lipids and lipoproteins: a randomized controlled trial. Am J Clin Nutr. 2016;103:341–7.

15. Chobanian AV, Bakris GL, Black HR, Cushman WC, Green LA, Izzo JL Jr, Jones DW, Materson BJ, Oparil S, Wright JT Jr, Roccella EJ, Joint National Committee on Prevention, Detection, Evaluation, and Treatment of High Blood Pressure. National Heart, Lung, and Blood Institute; National High Blood Pressure Education Program Coordinating Committee. Seventh report of the joint national committee on prevention, detection, evaluation, and treatment of high blood pressure. Hypertension. 2003;42:1206–52.

16. Cohen JFW, Lehnerd ME, Houser RF, Rimm EB. Dietary approaches to stop hypertension diet, weight status, and blood pressure among children and adolescents: national health and nutrition examination surveys 2003–2012. J Acad Nutr Diet. 2017;117:1437–1444 e2.

17. Conlin PR, Erlinger TP, Bohannon A, Miller ER 3rd, Appel LJ, Svetkey LP, Moore TJ. The DASH diet enhances the blood pressure response to losartan in hypertensive patients. Am J Hypertens. 2003;16:337–42.

18. Corsino L, Sotres-Alvarez D, Butera NM, Siega-Riz AM, Palacios C, Perez CM, Albrecht SS, Espinoza Giacinto RA, Perera MJ, Horn LV, Aviles-Santa ML. Association of the DASH dietary pattern with insulin resistance and diabetes in US Hispanic/Latino adults: results from the Hispanic Community Health Study/Study of Latinos (HCHS/SOL). BMJ Open Diabetes Res Care. 2017;5:e000402.

19. Davison B, Saeedi P, Black K, Harrex H, Haszard J, Meredith-Jones K, Quigg R, Skeaff S, Stoner L, Wong JE, Skidmore P. The association between parent diet quality and child dietary patterns in nine- to eleven-year-old children from Dunedin, New Zealand. Nutrients. 2017;9(5):483.

20. Djousse L, Ho YL, Nguyen XT, Gagnon DR, Wilson PWF, Cho K, Gaziano JM, VA Million Veteran Program. DASH score and subsequent risk of coronary artery disease: the findings from million veteran program. J Am Heart Assoc. 2018;7(9):e008089.

21. Eckel RH, Jakicic JM, Ard JD, De Jesus JM, Houston Miller N, Hubbard VS, Lee IM, Lichtenstein AH, Loria CM, Millen BE, Nonas CA, Sacks FM, Smith SC Jr, Svetkey LP, Wadden TA, Yanovski SZ, American College of Cardiology/American Heart Association Task Force on Practice Guidelines. 2013 AHA/ACC guideline on lifestyle management to reduce cardiovascular risk: a report of the American College of Cardiology/American Heart Association Task Force on Practice Guidelines. J Am Coll Cardiol. 2014;63:2960–84.

22. Elmer PJ, Obarzanek E, Vollmer WM, Simons-Morton D, Stevens VJ, Young DR, Lin PH, Champagne C, Harsha DW, Svetkey LP, Ard J, Brantley PJ, Proschan MA, Erlinger TP, Appel LJ, PREMIER Collaborative Research Group. Effects of comprehensive lifestyle modification on diet, weight, physical fitness, and blood pressure control: 18-month results of a randomized trial. Ann Intern Med. 2006;144:485–95.

23. Epstein DE, Sherwood A, Smith PJ, Craighead L, Caccia C, Lin PH, Babyak MA, Johnson JJ, Hinderliter A, Blumenthal JA. Determinants and consequences of adherence to the dietary approaches to stop hypertension diet in African-American and white adults with high blood pressure: results from the ENCORE trial. J Acad Nutr Diet. 2012;112:1763–73.

24. Estruch R, Ros E, Salas-Salvado J, Covas M, Corella D, Aros F, Gomez-Gracia E, Ruiz-Gutierrez V, Fiol M, Lapetra J, Lamuela-Raventos R, Serra-Majem L, Pinto X, Basora J, Munoz M, Sorli J, Martinez J, Fito M, Gea A, Hernan M, Martinez-Gonzalez M, Investigators PS. Primary prevention of cardiovascular disease with a Mediterranean diet supplemented with extra-virgin olive oil or nuts. N Engl J Med. 2018;378:e34.

25. Fryar CD, Ostchega Y, Hales CM, Zhang G, Kruszon-Moran D. Hypertension prevalence and control among adults: United States, 2015–2016. NCHS Data Brief, No. 289. Hyattsville: National Center for Health Statistics; 2017.

26. Fung TT, Hu FB, Wu K, Chiuve SE, Fuchs CS, Giovannucci E. The Mediterranean and Dietary Approaches to Stop Hypertension (DASH) diets and colorectal cancer. Am J Clin Nutr. 2010;92:1429–35.

27. Graudal NA, Hubeck-Graudal T, Jurgens G. Effects of low sodium diet versus high sodium diet on blood pressure, renin, aldosterone, catecholamines, cholesterol, and triglyceride. Cochrane Database Syst Rev. 2017;(4):CD004022.

28. He M, Tucker P, Irwin JD, Gilliland J, Larsen K, Hess P. Obesogenic neighbourhoods: the impact of neighbourhood restaurants and convenience stores on adolescents' food consumption behaviours. Public Health Nutr. 2012;15:2331–9.

29. Hertz RP, Unger AN, Cornell JA, Saunders E. Racial disparities in hypertension prevalence, awareness, and management. Arch Intern Med. 2005;165:2098–104.

30. Hirko KA, Willett WC, Hankinson SE, Rosner BA, Beck AH, Tamimi RM, Eliassen AH. Healthy dietary patterns and risk of breast cancer by molecular subtype. Breast Cancer Res Treat. 2016;155:579–88.

31. Jacobs S, Boushey CJ, Franke AA, Shvetsov YB, Monroe KR, Haiman CA, Kolonel LN, Le Marchand L, Maskarinec G. A priori-defined diet quality indices, biomarkers and risk for type 2 diabetes in five ethnic groups: the Multiethnic Cohort. Br J Nutr. 2017;118:312–20.

32. JNC-6. The sixth report of the Joint National Committee on prevention, detection, evaluation, and treatment of high blood pressure. Arch Intern Med. 1997;157:2413–46.

33. Jones NRV, Forouhi NG, Khaw KT, Wareham NJ, Monsivais P. Accordance to the dietary approaches to stop hypertension diet pattern and cardiovascular disease in a British, population-based cohort. Eur J Epidemiol. 2018;33:235–44.

34. Jones-Mclean E, Hu J, Greene-Finestone LS, De Groh M. A DASH dietary pattern and the risk of colorectal cancer in Canadian adults. Health Promot Chronic Dis Prev Can. 2015;35:12–20.

35. Lin PH, Allen JD, Li YJ, Yu M, Lien LF, Svetkey LP. Blood pressure-lowering mechanisms of the DASH dietary pattern. J Nutr Metab. 2012;2012:472396.

36. Lin PH, Yeh WT, Svetkey LP, Chuang SY, Chang YC, Wang C, Pan WH. Dietary intakes consistent with the DASH dietary pattern reduce blood pressure increase with age and risk for stroke in a Chinese population. Asia Pac J Clin Nutr. 2013;22:482–91.

37. Materson BJ, Reda DJ, Cushman WC, Massie BM, Freis ED, Kochar MS, Hamburger RJ, Fye C, Lakshman R, Gottdiener J, et al. Single-drug therapy for hypertension in men. A comparison of six antihypertensive agents with placebo. The Department of Veterans Affairs Cooperative Study Group on Antihypertensive Agents. N Engl J Med. 1993;328:914–21.

38. Mellen PB, Gao SK, Vitolins MZ, Goff DC Jr. Deteriorating dietary habits among adults with hypertension: DASH dietary accordance, NHANES 1988–1994 and 1999–2004. Arch Intern Med. 2008;168:308–14.

39. Miller WR, Rollnick S. Motivational interviewing: preparing people to change addictive behavior. New York: Guilford; 1991.

40. Moore L, Thompson F. Adults meeting fruit and vegetable intake recommendations-United States, 2013. MMWR Morb Mortal Wkly Rep. 2015;64(26):709. Accessed 30 Apr 2016.

41. Muntner P, Whelton PK. Using predicted cardiovascular disease risk in conjunction with blood pressure to guide antihypertensive medication treatment. J Am Coll Cardiol. 2017;69:2446–56.

42. Obarzanek E, Sacks FM, Vollmer WM, Bray GA, Miller ER 3rd, Lin PH, Karanja NM, Most-Windhauser MM, Moore TJ, Swain JF, Bales CW, Proschan MA, DASH Research Group. Effects on blood lipids of a blood pressure-lowering diet: the Dietary Approaches to Stop Hypertension (DASH) Trial. Am J Clin Nutr. 2001;74:80–9.

43. Odoms-Young A, Singleton CR, Springfield S, Mcnabb L, Thompson T. Retail environments as a venue for obesity prevention. Curr Obes Rep. 2016;5:184–91.
44. Pollak KI, Tulsky JA, Bravender T, Ostbye T, Lyna P, Dolor RJ, Coffman CJ, Bilheimer A, Lin PH, Farrell D, Bodner ME, Alexander SC. Teaching primary care physicians the 5 A's for discussing weight with overweight and obese adolescents. Patient Educ Couns. 2016;99:1620–5.
45. Prochaska JO, Diclemente CC. Stages and processes of self-change of smoking: toward an integrative model of change. J Consult Clin Psychol. 1983;51:390–5.
46. Prochaska JO, Velicer WF, Rossi JS, Goldstein MG, Marcus BH, Rakowski W, Fiore C, Harlow LL, Redding CA, Rosenbloom D. Stages of change and decisional balance for 12 problem behaviors. Health Psychol. 1994;13:39–46.
47. Rebholz CM, Crews DC, Grams ME, Steffen LM, Levey AS, Miller ER 3rd, Appel LJ, Coresh J. DASH (Dietary Approaches to Stop Hypertension) diet and risk of subsequent kidney disease. Am J Kidney Dis. 2016;68:853–61.
48. Rollnick S, Mason P, Butler C. Health behavior change: a guide for practitioners. Longdon: Church Livingstone; 1999.
49. Sacks FM, Svetkey LP, Vollmer WM, Appel LJ, Bray GA, Harsha D, Obarzanek E, Conlin PR, Miller ER 3rd, Simons-Morton DG, Karanja N, Lin PH, DASH-Sodium Collaborative Research Group. Effects on blood pressure of reduced dietary sodium and the Edinburgh; New York(DASH) diet. DASH-Sodium Collaborative Research Group. N Engl J Med. 2001;344:3–10.
50. Salehi-Abargouei A, Maghsoudi Z, Shirani F, Azadbakht L. Effects of Dietary Approaches to Stop Hypertension (DASH)-style diet on fatal or nonfatal cardiovascular diseases--incidence: a systematic review and meta-analysis on observational prospective studies. Nutrition. 2013;29:611–8.
51. Schneider L, Su LJ, Arab L, Bensen JT, Farnan L, Fontham ETH, Song L, Hussey J, Merchant AT, Mohler JL, Steck SE. Dietary patterns based on the Mediterranean diet and DASH diet are inversely associated with high aggressive prostate cancer in PCaP. Ann Epidemiol. 2018;29:16–22.e1.
52. Schwingshackl L, Bogensberger B, Hoffmann G. Diet quality as assessed by the healthy eating index, alternate healthy eating index, dietary approaches to stop hypertension score, and health outcomes: an updated systematic review and meta-analysis of cohort studies. J Acad Nutr Diet. 2018;118:74–100 e11.
53. Siervo M, Lara J, Chowdhury S, Ashor A, Oggioni C, Mathers JC. Effects of the Dietary Approach to Stop Hypertension (DASH) diet on cardiovascular risk factors: a systematic review and meta-analysis. Br J Nutr. 2015;113:1–15.
54. Smith SR, Klotman PE, Svetkey LP. Potassium chloride lowers blood pressure and causes natriuresis in older patients with hypertension. J Am Soc Nephrol. 1992;2:1302–9.
55. Steinberg D, Bennett GG, Svetkey L. The DASH diet, 20 years later. JAMA. 2017;317:1529–30.
56. Sun B, Williams JS, Svetkey LP, Kolatkar NS, Conlin PR. Beta2-adrenergic receptor genotype affects the renin-angiotensin-aldosterone system response to the Dietary Approaches to Stop Hypertension (DASH) dietary pattern. Am J Clin Nutr. 2010;92:444–9.
57. Svetkey LP, Pollak KI, Yancy WS Jr, Dolor RJ, Batch BC, Samsa G, Matchar DB, Lin PH. Hypertension improvement project: randomized trial of quality improvement for physicians and lifestyle modification for patients. Hypertension. 2009;54:1226–33.
58. Svetkey LP, Simons-Morton D, Vollmer WM, Appel LJ, Conlin PR, Ryan DH, Ard J, Kennedy BM. Effects of dietary patterns on blood pressure: subgroup analysis of the Dietary Approaches to Stop Hypertension (DASH) randomized clinical trial. Arch Intern Med. 1999;159:285–93.
59. Thomas SJ, Booth JN 3rd, Dai C, Li X, Allen N, Calhoun D, Carson AP, Gidding S, Lewis CE, Shikany JM, Shimbo D, Sidney S, Muntner P. Cumulative incidence of hypertension by 55 years of age in blacks and whites: the CARDIA study. J Am Heart Assoc. 2018;7(14):e007988.
60. Toro-Ramos T, Kim Y, Wood M, Randall J, Niejadlik K, Honcz J, Marrero D, Fawer A, Michaelides A. Efficacy of a mobile hypertension prevention delivery platform with human coaching. J Hum Hypertens. 2017;31(12):795–800.
61. USDA. Dietary guidelines for Americans, 2005. 6th ed. Washington, DC: U.S. Department of Health and Human Services and U.S. Department of Agriculture; 2005.
62. Vanstone M, Rewegan A, Brundisini F, Giacomini M, Kandasamy S, Dejean D. Diet modification challenges faced by marginalized and nonmarginalized adults with type 2 diabetes: a systematic review and qualitative meta-synthesis. Chronic Illn. 2017;13:217–35.
63. Vargas AJ, Neuhouser ML, George SM, Thomson CA, Ho GY, Rohan TE, Kato I, Nassir R, Hou L, Manson JE. Diet quality and colorectal cancer risk in the women's health initiative observational study. Am J Epidemiol. 2016;184:23–32.
64. Vollmer WM, Sacks FM, Ard J, Appel LJ, Bray GA, Simons-Morton DG, Conlin PR, Svetkey LP, Erlinger TP, Moore TJ, Karanja N, DASH-Sodium Collaborative Research Group. Effects of diet and sodium intake on blood pressure: subgroup analysis of the DASH-sodium trial. Ann Intern Med. 2001;135:1019–28.
65. Watson DL, Tharp RG. Self-directed behavior: self-modification for personal adjustment. Belmont: Wadsworth; 2002.

66. Whelton PK, Buring J, Borhani NO, Cohen JD, Cook N, Cutler JA, Kiley JE, Kuller LH, Satterfield S, Sacks FM, et al. The effect of potassium supplementation in persons with a high-normal blood pressure. Results from phase I of the Trials of Hypertension Prevention (TOHP). Trials of Hypertension Prevention (TOHP) Collaborative Research Group. Ann Epidemiol. 1995;5:85–95.

67. Whelton PK, Carey RM, Aronow WS, Casey DE Jr, Collins KJ, Dennison Himmelfarb C, Depalma SM, Gidding S, Jamerson KA, Jones DW, Maclaughlin EJ, Muntner P, Ovbiagele B, Smith SC Jr, Spencer CC, Stafford RS, Taler SJ, Thomas RJ, Williams KA Sr, Williamson JD, Wright JT Jr. 2017 ACC/AHA/AAPA/ABC/ACPM/AGS/APhA/ASH/ASPC/NMA/PCNA guideline for the prevention, detection, evaluation, and management of high blood pressure in adults: a report of the American College of Cardiology/American Heart Association task force on clinical practice guidelines. Circulation. 2018;138:e484–594.

68. Wright JD, Wang C-Y. Trends in intake of energy adn macronutrients in adults from 1999–2000 through 2007–2008. NCHS data brief. Hyattsville: National Center for Health Statistics; 2010.

Chapter 2
The Mediterranean Diet

Elena M. Yubero-Serrano, Francisco M. Gutierrez-Mariscal, Pablo Perez-Martinez, and Jose Lopez-Miranda

Keywords Mediterranean diet · Diet adherence · Cardiovascular disease · Oxidative stress

Key Points
- Since the "Seven Countries Study," numerous epidemiological studies support the health benefits and disease prevention effect of adherence to the Mediterranean diet.
- The Mediterranean dietary pattern is based on olive oil (mainly EVOO or VOO) as the main source of fat and provides an important source of minerals, vitamins, antioxidants, mono- and polyunsaturated fatty acids, and fiber.
- The Mediterranean diet exerts cardioprotective properties, effects on the incidence and control of the clinical features of metabolic syndrome, obesity or T2DM, neurodegenerative diseases, and aging.
- The health benefits of this diet are attributed to its high concentration in MUFA (oleic acid from EVOO) but also to the minor components (polyphenols and other compounds) of this oil, with antioxidant and anti-inflammatory capacity.
- Studies are required to fully elucidate the mechanism of the benefit on human health, especially of the minor components of EVOO.

Introduction

The Mediterranean diet is one of the best studied dietary patterns. Although this term refers to the dietary habits in a particular geographical location, the Mediterranean diet also needs to be considered as the result of sociocultural, political, religious, agricultural, and economic influences over time [1]. Since the Seven Countries Study associated the eating behaviors of Mediterranean countries with longevity and reduced risk of cardiovascular disease (CVD) compared to northern European countries and the USA over 25 years of follow-up [2], numerous epidemiological studies have supported the

E. M. Yubero-Serrano · F. M. Gutierrez-Mariscal · P. Perez-Martinez · J. Lopez-Miranda (✉)
Department of Lipids and Atherosclerosis Unit, Maimonides Institute for Biomedical Research in Cordoba, Reina Sofia University Hospital, University of Córdoba, Córdoba, Spain

CIBER Physiopathology of Obesity and Nutrition (CIBEROBN), Institute of Health Carlos III, Madrid, Spain
e-mail: jlopezmir@uco.es

© Springer Nature Switzerland AG 2020
J. Uribarri, J. A. Vassalotti (eds.), *Nutrition, Fitness, and Mindfulness*, Nutrition and Health,
https://doi.org/10.1007/978-3-030-30892-6_2

health benefits and disease prevention effects of adherence to the Mediterranean diet [3, 4]. This diet is a shared and dynamic cultural heritage that was recognized by UNESCO in 2010 [5]. Its consumption is associated with a decrease in the development of prevalent chronic diseases, particularly CVD and cancer [6, 7].

The proposed health benefits of the Mediterranean diet are mostly attributed to the consumption of traditional foods that encompass a wide variety of fresh and local and season products coupled with traditional culinary recipes. The Mediterranean diet defined as a dietary pattern is based on olive oil (mainly extra-virgin or virgin olive oil, EVOO and VOO, respectively) as the main source of fat, whole grains, legumes, fruits, vegetables, nuts, and fish, wine in moderation, and a moderate intake of lean, fresh meat, and dairy products, which provide an important source of minerals, vitamins, antioxidants, mono- and polyunsaturated fatty acids, and fiber [8]. The Mediterranean diet pattern is graphically represented as the "Mediterranean diet pyramid" including all food groups with adequate frequencies and quantities in the daily diet [8] (Fig. 2.1). Two indexes or scores are mainly used to facilitate the measurement of the adherence to the Mediterranean diet and, thus, to evaluate its associated health effects (Table 2.1): the Mediterranean Diet Score (MDS), a 0- to 9-point scale based on sample sex-specific medians of food groups, that presents potential limitations due its dependence on the habitual dietary characteristics of the sample [9] and the 14-item Mediterranean Diet Adherence Screener (MEDAS) that establishes adherence scores according to pre-defined normative criterion cutoff points for the consumption of specific food groups (pre-defined servings/day or servings/week) [10, 11].

The purpose of this chapter is to update the available evidence of the benefits of the Mediterranean diet in health through its impact on different chronic diseases.

Components of the Mediterranean Diet

Olive Oil as a Main Source of Fat

Olive oil is the primary source of dietary fat in the countries where olives are grown [12]. Historically, the healthy properties of the olive oil were attributed to its high proportion of monounsaturated fatty acids (MUFAs), namely, oleic acid (up to 80% of its total lipid composition) [13], one of the main characteristics that makes it unique compared to other oils. MUFAs have only one double bond which makes it more resistant to oxidation and a high stability and a long shelf life compared to PUFA-enriched oils [14]. Olive oil also contains minor components, mostly phenolic compounds (up to 1–2% of the total content) which contribute to its unique flavor and taste and distinguish it from other oils derived from seeds [15] (Table 2.2). Studies in humans and in animals (both in vivo and in vitro) have demonstrated that these phenolic compounds exhibit anti-inflammatory, antioxidant, and antithrombotic characteristics and, thereby, have the ability to reduce the risk of the development of chronic diseases [16, 17]. The physical methods used to produce olive oil preserve most of its antioxidant, anti-inflammatory, and antithrombotic qualities [18].

It is important to establish the type of olive oil, which depends in part on the production methods to obtain it, and determines not only its quality but also its taste and health properties. The first oil extracted, and produced using centrifugation and water only, is the so-called EVOO. It is the olive oil with the highest quality, considered as the fresh juice of the olive that preserves its high levels of natural antioxidants, vitamin E, and phenolic compounds. The VOO is also naturally obtained by the same process as EVOO although it has lower levels of minor components. Mechanical and subsequent pressings and refining processes involving heat and chemical solvents produce lowest-quality olive oils with loss of most of the healthy components.

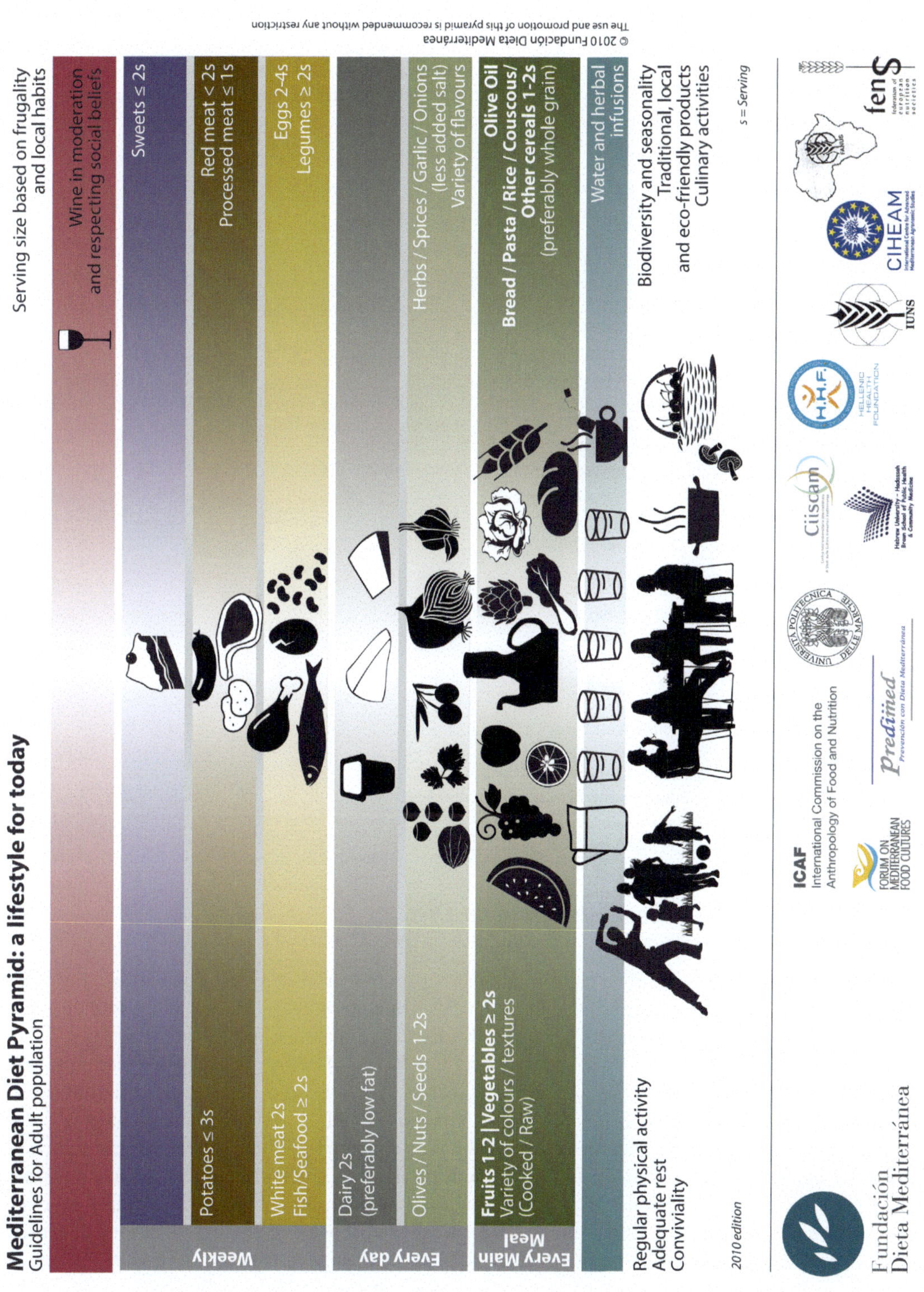

Fig. 2.1 Mediterranean diet pyramid [8]. It represents, for adult population, serving size based on frugality and local habits

Table 2.1 Main scores used in the measurement of the adherence to the Mediterranean diet

Name of score	Food components	Formula	Range of score
Mediterranean diet score (MDS-Trichopoulou)	*Beneficial foods*: 1. Vegetables 2. Fruit and nuts 3. Legumes 4. Cereals, bread, and potatoes 5. Fish 6. Ratio of monounsaturated fatty acids to saturated fatty acids 7. Moderate alcohol (10–50 g/day for men; 5–25 g/day for women) *Detrimental foods*: 1. Meat and poultry 2. Dairy products	Adding all points from positive items (higher than sex-specific median value) and negative items (lower than sex-specific median value)	0–9
Mediterranean Diet Adherence Screener (MEDAS)	1. Olive oil as main culinary fat 2. Olive oil ≥4 tablespoons/day 3. Vegetables ≥2 servings/day 4. Fruits ≥3 servings/day 5. Red or processed meats <1 serving/day 6. Butter, cream, margarine <1 serving/day 7. Sweet/carbonated beverages <1 serving/day 8. Wine ≥7 glasses/week 9. Legumes ≥3 servings/week 10. Fish or seafood ≥3 servings/week 11. Commercial bakery ≤2 servings/week 12. Nuts ≥3 serving/week 13. Poultry more than red meats 14. Use of *sofrito* sauce ≥2 servings/week	1 point allocated to positive responses; no points for negative responses	0–14

Other Components of the Mediterranean Diet

The Mediterranean diet is mainly a plant-food dietary pattern that fits a pyramid model [8] (Fig. 2.1). This pattern includes all food groups and the culinary techniques used in this diet along with the daily frequencies and quantities. Typically, plant-origin foods are situated at the base of the pyramid that represents their consumption every day and in several portions. They are cereals and legumes (preferably with whole foods because they are more fiber-rich), fruits, and vegetables, including fresh legumes, providing an important source of fiber, vitamins A and C, minerals, and antioxidant compounds [19]. Dairy products (yogurt, cheese, and other fermented products) should be consumed in moderate amounts because, despite their high concentration in calcium, they can be an important source of saturated fat. A reasonable consumption of nuts, seeds, and olives provides lipids, proteins, vitamins, minerals, and fiber [20]. Animal-origin foods and those rich in sugar and fats should be eaten in moderation and even in special occasions. Fish, shellfish, and white meat (poultry, turkey, or rabbit) can be consumed two to four servings per week providing high-quality protein and lipids. However, red meat is recommended less than two servings per week and processed meats intake less or equal to one serving per week [8].

Table 2.2 Principal EVOO components

Fatty acids
Oleic acid (C18:1) (55–83% of EVOO)
Linoleic acid (C18:2) (3.5–21% of EVOO)
Palmitic acid (C16:0) (7.5–20% of EVOO)
Stearic acid (C18:0) (0.5–5% of EVOO)
Linolenic acid (C18:3) (specifically alpha-linolenic acid, 0–1.5% of EVOO)
Unsaponifiable fraction
Polyphenols (18–37% of this fraction)
Flavonoids (*flavonols and anthocyanins*)
Phenolic acids and alcohols (*hydroxytyrosol, oleuropein, tyrosol, caffeic acid, ligstroside, vanillic acid*)
Sterols (triterpene, triterpene dialcohols, 4-methylsterols)
Tocopherols (2–3% of this fraction)
Alpha-, beta-, delta-, and gamma-tocopherols
Hydrocarbons (30–50% of this fraction)
Squalene
Beta-carotene

Pigments (chlorophylls and carotenoids)
EVOO extra-virgin olive oil (CX:Y), above indicates *C* carbon, *X* number of carbon atoms in the molecule, *Y* number of double bonds

The Mediterranean Diet in Health and Disease

The Cardioprotective Effect of the Mediterranean Diet

During the past decades, scientific evidence has demonstrated the cardioprotective effect of the Mediterranean diet by associating a high adherence to this diet with lower incidence of CVD [9, 21]. Accordingly, different intervention studies have demonstrated that consumption of this diet is associated with significant improvement in health status and reduction in all-cause, cardiovascular, and cancer mortality [22, 23]. In this sense, the primary prevention PREDIMED (Prevención con Dieta Mediterránea) trial including 7447 middle-aged people at high risk of CVD randomized to three diets: two Mediterranean diets, one supplemented with EVOO, and the other with nuts versus a control low-fat diet [24]. Following the initial publication, statistical reviewers concluded the relative reduction of 30% in the risk of first major CVD event (nonfatal myocardial infarction, nonfatal stroke, or cardiovascular death), after a median of 4.8 year's follow-up in both Mediterranean diet arms, could have been influenced by an effect size or even to problems with the integrity of randomization to the diets [25–27]. In response, the authors retracted the original manuscript, reanalyzed the data, and published a new report with similar results in terms of the Mediterranean diet effects [28].

Different pathophysiological mechanisms have been proposed by which the Mediterranean diet exerts its beneficial cardiovascular properties through anti-inflammatory, antioxidant, and antithrombotic effects, as well as by its action on endothelial dysfunction, blood pressure, and lipid profile.

The Mediterranean Diet Effects on Endothelial Function: Anti-inflammatory and Antioxidant Properties of the Diet

Endothelial dysfunction is characterized by enhanced expression and release into the circulation of inflammatory cytokines and adhesion molecules, decreased production of nitric oxide (NO), which maintains vascular homeostasis and plays a crucial role in the normal endothelial function, and increased production of reactive oxygen species. Indeed, one of the main mechanisms by which endothelium-dependent vasodilation is impaired is an increase in oxidative stress that inactivates NO [29].

A body of evidence supports a favorable effect of the Mediterranean diet on the vasomotor function of the endothelium. Accordingly, a 4-week period of consumption of a Mediterranean diet rich in EVOO was associated with an improvement in endothelial function versus a SFA-rich diet in hypercholesterolemic patients [30]. The same improvement was observed in elderly subjects after consumption of a Mediterranean diet, probably mediated by lower inflammation and oxidative stress and higher NO bioavailability, compared to other diets [31–33]. Moreover, this diet was able to reduce the endothelial microparticles concentration and to increase endothelial progenitor cell levels related to endothelial damage and regenerative capacity of the endothelium, respectively [34]. Results from the PREDIMED study showed that a Mediterranean diet rich in EVOO or nuts led to a reduction in C-reactive protein (CRP), interleukin-6 (IL-6), and other inflammatory biomarkers in subjects with high cardiovascular risk [35]. Similarly, patients were found to exhibit a reduction in the expression of pro-inflammatory and prothrombotic genes, after 3 months of a Mediterranean diet rich in EVOO compared to a Mediterranean diet rich in nuts or a control diet [36]. Similar findings were obtained during the postprandial state, where the Mediterranean diet also has anti-inflammatory effects [37, 38]. In addition to the high MUFA content, EVOO phenolic compounds of the Mediterranean diet are powerful antioxidants that have been shown to be effective treatment for the oxidative stress associated with several chronic diseases. Perez-Martinez et al. showed that consumption of a Mediterranean diet, rich in EVOO, reduced postprandial levels of lipid peroxide (LPO), protein carbonyl, and plasma hydrogen peroxide levels compared to a SFA-rich diet in metabolic syndrome subjects [39]. Similarly, this dietary pattern produced a greater postprandial decrease in plasma LPO and nitrotyrosine levels compared to other diets in elderly men and women [40].

The Mediterranean Diet Effects on Lipid Profile

Both total cholesterol (TC) and LDL-cholesterol levels are directly associated with CVD risk, while there is an inverse relationship with HDL-cholesterol [41]. Many studies have aimed to explore the effects of the fatty components of the diet on the lipid profile. The Mediterranean diet, due to its high MUFA concentration, has been shown to reduce TC, LDL-cholesterol, and the ratio TC/HDL-cholesterol when it is substituted for SFA [40, 42]. By design, most of the studies have focused on the influence of fasting lipids on CVD. However, it has become increasingly important to assess postprandial lipemia both for its relationship with pro-oxidative, prothrombotic, and pro-inflammatory biological changes as for a direct link to cardiovascular events [43]. When considering the effect of different dietary models on postprandial lipids, most of the research has been performed using the same (or very similar) meal base, enriched with different sources of fat. In this context, current evidence suggests that omega-3 leads to a low postprandial hypertriglyceridemia, but the amount of omega-3 necessary to cause such effect is difficult to maintain in a regular meal. However, a MUFA-rich fat and, in particular, phenolic compounds (provided by EVOO) provoke a sharper, earlier rise in triglyceride levels, followed by a faster lipid clearance, compared to SFA-rich meals, which produce a smaller increase in triglycerides [44].

The Mediterranean Diet on Metabolic Syndrome and Obesity

The metabolic syndrome (MetS) is a cluster of risk factors that reflects mainly overnutrition and sedentary lifestyle. In 2001, the National Cholesterol Education Program Adult Treatment Panel III (NCEP-ATP III) [45] proposed the presence of three of the following five factors to define

MetS: abdominal obesity (highly correlated with insulin resistance), reduced HDL-cholesterol, elevated triglycerides, elevated blood pressure, and elevated fasting glucose. In 2005, the International Diabetes Federation (IDF) set up a novel criterion for the assessment of MetS, which compromises central obesity as the principal characteristic pairing with two of the four criteria described by NCEP-ATP III [46]. Patients with MetS are at risk for type 2 diabetes mellitus (T2DM) and CVD [47]. In fact, this syndrome is associated with increased morbidity and all-cause mortality [48]. The pr of MetS in adults is estimated at 25% of the population [49] and is increasing to epidemic proportions, making it an important worldwide public health problem. The cause of MetS is multifactorial implicating a complex interaction between genetic background, hormones, and nutrition [50]. Accordingly, investigators have concluded that lifestyle modifications, such as increased physical activity, weight loss, or adherence to a healthy eating such as the Mediterranean dietary pattern, should be associated with reversal of MetS or improvement in its components [51].

Recent evidence highlights the protective effect of the Mediterranean diet on components of MetS [52]. The benefits associated with this diet might be due mainly to its well-described and documented antioxidant and anti-inflammatory properties [53]. The ATTICA study demonstrated 20% decrease in the risk of developing MetS with Mediterranean diet adherence for 3042 Greek subjects without CVD or diabetes, who lived in the Athens province for which the study is named. The authors suggested a relationship between the Mediterranean diet and an increase in antioxidant capacity accompanied by low oxidized LDL-cholesterol concentrations as potential mechanisms for the beneficial risk reduction [54]. The diminishing risk for MetS associated with adherence to the Mediterranean diet was also shown in another cohort study carried out by Tortosa et al. during a 6-year follow-up [55]. These beneficial Mediterranean diet effects have been attributed, at least in part, to its fat composition, specifically to the content in MUFA. Previously, the LIPGENE study, a large pan-European isocaloric dietary intervention study of MetS subjects, showed that diets with SFA replacement with MUFA or low-fat, high amount of complex carbohydrate, had an effective improvement of insulin sensitivity [56], postprandial inflammatory status [57], and oxidative stress [39], as well as improvement in endothelial function [58]. Especially interesting are studies of non-Mediterranean populations, such as the 7-year follow-up investigation of the Framingham Heart Study Offspring Cohort of 1918 US participants that revealed a reduced incidence of MetS, including reduced abdominal obesity and enhanced insulin resistance, associated with adherence to the Mediterranean diet [59]. More recently, two clinical trials have explored the effect of the Mediterranean diet on MetS patients at risk of CVD. The first is in the context of the PREDIMED study [28]. This study showed that a Mediterranean diet supplemented with nuts reversed MetS more than a low-fat diet, in the context of primary prevention of CVD, after the first year of follow-up [60]. In fact, the Mediterranean diet, either supplemented with EVOO oil or nuts, was not associated with the onset of MetS but with its regression [61]. The second trial is the CORDIOPREV (CORonary Diet Intervention with Olive oil and cardiovascular PREVention) study that included 1002 patients with coronary artery disease (CAD) in the context of secondary prevention of CVD [62]. Results from the CORDIOPREV study demonstrated that in patients with MetS, the polymorphism at the TNF-alpha gene interacts with the Mediterranean diet to influence triglyceride metabolism and inflammation status, showing that the detrimental profile associated with G/G genotype improved after 1 year of dietary intervention [63]. The results from CORDIOPREV study support the mechanism that Mediterranean diet consumption might play a contributing role in triggering lipid metabolism by interacting with the rs3764261 SNP at CETP gene locus in MetS patients [64]. In summary, these results support the important role of the Mediterranean diet in personalized treatment of patients with MetS. Adherence to the Mediterranean diet has a great impact on the individual components of the MetS. In fact, the Mediterranean diet could be considered the first step in the clinical management of patients with MetS [19, 65].

Impact of the Mediterranean Diet on Type 2 Diabetes Mellitus

Type 2 diabetes mellitus (T2DM) is difficult to prevent and control. Lifestyle modifications, particularly, a healthy diet, are well established as beneficial in the treatment of T2DM. The Mediterranean diet is one of the most widely investigated dietary patterns hypothesized to be effective in the management and prevention of T2DM and, in turn, the reduction of T2DM complications [66]. In fact, Martinez-Gonzalez et al. found in a prospective cohort study that high adherence to the Mediterranean diet was associated with reduction in the development of T2DM [67]. These findings were also confirmed in other prospective cohort studies (TOSCA.IT and EPIC-Potsdam [4, 21]) and in intervention dietary clinical trials, including the SUN cohort, PREDIMED, and CORDIOPREV studies [21, 68, 69].

The health benefits of the Mediterranean diet on T2DM could be attributed to the anti-inflammatory and high antioxidant properties of the diet [2] and improvement in glycemic control and endothelial function [70]. For example, EVOO prevents insulin resistance, metabolic syndrome, or obesity and might lead to better lipid profiles not only due to the high MUFA content but also attributed to other minor components of this oil. Although the adherence to this diet improves β-cell function, it is tissue-specific, producing an increase of insulin sensitivity in T2DM patients who have muscle insulin resistance [69]. The Mediterranean diet consumption is also associated with higher adiponectin [71], lower advanced glycation end products levels, modulation of the glycotoxin metabolism, and also a lower glycemic index, which may also partly explain the beneficial effects on glucose control, hyperinsulinemia and insulin resistance, and, ultimately, the reduced T2DM risk [72, 73].

Impact of the Mediterranean Diet on Kidney Disease

Patients with chronic kidney disease (CKD) are at high risk of CVD complications. In the last decade, different dietary strategies have been proposed in the approach to prevent CKD and delay the need for dialysis. Mainly, these dietary recommendations are focused on changes of energy and protein and the restriction of single micronutrients (sodium, potassium, and phosphorus) consumption [74].

Recently, the application of a Mediterranean diet was shown to have a favorable effect, at least, in the earlier stages of CKD, establishing a relationship between this diet and markers related to kidney function (a reduction of albuminuria, glomerular filtration rate decline, and serum levels of urea and creatinine) [75]. Of note, these health benefits do not result from a single component of the Mediterranean diet, but the whole diet model is responsible. In this sense, protein content in the Mediterranean diet aligns with the recommended protein intake for CKD (~0.8 g/kg/day) where the main source comes from vegetables, fish, and white meat providing, compared to red meat, lower dietary sodium, phosphate, and potassium [76, 77]. Moreover, the lipid-derived energy of the Mediterranean diet is mainly due to oleic acid from EVOO (50% MUFA of the total fat), highly associated with a lower risk of both CVD and all-cause mortality. The low consumption of red or processed meat determines a low SFA intake, not exceeding 7–8%, contributing to the beneficial effect of this diet since SFA is associated with pro-inflammatory and pro-oxidant properties [78]. This, together with other favorable effects of the Mediterranean diet, described previously, provides mechanistic pathways to explain reduction of renal function decline and improved survival in CKD patients who have high adherence to a Mediterranean diet.

Impact of the Mediterranean Diet on Neurodegenerative Diseases

Neurodegenerative disorders constitute the most prevalent among age-related diseases, and according to the World Health Organization (WHO), around 50 million people have dementia [79]. By 2050, it is projected that Alzheimer's disease (AD) will affect 13.8 million worldwide [80]. Neurodegenerative diseases share mitochondrial dysfunction and increases in oxidative stress as common features [81]. Parkinson's disease (PD) is estimated to be the second most prevalent neurodegenerative disorder, so that by the age of 85 years, half of the population develops PD signs [82]. Since no curative therapies are available for neurodegenerative diseases, the current focus is on prevention. Accordingly, lifestyle and health behaviors, such as diet, are the more relevant preventative therapies [83]. Due to the antioxidant, cardioprotective, and anti-inflammatory properties of the Mediterranean diet, investigators hypothesized it to be protective for neurodegenerative diseases.

Among protective modifiable lifestyle factors against AD and cognitive decline, the Mediterranean diet is one of the more extensively studied in the literature [84]. Several prospective cohort and case-control studies suggest an association between adherence to the Mediterranean diet and improved AD, dementia, and cognitive function outcomes, although in some studies the findings were inconclusive [23]. A meta-analysis published in 2014 showed that people in the highest Mediterranean diet tertile had up to 33% lower risk of AD compared to the lowest tertile, with an increased protective effect against the progression of dementia with greater Mediterranean diet adherence, suggesting a dose response [85]. These findings highlight the necessity for additional investigation of the Mediterranean diet and dementia-related diseases. More recently, the results from a population of 1865 individuals of the HELIAD (Hellenic Longitudinal Investigation of Aging and Diet) study showed that greater adherence to the Mediterranean diet was associated with decreased risk of dementia and better cognition, with a strong association for memory [86].

Regarding other neurodegenerative diseases, there is only limited evidence of an association between dietary patterns and onset of the diseases. In the case of PD, most of the literature has focused on individual foods rather than on dietary patterns. The studies have revealed no consistent findings regarding the protective effect of the Mediterranean diet on PD. In a recent case-control PD study in Italy, there was no difference between the groups in terms of overall Mediterranean diet adherence [87]. In contrast, another case-control study performed in the USA showed that adherence to the Mediterranean diet was inversely associated with the odds of PD and also was directly associated with a later age of PD onset [88]. A recent study by Agarwal et al., published in 2018 on a population of 706 participants from the Rush Memory and Aging Project (MAP), showed a moderate protective association for the Mediterranean diet and development of PD and progression of the parkinsonian signs [89]. The authors found the strongest association of positive outcomes with the adherence to MIND (Mediterranean-DASH Diet Intervention for Neurodegenerative Delay) diet, which emphasizes foods and nutrients that have shown to protect the brain with aging in previous studies [90, 91].

The potential mechanisms which might be involved in the protective effects of the Mediterranean diet on neurodegenerative diseases have been investigated using animal and in vitro models. These studies have explored the specific components of the Mediterranean diet with neuroprotective effect. In this context, polyphenols found in EVOO and red wine have been of particular interest, with evidence suggesting that they could act as "caloric restriction mimickers," activating similar sirtuin pathways as caloric restriction diets [92]. A recent in vitro study has demonstrated protective properties of resveratrol on PC12 cells from the apoptotic action of Aβ23–Aβ35 peptides [93].

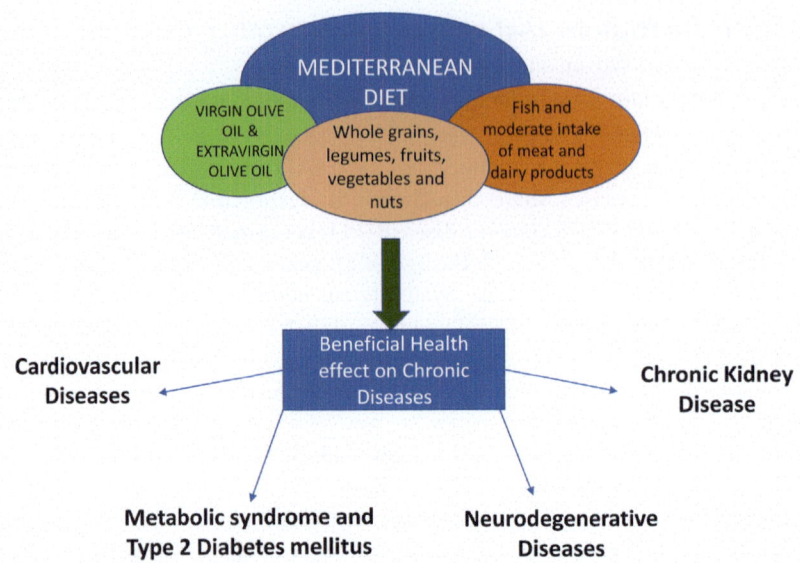

Fig. 2.2 Health benefits by Mediterranean diet. The scheme represents the mainly chronic diseases with documented evidence for the beneficial effects of the Mediterranean diet

Conclusions

Growing evidence indicates that adherence to a Mediterranean diet is associated with benefits on human health, particularly reducing the incidence and development of different chronic diseases. This fact is not only attributed to its high concentration in MUFA (oleic acid from EVOO) but also to the minor components (polyphenols and other compounds) of this oil, with antioxidant and anti-inflammatory capacity. In addition, the Mediterranean diet is also associated with limited intake of pro-inflammatory simple carbohydrates, SFA, and processed meats. All of this confers the Mediterranean diet with cardioprotective properties, slowing down the earlier stages of the development of atherosclerosis, producing a favorable lipid profile, decreasing blood pressure, and shortening postprandial lipemia, effects on the incidence and control of the clinical features of metabolic syndrome, obesity or T2DM and neurodegenerative diseases, and aging (Fig. 2.2). Although the current review provides strong evidence for the beneficial effects derived from a Mediterranean diet consumption in humans, more studies are required to fully elucidate the mechanism of the benefit, especially of the minor components of EVOO on human health. In this sense, it would be particularly interesting to evaluate whether it is one or more phenolic compounds, which cause these effects, or if they are the consequence of a synergic effect of the total phenolic fraction.

References

1. Dernini S, Berry E, Serra-Majem L, La Vecchia C, Capone R, Medina FX, Aranceta J, Belahsen R, Burlingame B, Giorgio C, Corella D, Donini L, Lairon D, Meybeck A, Pekcan G, Piscopo S, Yngve A, Trichopoulou A. Med diet 4.0: the Mediterranean diet with four sustainable benefits. 2016;20. https://doi.org/10.1017/S1368980016003177.
2. Villani A, Sultana J, Doecke J, Mantzioris E. Differences in the interpretation of a modernized Mediterranean diet prescribed in intervention studies for the management of type 2 diabetes: how closely does this align with a traditional Mediterranean diet? Eur J Nutr. 2018; https://doi.org/10.1007/s00394-018-1757-3.
3. Martinez-Gonzalez MA, Bes-Rastrollo M. Dietary patterns, Mediterranean diet, and cardiovascular disease. Curr Opin Lipidol. 2014;25(1):20–6. https://doi.org/10.1097/MOL.0000000000000044.

4. Vitale M, Masulli M, Calabrese I, Rivellese AA, Bonora E, Signorini S, Perriello G, Squatrito S, Buzzetti R, Sartore G, Babini AC, Gregori G, Giordano C, Clemente G, Grioni S, Dolce P, Riccardi G, Vaccaro O, Group TIS. Impact of a Mediterranean dietary pattern and its components on cardiovascular risk factors, glucose control, and body weight in people with type 2 diabetes: a real-life study. Nutrients. 2018;10(8). https://doi.org/10.3390/nu10081067.

5. UNESCO. Representative list of the intangible cultural heritage of humanity. 2010. http://www.unesco.org/culture/ich/en/RL/00394. Accessed April 2011.

6. Coni E, Di Benedetto R, Di Pasquale M, Masella R, Modesti D, Mattei R, Carlini EA. Protective effect of oleuropein, an olive oil biophenol, on low density lipoprotein oxidizability in rabbits. Lipids. 2000;35(1):45–54.

7. Keys A, Aravanis C, Van Buchem H, et al. The diet and all-causes death rate in the Seven Countries Study. Lancet. 1981;2(8237):58–61.

8. Bach-Faig A, Berry EM, Lairon D, Reguant J, Trichopoulou A, Dernini S, Medina FX, Battino M, Belahsen R, Miranda G, Serra-Majem L, Mediterranean Diet Foundation Expert G. Mediterranean diet pyramid today. Science and cultural updates. Public Health Nutr. 2011;14(12A):2274–84. https://doi.org/10.1017/S1368980011002515.

9. Trichopoulou A, Costacou T, Bamia C, Trichopoulos D. Adherence to a Mediterranean diet and survival in a Greek population. N Engl J Med. 2003;348(26):2599–608. https://doi.org/10.1056/NEJMoa025039.

10. Schroder H, Fito M, Estruch R, Martinez-Gonzalez MA, Corella D, Salas-Salvado J, Lamuela-Raventos R, Ros E, Salaverria I, Fiol M, Lapetra J, Vinyoles E, Gomez-Gracia E, Lahoz C, Serra-Majem L, Pinto X, Ruiz-Gutierrez V, Covas MI. A short screener is valid for assessing Mediterranean diet adherence among older Spanish men and women. J Nutr. 2011;141(6):1140–5. https://doi.org/10.3945/jn.110.135566.

11. Martinez-Gonzalez MA, Fernandez-Jarne E, Serrano-Martinez M, Marti A, Martinez JA, Martin-Moreno JM. Mediterranean diet and reduction in the risk of a first acute myocardial infarction: an operational healthy dietary score. Eur J Nutr. 2002;41(4):153–60. https://doi.org/10.1007/s00394-002-0370-6.

12. Visioli F, Poli A, Gall C. Antioxidant and other biological activities of phenols from olives and olive oil. Med Res Rev. 2002;22(1):65–75.

13. Tripoli E, Giammanco M, Tabacchi G, Di Majo D, Giammanco S, La Guardia M. The phenolic compounds of olive oil: structure, biological activity and beneficial effects on human health. Nutr Res Rev. 2005;18(1):98–112.

14. Owen RW, Mier W, Giacosa A, Hull WE, Spiegelhalder B, Bartsch H. Phenolic compounds and squalene in olive oils: the concentration and antioxidant potential of total phenols, simple phenols, secoiridoids, lignansand squalene. Food Chem Toxicol. 2000;38(8):647–59.

15. Fito M, de la Torre R, Farre-Albaladejo M, Khymenetz O, Marrugat J, Covas MI. Bioavailability and antioxidant effects of olive oil phenolic compounds in humans: a review. Annali dell'Istituto superiore di sanita. 2007;43(4):375–81.

16. Covas M, Nyyssonen K, Poulsen H, Kaikkonen J, Zunft H, Kiesewetter H, Gaddi A, de la Torre R, Mursu J, Baumler H, Nascetti S, Salonen J, Fito M, Virtanen J, Marrugat J. The effect of polyphenols in olive oil on heart disease risk factors: a randomized trial. Ann Intern Med. 2006;145:333–41.

17. Camargo A, Ruano J, Fernandez JM, Parnell LD, Jimenez A, Santos-Gonzalez M, Marin C, Perez-Martinez P, Uceda M, Lopez-Miranda J, Perez-Jimenez F. Gene expression changes in mononuclear cells in patients with metabolic syndrome after acute intake of phenol-rich virgin olive oil. BMC Genomics. 2010;11:253.

18. Corona G, Spencer JP, Dessi MA. Extra virgin olive oil phenolics: absorption, metabolism, and biological activities in the GI tract. Toxicol Ind Health. 2009;25(4–5):285–93. https://doi.org/10.1177/0748233709102951.

19. Sofi F, Cesari F, Abbate R, Gensini GF, Casini A. Adherence to Mediterranean diet and health status: meta-analysis. BMJ. 2008;337:a1344. https://doi.org/10.1136/bmj.a1344.

20. Sabate J, Ros E, Salas-Salvado J. Nuts: nutrition and health outcomes. Preface. Br J Nutr. 2006;96(Suppl 2):S1–2.

21. Galbete C, Kroger J, Jannasch F, Iqbal K, Schwingshackl L, Schwedhelm C, Weikert C, Boeing H, Schulze MB. Nordic diet, Mediterranean diet, and the risk of chronic diseases: the EPIC-Potsdam study. BMC Med. 2018;16(1):99. https://doi.org/10.1186/s12916-018-1082-y.

22. Martinez-Gonzalez MA, Martin-Calvo N. Mediterranean diet and life expectancy; beyond olive oil, fruits, and vegetables. Curr Opin Clin Nutr Metab Care. 2016;19(6):401–7. https://doi.org/10.1097/MCO.0000000000000316.

23. Sofi F, Macchi C, Abbate R, Gensini GF, Casini A. Mediterranean diet and health. Biofactors. 2013;39(4):335–42. https://doi.org/10.1002/biof.1096.

24. Estruch R, Ros E, Salas-Salvado J, Covas MI, Corella D, Aros F, Gomez-Gracia E, Ruiz-Gutierrez V, Fiol M, Lapetra J, Lamuela-Raventos RM, Serra-Majem L, Pinto X, Basora J, Munoz MA, Sorli JV, Martinez JA, Martinez-Gonzalez MA, Investigators PS. Primary prevention of cardiovascular disease with a Mediterranean diet. N Engl J Med. 2013;368(14):1279–90. https://doi.org/10.1056/NEJMoa1200303.

25. Estruch R, Ros E, Salas-Salvado J, Covas MI, Corella D, Aros F, Gomez-Gracia E, Ruiz-Gutierrez V, Fiol M, Lapetra J, Lamuela-Raventos RM, Serra-Majem L, Pinto X, Basora J, Munoz MA, Sorli JV, Martinez JA, Martinez-Gonzalez MA. Retraction and republication: primary prevention of cardiovascular disease with a Mediterranean diet. N Engl J Med 2013. 2018a;368:1279–90. N Engl J Med. 378(25):2441–2442. https://doi.org/10.1056/NEJMc1806491.

26. Correia LCL. Primary prevention of cardiovascular disease with a Mediterranean diet supplemented with extra-virgin olive oil or nuts. N Engl J Med. 2018;379(14):1387. https://doi.org/10.1056/NEJMc1809971.
27. Stewart RAH. Primary prevention of cardiovascular disease with a Mediterranean diet supplemented with extra-virgin olive oil or nuts. N Engl J Med. 2018;379(14):1388. https://doi.org/10.1056/NEJMc1809971.
28. Estruch R, Ros E, Salas-Salvado J, Covas MI, Corella D, Aros F, Gomez-Gracia E, Ruiz-Gutierrez V, Fiol M, Lapetra J, Lamuela-Raventos RM, Serra-Majem L, Pinto X, Basora J, Munoz MA, Sorli JV, Martinez JA, Fito M, Gea A, Hernan MA, Martinez-Gonzalez MA, Investigators PS. Primary prevention of cardiovascular disease with a Mediterranean diet supplemented with extra-virgin olive oil or nuts. N Engl J Med. 2018b;378(25):e34. https://doi.org/10.1056/NEJMoa1800389.
29. Higashi Y, Noma K, Yoshizumi M, Kihara Y. Endothelial function and oxidative stress in cardiovascular diseases. Circ J. 2009;73(3):411–8.
30. Fuentes F, Lopez-Miranda J, Sanchez E, Sanchez F, Paez J, Paz-Rojas E, Marin C, Gomez P, Jimenez-Pereperez J, Ordovas JM, Perez-Jimenez F. Mediterranean and low-fat diets improve endothelial function in hypercholesterolemic men. Ann Intern Med. 2001;134(12):1115–9.
31. Yubero-Serrano EM, Delgado-Casado N, Delgado-Lista J, Perez-Martinez P, Tasset-Cuevas I, Santos-Gonzalez M, Caballero J, Garcia-Rios A, Marin C, Gutierrez-Mariscal FM, Fuentes F, Villalba JM, Tunez I, Perez-Jimenez F, Lopez-Miranda J. Postprandial antioxidant effect of the Mediterranean diet supplemented with coenzyme Q10 in elderly men and women. Age (Dordr). 2011a;33(4):579–90. https://doi.org/10.1007/s11357-010-9199-8.
32. Yubero-Serrano EM, Gonzalez-Guardia L, Rangel-Zuniga O, Delgado-Casado N, Delgado-Lista J, Perez-Martinez P, Garcia-Rios A, Caballero J, Marin C, Gutierrez-Mariscal FM, Tinahones FJ, Villalba JM, Tunez I, Perez-Jimenez F, Lopez-Miranda J. Postprandial antioxidant gene expression is modified by Mediterranean diet supplemented with coenzyme Q(10) in elderly men and women. Age (Dordr). 2013;35(1):159–70. https://doi.org/10.1007/s11357-011-9331-4.
33. Yubero-Serrano EM, Gonzalez-Guardia L, Rangel-Zuniga O, Delgado-Lista J, Gutierrez-Mariscal FM, Perez-Martinez P, Delgado-Casado N, Cruz-Teno C, Tinahones FJ, Villalba JM, Perez-Jimenez F, Lopez-Miranda J. Mediterranean diet supplemented with coenzyme Q10 modifies the expression of proinflammatory and endoplasmic reticulum stress-related genes in elderly men and women. J Gerontol A Biol Sci Med Sci. 2012;67(1):3–10. https://doi.org/10.1093/gerona/glr167.
34. Marin C, Ramirez R, Delgado-Lista J, Yubero-Serrano EM, Perez-Martinez P, Carracedo J, Garcia-Rios A, Rodriguez F, Gutierrez-Mariscal FM, Gomez P, Perez-Jimenez F, Lopez-Miranda J. Mediterranean diet reduces endothelial damage and improves the regenerative capacity of endothelium. Am J Clin Nutr. 2011;93(2):267–74. https://doi.org/10.3945/ajcn.110.006866.
35. Estruch R. Anti-inflammatory effects of the Mediterranean diet: the experience of the PREDIMED study. Proc Nutr Soc. 2010;69(3):333–40. https://doi.org/10.1017/S0029665110001539.
36. Llorente-Cortes V, Estruch R, Mena MP, Ros E, Gonzalez MA, Fito M, Lamuela-Raventos RM, Badimon L. Effect of Mediterranean diet on the expression of pro-atherogenic genes in a population at high cardiovascular risk. Atherosclerosis. 2010;208(2):442–50. https://doi.org/10.1016/j.atherosclerosis.2009.08.004.
37. Jimenez-Gomez Y, Lopez-Miranda J, Blanco-Colio LM, Marin C, Perez-Martinez P, Ruano J, Paniagua JA, Rodriguez F, Egido J, Perez-Jimenez F. Olive oil and walnut breakfasts reduce the postprandial inflammatory response in mononuclear cells compared with a butter breakfast in healthy men. Atherosclerosis. 2009;204(2):e70–6. https://doi.org/10.1016/j.atherosclerosis.2008.09.011.
38. Konstantinidou V, Khymenets O, Fito M, De La Torre R, Anglada R, Dopazo A, Covas MI. Characterization of human gene expression changes after olive oil ingestion: an exploratory approach. Folia Biol (Praha). 2009;55(3):85–91.
39. Perez-Martinez P, Garcia-Quintana JM, Yubero-Serrano EM, Tasset-Cuevas I, Tunez I, Garcia-Rios A, Delgado-Lista J, Marin C, Perez-Jimenez F, Roche HM, Lopez-Miranda J. Postprandial oxidative stress is modified by dietary fat: evidence from a human intervention study. Clin Sci (Lond). 2010a;119(6):251–61. https://doi.org/10.1042/CS20100015.
40. Yubero-Serrano EM, Garcia-Rios A, Delgado-Lista J, Delgado-Casado N, Perez-Martinez P, Rodriguez-Cantalejo F, Fuentes F, Cruz-Teno C, Tunez I, Tasset-Cuevas I, Tinahones FJ, Perez-Jimenez F, Lopez-Miranda J. Postprandial effects of the Mediterranean diet on oxidant and antioxidant status in elderly men and women. J Am Geriatr Soc. 2011b;59(5):938–40. https://doi.org/10.1111/j.1532-5415.2011.03381.x.
41. Rader DJ, Alexander ET, Weibel GL, Billheimer J, Rothblat GH. The role of reverse cholesterol transport in animals and humans and relationship to atherosclerosis. J Lipid Res. 2009;50(Suppl):S189–94. https://doi.org/10.1194/jlr.R800088-JLR200.
42. Ramirez-Tortosa MC, Suarez A, Gomez MC, Mir A, Ros E, Mataix J, Gil A. Effect of extra-virgin olive oil and fish-oil supplementation on plasma lipids and susceptibility of low-density lipoprotein to oxidative alteration in free-living Spanish male patients with peripheral vascular disease. Clin Nutr. 1999;18(3):167–74. https://doi.org/10.1054/clnu.1999.0025.

43. Kolovou GD, Mikhailidis DP, Kovar J, Lairon D, Nordestgaard BG, Ooi TC, Perez-Martinez P, Bilianou H, Anagnostopoulou K, Panotopoulos G. Assessment and clinical relevance of non-fasting and postprandial triglycerides: an expert panel statement. Curr Vasc Pharmacol. 2011;9(3):258–70.

44. Sanders TA, de Grassi T, Miller GJ, Morrissey JH. Influence of fatty acid chain length and cis/trans isomerization on postprandial lipemia and factor VII in healthy subjects (postprandial lipids and factor VII). Atherosclerosis. 2000;149(2):413–20.

45. Expert Panel on Detection E, Treatment of High Blood Cholesterol in A. Executive summary of the third report of the National Cholesterol Education Program (NCEP) expert panel on detection, evaluation, and treatment of high blood cholesterol in adults (adult treatment panel III). JAMA. 2001;285(19):2486–97.

46. Zimmet P, Magliano D, Matsuzawa Y, Alberti G, Shaw J. The metabolic syndrome: a global public health problem and a new definition. J Atheroscler Thromb. 2005;12(6):295–300.

47. Schmidt C, Bergstrom GM. The metabolic syndrome predicts cardiovascular events: results of a 13-year follow-up in initially healthy 58-year-old men. Metab Syndr Relat Disord. 2012;10(6):394–9. https://doi.org/10.1089/met.2012.0048.

48. Mottillo S, Filion KB, Genest J, Joseph L, Pilote L, Poirier P, Rinfret S, Schiffrin EL, Eisenberg MJ. The metabolic syndrome and cardiovascular risk a systematic review and meta-analysis. J Am Coll Cardiol. 2010;56(14):1113–32. https://doi.org/10.1016/j.jacc.2010.05.034.

49. Beltran-Sanchez H, Harhay MO, Harhay MM, McElligott S. Prevalence and trends of metabolic syndrome in the adult U.S. population, 1999-2010. J Am Coll Cardiol. 2013;62(8):697–703. https://doi.org/10.1016/j.jacc.2013.05.064.

50. Perez-Martinez P, Lopez-Miranda J. Editorial: nutritional therapy in metabolic syndrome. Curr Vasc Pharmacol. 2013;11(6):838–41.

51. Perez-Martinez P, Mikhailidis DP, Athyros VG, Bullo M, Couture P, Covas MI, de Koning L, Delgado-Lista J, Diaz-Lopez A, Drevon CA, Estruch R, Esposito K, Fito M, Garaulet M, Giugliano D, Garcia-Rios A, Katsiki N, Kolovou G, Lamarche B, Maiorino MI, Mena-Sanchez G, Munoz-Garach A, Nikolic D, Ordovas JM, Perez-Jimenez F, Rizzo M, Salas-Salvado J, Schroder H, Tinahones FJ, de la Torre R, van Ommen B, Wopereis S, Ros E, Lopez-Miranda J. Lifestyle recommendations for the prevention and management of metabolic syndrome: an international panel recommendation. Nutr Rev. 2017;75(5):307–26. https://doi.org/10.1093/nutrit/nux014.

52. Chiva-Blanch G, Badimon L. Effects of polyphenol intake on metabolic syndrome: current evidences from human trials. Oxidative Med Cell Longev. 2017;2017:5812401. https://doi.org/10.1155/2017/5812401.

53. Grosso G, Mistretta A, Marventano S, Purrello A, Vitaglione P, Calabrese G, Drago F, Galvano F. Beneficial effects of the Mediterranean diet on metabolic syndrome. Curr Pharm Des. 2014;20(31):5039–44.

54. Panagiotakos DB, Pitsavos C, Chrysohoou C, Skoumas J, Tousoulis D, Toutouza M, Toutouzas P, Stefanadis C. Impact of lifestyle habits on the prevalence of the metabolic syndrome among Greek adults from the ATTICA study. Am Heart J. 2004;147(1):106–12.

55. Tortosa A, Bes-Rastrollo M, Sanchez-Villegas A, Basterra-Gortari FJ, Nunez-Cordoba JM, Martinez-Gonzalez MA. Mediterranean diet inversely associated with the incidence of metabolic syndrome: the SUN prospective cohort. Diabetes Care. 2007;30(11):2957–9. https://doi.org/10.2337/dc07-1231.

56. Tierney AC, McMonagle J, Shaw DI, Gulseth HL, Helal O, Saris WH, Paniagua JA, Golabek-Leszczynska I, Defoort C, Williams CM, Karsltrom B, Vessby B, Dembinska-Kiec A, Lopez-Miranda J, Blaak EE, Drevon CA, Gibney MJ, Lovegrove JA, Roche HM. Effects of dietary fat modification on insulin sensitivity and on other risk factors of the metabolic syndrome--LIPGENE: a European randomized dietary intervention study. Int J Obes. 2011;35(6):800–9. https://doi.org/10.1038/ijo.2010.209.

57. Cruz-Teno C, Perez-Martinez P, Delgado-Lista J, Yubero-Serrano EM, Garcia-Rios A, Marin C, Gomez P, Jimenez-Gomez Y, Camargo A, Rodriguez-Cantalejo F, Malagon MM, Perez-Jimenez F, Roche HM, Lopez-Miranda J. Dietary fat modifies the postprandial inflammatory state in subjects with metabolic syndrome: the LIPGENE study. Mol Nutr Food Res. 2012;56(6):854–65. https://doi.org/10.1002/mnfr.201200096.

58. Perez-Martinez P, Moreno-Conde M, Cruz-Teno C, Ruano J, Fuentes F, Delgado-Lista J, Garcia-Rios A, Marin C, Gomez-Luna MJ, Perez-Jimenez F, Roche HM, Lopez-Miranda J. Dietary fat differentially influences regulatory endothelial function during the postprandial state in patients with metabolic syndrome: from the LIPGENE study. Atherosclerosis. 2010b;209(2):533–8. https://doi.org/10.1016/j.atherosclerosis.2009.09.023.

59. Rumawas ME, Meigs JB, Dwyer JT, McKeown NM, Jacques PF. Mediterranean-style dietary pattern, reduced risk of metabolic syndrome traits, and incidence in the Framingham Offspring Cohort. Am J Clin Nutr. 2009;90(6):1608–14. https://doi.org/10.3945/ajcn.2009.27908.

60. Salas-Salvado J, Fernandez-Ballart J, Ros E, Martinez-Gonzalez MA, Fito M, Estruch R, Corella D, Fiol M, Gomez-Gracia E, Aros F, Flores G, Lapetra J, Lamuela-Raventos R, Ruiz-Gutierrez V, Bullo M, Basora J, Covas MI, Investigators PS. Effect of a Mediterranean diet supplemented with nuts on metabolic syndrome status: one-year results of the PREDIMED randomized trial. Arch Intern Med. 2008;168(22):2449–58. https://doi.org/10.1001/archinte.168.22.2449.

61. Babio N, Toledo E, Estruch R, Ros E, Martinez-Gonzalez MA, Castaner O, Bullo M, Corella D, Aros F, Gomez-Gracia E, Ruiz-Gutierrez V, Fiol M, Lapetra J, Lamuela-Raventos RM, Serra-Majem L, Pinto X, Basora J, Sorli JV, Salas-Salvado J, Investigators PS. Mediterranean diets and metabolic syndrome status in the PREDIMED randomized trial. CMAJ. 2014;186(17):E649–57. https://doi.org/10.1503/cmaj.140764.
62. Delgado-Lista J, Perez-Martinez P, Garcia-Rios A, Alcala-Diaz JF, Perez-Caballero AI, Gomez-Delgado F, Fuentes F, Quintana-Navarro G, Lopez-Segura F, Ortiz-Morales AM, Delgado-Casado N, Yubero-Serrano EM, Camargo A, Marin C, Rodriguez-Cantalejo F, Gomez-Luna P, Ordovas JM, Lopez-Miranda J, Perez-Jimenez F. CORonary Diet Intervention with Olive oil and cardiovascular PREVention study (the CORDIOPREV study): rationale, methods, and baseline characteristics: a clinical trial comparing the efficacy of a Mediterranean diet rich in olive oil versus a low-fat diet on cardiovascular disease in coronary patients. Am Heart J. 2016;177:42–50. https://doi.org/10.1016/j.ahj.2016.04.011.
63. Gomez-Delgado F, Alcala-Diaz JF, Garcia-Rios A, Delgado-Lista J, Ortiz-Morales A, Rangel-Zuniga O, Tinahones FJ, Gonzalez-Guardia L, Malagon MM, Bellido-Munoz E, Ordovas JM, Perez-Jimenez F, Lopez-Miranda J, Perez-Martinez P. Polymorphism at the TNF-alpha gene interacts with Mediterranean diet to influence triglyceride metabolism and inflammation status in metabolic syndrome patients: from the CORDIOPREV clinical trial. Mol Nutr Food Res. 2014;58(7):1519–27. https://doi.org/10.1002/mnfr.201300723.
64. Garcia-Rios A, Alcala-Diaz JF, Gomez-Delgado F, Delgado-Lista J, Marin C, Leon-Acuna A, Camargo A, Rodriguez-Cantalejo F, Blanco-Rojo R, Quintana-Navarro G, Ordovas JM, Perez-Jimenez F, Lopez-Miranda J, Perez-Martinez P. Beneficial effect of CETP gene polymorphism in combination with a Mediterranean diet influencing lipid metabolism in metabolic syndrome patients: CORDIOPREV study. Clin Nutr. 2018;37(1):229–34. https://doi.org/10.1016/j.clnu.2016.12.011.
65. Chrysohoou C, Panagiotakos DB, Pitsavos C, Das UN, Stefanadis C. Adherence to the Mediterranean diet attenuates inflammation and coagulation process in healthy adults: the ATTICA study. J Am Coll Cardiol. 2004;44(1):152–8. https://doi.org/10.1016/j.jacc.2004.03.039.
66. Schwingshackl L, Chaimani A, Hoffmann G, Schwedhelm C, Boeing H. A network meta-analysis on the comparative efficacy of different dietary approaches on glycaemic control in patients with type 2 diabetes mellitus. Eur J Epidemiol. 2018;33(2):157–70. https://doi.org/10.1007/s10654-017-0352-x.
67. Martinez-Gonzalez MA, de la Fuente-Arrillaga C, Nunez-Cordoba JM, Basterra-Gortari FJ, Beunza JJ, Vazquez Z, Benito S, Tortosa A, Bes-Rastrollo M. Adherence to Mediterranean diet and risk of developing diabetes: prospective cohort study. BMJ. 2008;336(7657):1348–51. https://doi.org/10.1136/bmj.39561.501007.BE.
68. Martinez-Gonzalez MA, Salas-Salvado J, Estruch R, Corella D, Fito M, Ros E, Predimed I. Benefits of the Mediterranean diet: insights from the PREDIMED study. Prog Cardiovasc Dis. 2015;58(1):50–60. https://doi.org/10.1016/j.pcad.2015.04.003.
69. Blanco-Rojo R, Alcala-Diaz JF, Wopereis S, Perez-Martinez P, Quintana-Navarro GM, Marin C, Ordovas JM, van Ommen B, Perez-Jimenez F, Delgado-Lista J, Lopez-Miranda J. The insulin resistance phenotype (muscle or liver) interacts with the type of diet to determine changes in disposition index after 2 years of intervention: the CORDIOPREV-DIAB randomised clinical trial. Diabetologia. 2015; https://doi.org/10.1007/s00125-015-3776-4.
70. Torres-Pena JD, Garcia-Rios A, Delgado-Casado N, Gomez-Luna P, Alcala-Diaz JF, Yubero-Serrano EM, Gomez-Delgado F, Leon-Acuna A, Lopez-Moreno J, Camargo A, Tinahones FJ, Delgado-Lista J, Ordovas JM, Perez-Martinez P, Lopez-Miranda J. Mediterranean diet improves endothelial function in patients with diabetes and prediabetes: a report from the CORDIOPREV study. Atherosclerosis. 2018;269:50–6. https://doi.org/10.1016/j.atherosclerosis.2017.12.012.
71. Mantzoros CS, Williams CJ, Manson JE, Meigs JB, Hu FB. Adherence to the Mediterranean dietary pattern is positively associated with plasma adiponectin concentrations in diabetic women. Am J Clin Nutr. 2006;84(2):328–35. https://doi.org/10.1093/ajcn/84.1.328.
72. Lopez-Moreno J, Quintana-Navarro GM, Camargo A, Jimenez-Lucena R, Delgado-Lista J, Marin C, Tinahones FJ, Striker GE, Roche HM, Perez-Martinez P, Lopez-Miranda J, Yubero-Serrano EM. Dietary fat quantity and quality modifies advanced glycation end products metabolism in patients with metabolic syndrome. Mol Nutr Food Res. 2017;61(8). https://doi.org/10.1002/mnfr.201601029.
73. Lopez-Moreno J, Quintana-Navarro GM, Delgado-Lista J, Garcia-Rios A, Delgado-Casado N, Camargo A, Perez-Martinez P, Striker GE, Tinahones FJ, Perez-Jimenez F, Lopez-Miranda J, Yubero-Serrano EM. Mediterranean diet reduces serum advanced glycation end products and increases antioxidant defenses in elderly adults: a randomized controlled trial. J Am Geriatr Soc. 2016;64(4):901–4. https://doi.org/10.1111/jgs.14062.
74. Campbell KL, Carrero JJ. Diet for the management of patients with chronic kidney disease; it is not the quantity, but the quality that matters. J Ren Nutr. 2016;26(5):279–81. https://doi.org/10.1053/j.jrn.2016.07.004.
75. Khatri M, Moon YP, Scarmeas N, Gu Y, Gardener H, Cheung K, Wright CB, Sacco RL, Nickolas TL, Elkind MS. The association between a Mediterranean-style diet and kidney function in the Northern Manhattan Study cohort. Clin J Am Soc Nephrol. 2014;9(11):1868–75. https://doi.org/10.2215/CJN.01080114.

76. Haring B, Selvin E, Liang M, Coresh J, Grams ME, Petruski-Ivleva N, Steffen LM, Rebholz CM. Dietary protein sources and risk for incident chronic kidney disease: results from the atherosclerosis risk in communities (ARIC) study. J Ren Nutr. 2017;27(4):233–42. https://doi.org/10.1053/j.jrn.2016.11.004.
77. Tektonidis TG, Akesson A, Gigante B, Wolk A, Larsson SC. A Mediterranean diet and risk of myocardial infarction, heart failure and stroke: a population-based cohort study. Atherosclerosis. 2015;243(1):93–8. https://doi.org/10.1016/j.atherosclerosis.2015.08.039.
78. Kushi LH, Lenart EB, Willett WC. Health implications of Mediterranean diets in light of contemporary knowledge. 1. Plant foods and dairy products. Am J Clin Nutr. 1995;61(6 Suppl):1407S–15S. https://doi.org/10.1093/ajcn/61.6.1407S.
79. Group GBDNDC. Global, regional, and national burden of neurological disorders during 1990-2015: a systematic analysis for the Global Burden of Disease Study 2015. Lancet Neurol. 2017;16(11):877–97. https://doi.org/10.1016/S1474-4422(17)30299-5.
80. Hebert LE, Weuve J, Scherr PA, Evans DA. Alzheimer disease in the United States (2010-2050) estimated using the 2010 census. Neurology. 2013;80(19):1778–83. https://doi.org/10.1212/WNL.0b013e31828726f5.
81. Ma D, Stokes K, Mahngar K, Domazet-Damjanov D, Sikorska M, Pandey S. Inhibition of stress induced premature senescence in presenilin-1 mutated cells with water soluble Coenzyme Q10. Mitochondrion. 2014;17:106–15.
82. Buchman AS, Wilson RS, Shulman JM, Leurgans SE, Schneider JA, Bennett DA. Parkinsonism in older adults and its association with adverse health outcomes and neuropathology. J Gerontol A Biol Sci Med Sci. 2016;71(4):549–56. https://doi.org/10.1093/gerona/glv153.
83. Gardener H, Caunca MR. Mediterranean diet in preventing neurodegenerative diseases. Curr Nutr Rep. 2018;7(1):10–20. https://doi.org/10.1007/s13668-018-0222-5.
84. Baumgart M, Snyder HM, Carrillo MC, Fazio S, Kim H, Johns H. Summary of the evidence on modifiable risk factors for cognitive decline and dementia: a population-based perspective. Alzheimers Dement. 2015;11(6):718–26. https://doi.org/10.1016/j.jalz.2015.05.016.
85. Singh B, Parsaik AK, Mielke MM, Erwin PJ, Knopman DS, Petersen RC, Roberts RO. Association of Mediterranean diet with mild cognitive impairment and Alzheimer's disease: a systematic review and meta-analysis. J Alzheimers Dis. 2014;39(2):271–82. https://doi.org/10.3233/JAD-130830.
86. Anastasiou CA, Yannakoulia M, Kosmidis MH, Dardiotis E, Hadjigeorgiou GM, Sakka P, Arampatzi X, Bougea A, Labropoulos I, Scarmeas N. Mediterranean diet and cognitive health: initial results from the hellenic longitudinal investigation of ageing and diet. PLoS One. 2017;12(8):e0182048. https://doi.org/10.1371/journal.pone.0182048.
87. Cassani E, Barichella M, Ferri V, Pinelli G, Iorio L, Bolliri C, Caronni S, Faierman SA, Mottolese A, Pusani C, Monajemi F, Pasqua M, Lubisco A, Cereda E, Frazzitta G, Petroni ML, Pezzoli G. Dietary habits in Parkinson's disease: adherence to Mediterranean diet. Parkinsonism Relat Disord. 2017;42:40–6. https://doi.org/10.1016/j.parkreldis.2017.06.007.
88. Alcalay RN, Gu Y, Mejia-Santana H, Cote L, Marder KS, Scarmeas N. The association between Mediterranean diet adherence and Parkinson's disease. Mov Disord. 2012;27(6):771–4. https://doi.org/10.1002/mds.24918.
89. Agarwal P, Wang Y, Buchman AS, Holland TM, Bennett DA, Morris MC. MIND diet associated with reduced incidence and delayed progression of ParkinsonismA in old age. J Nutr Health Aging. 2018;22(10):1211–5. https://doi.org/10.1007/s12603-018-1094-5.
90. Morris MC, Tangney CC, Wang Y, Sacks FM, Barnes LL, Bennett DA, Aggarwal NT. MIND diet slows cognitive decline with aging. Alzheimers Dement. 2015a;11(9):1015–22. https://doi.org/10.1016/j.jalz.2015.04.011.
91. Morris MC, Tangney CC, Wang Y, Sacks FM, Bennett DA, Aggarwal NT. MIND diet associated with reduced incidence of Alzheimer's disease. Alzheimers Dement. 2015b;11(9):1007–14. https://doi.org/10.1016/j.jalz.2014.11.009.
92. Rigacci S, Stefani M Nutraceutical properties of olive oil polyphenols. An itinerary from cultured cells through animal models to humans. Int J Mol Sci. 2016;17(6). https://doi.org/10.3390/ijms17060843.
93. Feng X, Liang N, Zhu D, Gao Q, Peng L, Dong H, Yue Q, Liu H, Bao L, Zhang J, Hao J, Gao Y, Yu X, Sun J. Resveratrol inhibits beta-amyloid-induced neuronal apoptosis through regulation of SIRT1-ROCK1 signaling pathway. PLoS One. 2013;8(3):e59888. https://doi.org/10.1371/journal.pone.0059888.

Chapter 3
Plant-Based Nutrition

Hena N. Patel and Kim Allan Williams Sr.

Keywords Plant-based nutrition · Cardiovascular disease · Healthy diet · Dietary patterns · Plant-based foods · Plant-based whole foods · Macronutrients · Micronutrients · Bioactive compounds

---

Key Points
- Multiple professional health societies have endorsed plant-predominant dietary patterns in recent years.
- Plant-based diets can benefit heart health by significantly reducing the risk factors that contribute to heart disease.
- Plant-based nutrition can prevent CVD risk factors, including diabetes and high blood pressure, as well as cardiac events.
- Animal-based food is not a necessary source of protein. With careful planning, plant proteins can provide adequate amounts of essential and nonessential amino acids.
- Physicians should be well informed with nutrition concepts to appropriately educate patients and staff about healthy, whole, plant-based foods.

Mechanism of Action

Coronary artery disease (CAD) is a largely preventable condition characterized by atherosclerotic plaques, resulting from an excessive, inflammatory fibro-proliferative response to various forms of insult to the vascular endothelial cell (VEC) lining the coronary arteries [18]. CAD risk factors such as tobacco use, dyslipidemia, hypertension, and type 2 diabetes mellitus (T2DM) have all been found to cause VEC injury and dysfunction leading to atherogenesis, atherosclerosis, or atherothrombotic CAD [18]. The three main stages of atherogenesis that lead to atherosclerosis include VEC injury, LDL oxidation, and macrophage activation [10]. VEC function regulates vascular homeostasis, and it contributes to the pathogenesis and clinical expression of CAD [66]. Studies suggest that plant-based nutrition may decrease CAD mortality by interrupting or reversing the atherogenic process [19, 51]. One potential mechanism by which plant-based nutrition promotes health is through the positive effects of polyphenols on endothelial cell function [66]. Individuals with the largest intake of polyphenols are shown to have modestly reduced CAD risk [29, 48]. Polyphenols also limit platelet adhesion

---

H. N. Patel · K. A. Williams Sr. (✉)
Department of Cardiology, Rush University Medical Center, Chicago, IL, USA
e-mail: Kim_a_williams@rush.edu

© Springer Nature Switzerland AG 2020
J. Uribarri, J. A. Vassalotti (eds.), *Nutrition, Fitness, and Mindfulness*, Nutrition and Health,
https://doi.org/10.1007/978-3-030-30892-6_3

and aggregation, which can precipitate acute coronary syndromes after plaque rupture [48]. Lastly, polyphenols also have beneficial effects on LDL oxidation [12, 25].

Red meat is an established risk factor for heart disease. The prospective Nurses' Health Study reported that higher intakes of red meat were significantly associated with an elevated risk of heart disease [8]. This conclusion was later confirmed in a cohort of male physicians, with men in the highest quintile for red meat consumption having a 24% increase in risk of heart failure compared with those in the lowest quintile [5]. Studies in animals and humans suggest a mechanistic link between intestinal microbial metabolism of nutrients in red meat (choline and L-carnitine) and CAD through the production of a pro-atherosclerotic metabolite called trimethylamine N-oxide (TMAO) [41]. Omnivorous individuals produce more TMAO compared with consumers of primarily plant-based diets [61], and elevated TMAO levels are predictors of CAD [73]. TMAO produced from red meat nutrients may play a role in promoting atherosclerosis by activating macrophages and foam cells [68].

Emerging evidence suggests that increased atheroma burden and unstable plaque formation may be associated with type 2 immunity [70]. The mammalian oligosaccharide galactose α-1,3-galactose (α-Gal) is the target allergen of delayed anaphylaxis to red meat. A recent study demonstrated that IgE sensitization to α-Gal is associated with CAD, identifying a potentially modifiable risk factor for atherosclerotic coronary disease [70].

Plant-Based Dietary Patterns and CVD Risk Factors

Randomized controlled trials and epidemiological studies indicate that plant-based diets, particularly vegan diets, are associated with significant improvement in CVD events, lowering risk factors such as T2DM and hypertension [24], decreasing symptomatic and scintigraphic myocardial ischemia and regression of CAD [50], thus revolutionizing our understanding about heart-healthy food patterns and the biological mechanisms linking dietary factors and CVD [65].

Diabetes Mellitus

The leading cause of death for patients with diabetes is CVD, and the relative risk for CVD mortality and morbidity is 2.5–5 times higher in adults with diabetes, compared to those without diabetes [3]. Multiple studies have shown the beneficial effects of plant-based nutrition in diabetes prevention and treatment. The longitudinal Adventist Health Study-2 demonstrated the lowest risk of developing diabetes in vegans, followed by lacto-ovo vegetarians, pesco-vegetarians, and semi-vegetarians, compared to non-vegetarians [63]. Similarly, analysis from the large prospective Adventist Health Study-2, which included a 2-year follow-up of over 41,000 subjects, found that the incidence of diabetes was lowest in vegans compared with non-vegetarians [62]. In a prospective study of older women initially free of diabetes, total grain, whole-grain, total dietary fiber, cereal fiber, and dietary magnesium intake showed strong inverse associations with incidence of diabetes after adjustment for potential non-dietary confounding variables [45]. Similarly, the Nurses' Health Study demonstrated a lower T2DM incidence for ascending quintiles of intake of cereal fiber and the ratio of polyunsaturated fat intake to saturated fat intake, along with a higher incidence for ascending quartiles of trans fat intake and glycemic load [59]. In the same cohort, nut consumption was inversely associated with risk of T2DM [34] after adjustment for other clinical and dietary factors. Analysis of 3 studies that followed more than 200,000 male and female health professionals across the USA for more than 20 years found that a diet emphasizing plant foods and low in animal foods was associated with an approximately 20% reduction in the risk of T2DM [55].

Plant-based diets are also more effective in reducing body weight and improving glycemic control than non-vegetarian diets in diabetes treatment [1]. A recent meta-analysis of controlled trials found that vegetarian diets significantly improved glycemic control in diabetics [74, 76]. In fact, adherence to plant-based nutrition reduced HbA1c by an average of 0.4 points in comparison with conventional diets [74, 76]. Exercise further augments these benefits [37].

Currently, both the Canadian and American Diabetes Associations include plant-based diets among several recommended dietary patterns for individuals with T2DM [44, 54].

Hypertension

Approximately 75 million Americans, or over a third of the population, have hypertension (HTN), using the threshold for detection 140/90 mm Hg [39]. Hypertension is a well-established risk factor for CVD and can significantly increase the risk of death from stroke and CVD [7]. A large analysis of population-based studies between 1990 and 2015 found that 14% of all deaths and 143 million life-years of disability were attributable to HTN [23]. Multiple studies have shown that increased fruit and vegetable consumption and reduced sodium intake can decrease both systolic and diastolic blood pressure [4, 35]. For instance, the Coronary Artery Risk Development in Young Adults HTN sub-study, which followed young adults over 15 years, found that intake of plant-based foods was inversely related to the incidence of elevated BP, while red meat and processed meat were associated with elevated blood pressure [60]. Similarly, a large prospective study of three longitudinal cohorts, from the Nurses' Health Study, Nurses' Health Study II, and the Health Professionals Follow-Up Study, found that intake of even one daily serving of animal products was associated with a 30% increased risk of HTN [9]. A meta-analysis from 2013 that included 7 randomized trials and 32 observational studies also found that vegetarian diets were associated with lowered blood pressure levels, compared with non-vegetarian diets [74, 76]. A more recent prospective study of over 4000 individuals found that those who followed a vegetarian diet had a 34% lower risk for HTN, compared with their omnivorous counterparts, even after adjusting for insulin resistance, inflammation, and obesity [13]. Conversely, vegetarian diets are related to reductions in both systolic and diastolic blood pressure, in comparison with animal-based diets [76]. These outcome measurements were independent of sodium intake, body weight, and exercise levels. A reduction in systolic blood pressure by 5 mmHg results in an estimated 7% reduction in all-cause mortality, 9% reduction in mortality from coronary heart disease, and 14% reduction in mortality from stroke [38, 74, 76]. Thus, the benefits of plant-based nutrition for HTN are clearly established.

Cholesterol

According to recent data, nearly 95 million American adults have high total cholesterol [39, 47], and 78 million have elevated levels of low-density lipoprotein cholesterol (LDL-C) [39]. Even more concerning, approximately 7% of children aged 9–16 years also have high LDL-C [39]. Over one-third of all CVD cases are due to elevated LDL-C levels [39], and every 1% reduction in LDL-C reduces the risk for a major cardiac event by approximately 1% [39]. Along with exercise, diet can lower LDL-C levels by 30–40% in individuals with or at risk for CVD [39, 50]. Dietary patterns strongly affect plasma LDL-C levels; thus, nutrition is a key component of disease prevention and management.

Consumption of saturated fat, trans fats, and dietary cholesterol, primarily from animal products in the American diet, leads to an increase in serum cholesterol concentration. However, replacing dietary saturated fats with plant-based products can reduce the risk of CVD by approximately 30%, similar to the effects of statin therapy [32, 49]. Several observational studies showed lower levels of total and

LDL-C in vegetarians versus non-vegetarians, with the lowest lipid levels found in vegans [33, 39]. These observations have been confirmed by randomized clinical trials. A recent meta-analysis of ten randomized trials demonstrated significant reductions in total cholesterol and LDL-C levels from plant-based dietary patterns [67]. A subsequent meta-analysis of randomized trials confirmed that these beneficial effects lasted in the long-term setting [75].

Cerebrovascular Accident

Cerebrovascular disease is estimated to be the second leading cause of death after CVD worldwide [21]. In the USA, nearly 795,000 strokes occur annually [7]. A meta-analysis of prospective studies found an inverse association between the risk of stroke and vegetable and fruit consumption [30], while red meat (especially processed meat) was associated with significantly increased risks for stroke [71]. A recent dose-response meta-analysis showed that adding an additional serving of meat into one's diet increased the chances of ischemic stroke by 24% [72]. Conversely, adhering to a predominantly plant-based diet has been found to reduce the mortality and morbidity from CVD, including stroke. Data from Nurses' Health Study, comprising a cohort of more than 70,000 women followed over for 20 years, demonstrated that women who adhered the most to a plant-based diet (PBD) were at lower risk of incident CVD and stroke compared with those that adhered the least (relative risk [RR], 0.71; 95% CI, 0.62 to 0.82; $p < 0.0001$ for CHD; RR, 0.87; 95% CI, 0.73 to 1.02; $p = 0.03$ for stroke). Importantly, CVD mortality was significantly lower among women with the highest consumption of a PBD (RR, 0.61; 95% CI, 0.49 to 0.76; $p < 0.0001$) [26]. Similarly, the PREDIMED trial, a large primary prevention trial, found that the Mediterranean diet reduced CVD events, defined as nonfatal acute myocardial infarction, nonfatal stroke, or cardiovascular death, by 30% compared with controls [20]. Thus, plant-based dietary patterns may provide benefits in lowering both the risk of cerebrovascular morbidity and stroke mortality.

Chronic Kidney Disease

Chronic kidney disease (CKD) is a progressive disease characterized by gradual loss of kidney function, often leading to kidney failure over time. The prevalence of CKD is growing, particularly in those over age 60 years. Approximately 30 million American adults have CKD, and another 1 in 3 is at risk for developing it [53]. Furthermore, CKD increases the risk of CVD by 30% [53]. Studies have shown that plant-based nutrition is beneficial for both preserving and improving kidney function (Table 3.1). Plant-based diets are suggested to provide endothelial protection, control high blood pressure, delay progression of CKD, and decrease proteinuria.

However, plant-based proteins were traditionally viewed as nutritionally inadequate and potentially even dangerous for patients with CKD. In particular, there are concerns that predominantly plant-based diets, while low in protein, may be rich in potassium and phosphorus. Although many of these concerns have been debunked, they have limited use of plant-based nutrition in this patient population.

Dietary interventions focused on reducing the consumption of nutrients such as protein, phosphorus, and sodium have been linked to improved outcomes in CKD, particularly in those with moderate to severe disease. Protein derived from plant sources may have less adverse effects on the metabolic risk factors in CKD, compared with animal-derived proteins [36]. Plant-based proteins also provide added benefits of reduced serum phosphate levels, which lower fibroblast growth factor 23 (FGF23) induction, as well as reduced metabolic acidosis and systemic blood pressure. Although plant-based

Table 3.1 Overview of the advantages and disadvantages of plant-based diets for management of CKD patients

Criteria	Advantage	Disadvantage
Protein quality	Meets EAR and RDA Avoids protein overload Can be adjusted up or down to meet desired needs	Dietary planning may be necessary in patients with unusually high protein requirements
Protein quality	More than adequate in a balanced diet	Cannot depend on 1 or 2 staple foods
Blood pressure	Improved	None
Phosphate	Improved	None
Metabolic acidosis	Improved	None
Uremic toxins	Likely improved	None
Potassium	Plant foods increase bowel movements and potassium excretion	Plant foods contain potassium
Microbiome	Improved gut barrier, reduced inflammation, and CKD progression	None
Diabetes	Improved	None
Heart disease	Improved	None

Source: Joshi et al. [36]; published online ahead of print

proteins contain more phosphorus, they are stored in a nonabsorbable form as phytate. Consequently, phosphorus in plant proteins is only 30–50% bioavailable because humans lack the enzyme phytase, whereas animal proteins are approximately 70% bioavailable [52]. Thus, advising patients with CKD to consume more animal-based proteins may actually worsen serum phosphorus levels, promoting CKD progression and worsening secondary hyperparathyroidism. Studies of CKD have shown that serum phosphorus levels worsened when protein was derived from animal-based diets and improved with plant-based sources [46, 56].

Potassium can also be safely included in the renal diet. Legumes typically have a higher potassium-to-protein ratio than equal amounts of protein from animal meats. However, legumes also contain other beneficial nutrients. Substituting higher potassium plant proteins (i.e., tofu) with nuts or soybeans is simple modification to safely satisfy the renal diet.

While intake of individual micronutrients may play an important role in CKD outcomes, it can not only be difficult to quantify them in population-based studies but also overwhelming to address multiple micronutrients when targeting dietary modifications as a means to slow CKD progression. Instead, emphasizing healthful dietary patterns may be more efficacious. Both the Dietary Approaches to Stop Hypertension (DASH) diet and the Mediterranean diet have been associated with favorable CKD outcomes. A subgroup analysis from the Nurses' Health Study found that adherence to a DASH-type dietary pattern was associated with lower odds of declining estimated glomerular filtration rate (eGFR) compared with those consuming a non-DASH diet [43]. Similarly, a recent study showed that adherence with a Mediterranean diet was associated with a significantly reduced risk of developing CKD [40]. The authors performed an observational, community-based prospective study to assess the association of adherence to the Mediterranean diet on long-term kidney function. In adjusted models, every 1-point increase in the Mediterranean diet score was associated with decreased odds of incident eGFR <60 ml/min/1.73 m^2 and decreased odds of being in the upper quartile of eGFR decline. Another recent study suggested that a plant-based dietary pattern high in fruits, vegetables, and fish was associated with a lower risk of mortality in CKD patients, compared with a general diet [27].

Thus, plant-based diets may exhibit beneficial metabolic effects in patients with CKD and should be encouraged as part of effective management of CKD [36]. Accordingly, the National Kidney Foundation recommends vegetarianism, or part-time vegetarian diet, as being beneficial to CKD patients. As most data in this population have been obtained from small observational and translational studies, future trials are needed to establish their efficacy in improving outcomes in patients with CKD.

Diet Quality

Nutrient deficiency is a primary concern for many people when considering plant-based nutrition. However, the Academy of Nutrition and Dietetics states that "vegetarian diets, including total vegetarian or vegan diets, are healthful, nutritionally adequate, and may provide health benefits in the prevention and treatment of certain diseases [14]."

Protein

One of the greatest concerns about consuming a predominantly plant-based diet is whether it can provide enough protein. Generally, patients on a plant-based diet are not at risk for protein deficiency as all essential nutrients are available in plants, though in varying amounts [77]. Importantly, these essential amino acids can be obtained by consuming various combinations of plant-based foods. Thus, a well-balanced, plant-based diet will provide adequate amounts of essential amino acids and prevent protein deficiency [77].

Vitamin B12

Vitamin B12 is needed for blood formation and cell division, and its deficiency can lead to macrocytic anemia and irreversible nerve damage. This nutrient is not produced by plants nor animals but rather by bacteria [17]. Consumers of plant-based diets are strongly advised to supplement with vitamin B12 but with limited doses in male ex-smokers due to the association with increased lung cancer risk [11].

Iron

Although iron is abundant in plant-based diets, heme iron absorption from animal foods may be higher than non-heme iron absorption from plant foods. Nonetheless, hemoglobin concentrations and the risk of iron deficiency are similar for vegans compared with omnivores and other vegetarians [14, 69]. Additionally, consumers of plant-based diets often consume large amounts of food rich in vitamin C, improving the absorption on non-heme iron.

Zinc

Zinc is an important mineral for normal growth and development, cellular integrity, and maintaining a healthy immune system [31]. Vegetarians are often considered to be at risk for zinc deficiency due to impaired absorption when bound to certain plant components, such as phytates. However, a sensitive marker to measure zinc status in humans has not been well established, and the effects of marginal zinc intakes are poorly understood [31]. Although vegans have lower zinc intake than omnivores, they do not differ from the non-vegetarians in functional immunocompetence [28]. It appears that there may be facilitators of zinc absorption and compensatory mechanisms to help vegetarians adapt to a lower intake of zinc [28].

Calcium and Vitamin D

Calcium intake can be adequate in a well-balanced, carefully planned plant-based diet. Studies have shown that fracture risk is similar for vegetarians and non-vegetarians. Bone health has traditionally been associated with calcium intake; however mounting data suggest that neither calcium nor dairy reduce the risk of fractures. Rather, the key to bone health is adequate vitamin D intake [22, 42, 58]. The EPIC-Oxford study revealed that vegans had the lowest mean intake of vitamin D (0.88 µg/d), a value one-fourth the mean intake of omnivores [15]. Vitamin D2, the form typically consumed by vegans, is less bioavailable than the animal-derived vitamin D3 [64]. However, vitamin D deficiency is common in the general population. Plant-based products, such as soy milk and cereal grains, may be fortified to provide an adequate source of vitamin D.

Fatty Acids

There are two identified essential fatty acids – linoleic acid (LA) and alpha-linolenic acid (an omega-3 fatty acid). Three other fatty acids are only conditionally essential (may become inadequate during severe stress, including severe sepsis, burns, and catabolic distress) and include palmitoleic acid (a monounsaturated fatty acid), lauric acid (a saturated fatty acid), and gamma-linolenic acid (an omega-6 fatty acid). Essential fatty acids play a role in stimulating growth and reproduction, wound healing, neural development, and the health and growth of the hair and skin [16]. Consequently, clinical signs associated with deficiencies in these essential fatty acids include a dry, scaly rash, hair loss, soft or brittle nails, restricted growth and development in children, increased susceptibility to infection, and poor wound healing [16]. Predominantly plant-based diets generally lack the long-chain omega-3 fats, eicosapentaenoic acid (EPA), and docosahexaenoic acid (DHA) but can be formed by conversion of the plant-based n-3 fatty acid α-linolenic acid, though with low efficiency [61, 68]. Compared with omnivores, vegetarians, and especially vegans, tend to have lower blood concentrations of EPA and DHA [57]. However, DHA can be obtained from microalgae supplements containing DHA and from foods fortified with DHA. EPA can be obtained from the retro-conversion of DHA in the body. Additionally, oil from brown algae, or kelp, is also a good source of EPA [57].

Implementation in Clinical Practice

Multiple professional health organizations have endorsed plant-predominant dietary patterns in recent guidelines, including the 2018 American Association of Clinical Endocrinologists, the 2015 USDA Dietary Guidelines, and the 2018 American Diabetes Association guidelines. The dietary guidelines of Brazil, Germany, Sweden, Qatar, and the Netherlands and the Nordic Nutrition Recommendations also recommend a more plant-based diet for both health and environmental sustainability. In addition, the American Institute for Cancer Research also suggests plant-based nutrition as a cancer prevention strategy. Lastly, the proposed 2018 Canada's Food Guide also states that a shift toward plant-based nutrition is needed.

In addition to health benefits, plant-based dietary patterns have been shown to significantly improve quality of life and overall well-being [38]. Nevertheless, shifting dietary patterns can be challenging. Focusing on attainable and measurable short-term benefits is crucial to guide dietary choices toward plant-based habits in the long term [39]. For instance, individuals may experience weight loss twice as fast on an unrestricted vegan diet, compared with a conventional calorie-restricted diet [6, 39]. Experiencing these short-term gains may help people adhere to their new dietary patterns in the long term.

While nutritional counseling, a medically necessary preventive service for individuals with CVD risk factors, the time constraints of office visits often limit physicians from providing effective dietary counseling. Registered dieticians (RDs) are members of the healthcare team who can bridge this gap and help improve patient outcomes [2]. Working in a coordinated, multidisciplinary team effort with physicians, RDs obtain detailed assessments of overall nutritional status and physical activity to tailor individualized diet, counseling, and/or specialized nutrition therapies. RDs spend significant time discussing the patient's diet and lifestyle – including how food is prepared, how the family eats, and fast-food habits – and work with the patient to develop sustainable healthy meal plans, which most physicians are usually not able to cover in a standard appointment. However, medical nutrition therapy has been problematic in that a whole-food, plant-based diet, which is the optimal nutrition pattern for reduction of CV risk factors and disease, was rejected by RDs until relatively recently [14]. Commonly expressed concerns about protein quantity and quality have been shown to be unfounded and were not biochemically logical in that the largest land mammals (e.g., horses, elephants, cows) are vegetarian species and are not protein deficient. But widespread recognition and adoption of the American Dietetic Association position have been limited, and the resulting conflicting dietary recommendations given to patients become a barrier to progress.

Furthermore, though medical nutrition therapy has been integrated into the treatment guidelines for a number of chronic diseases, adequate reimbursement for dietitian services is still a challenge for many practices. Currently, Medicare Part B only covers medical nutrition therapy services for Medicare beneficiaries who meet at least one of the following conditions: diabetes, kidney disease, or kidney transplant in the last 36 months.

In summary, there is substantial evidence from multiple observational studies and clinical trials supporting the beneficial effects of plant-based dietary patterns for CVD and overall health. Thus, plant-based nutrition should be recommended as an essential part of the overall CVD prevention and management care plan.

References

1. Acar J, Cormier B, Grimberg D, Kawthekar G, Iung B, Scheuer B, Farah E. Diagnosis of left atrial thrombi in mitral stenosis--usefulness of ultrasound techniques compared with other methods. Eur Heart J. 1991;12(suppl B):70–6. https://doi.org/10.1093/eurheartj/12.suppl_B.70.
2. Agee MD, Gates Z, Irwin PM. Effect of medical nutrition therapy for patients with type 2 diabetes in a low-/no-cost clinic: a propensity score–matched cohort study. Diabetes Spectr. 2018;31(1):83–9. https://doi.org/10.2337/ds16-0077.
3. Alvarez CA, Lingvay I, Vuylsteke V, Koffarnus RL, McGuire DK. Cardiovascular risk in diabetes mellitus: complication of the disease or of antihyperglycemic medications. Clin Pharmacol Ther. 2015;98(2):145–61. https://doi.org/10.1002/cpt.143.
4. Appel LJ, Moore TJ, Obarzanek E, Vollmer WM, Svetkey LP, Sacks FM, Bray GA, et al. A clinical trial of the effects of dietary patterns on blood pressure. N Engl J Med. 1997;336(16):1117–24. https://doi.org/10.1056/NEJM199704173361601.
5. Ashaye A, Gaziano J, Djoussé L. Red meat consumption and risk of heart failure in male physicians. Nutr Metab Cardiovasc Dis. 2011;21(12):941–6. https://doi.org/10.1016/j.numecd.2010.03.009.

6. Barnard RJ, DiLauro SC, Inkeles SB. Effects of intensive diet and exercise intervention in patients taking cholesterol-lowering drugs. Am J Cardiol. 1997;79(8):1112–4.
7. Benjamin EJ, Blaha MJ, Chiuve SE, Cushman M, Das SR, Deo R, de Ferranti SD, et al. Heart disease and stroke statistics—2017 update: a report from the American Heart Association. Circulation. 2017;135(10):e146–603. https://doi.org/10.1161/CIR.0000000000000485.
8. Bernstein AM, Sun Q, Hu FB, Stampfer MJ, Manson JE, Willett WC. Major dietary protein sources and risk of coronary heart disease in women. Circulation. 2010;122(9):876–83. https://doi.org/10.1161/CIRCULATIONAHA.109.915165.
9. Borgi L, Curhan GC, Willett WC, Hu FB, Satija A, Forman JP. Long-term intake of animal flesh and risk of developing hypertension in three prospective cohort studies. J Hypertens. 2015;33(11):2231–8. https://doi.org/10.1097/HJH.0000000000000722.
10. Boyle J. Macrophage activation in atherosclerosis: pathogenesis and pharmacology of plaque rupture. Curr Vasc Pharmacol. 2005;3(1):63–8. https://doi.org/10.2174/1570161052773861.
11. Brasky TM, White E, Chen C-L. Long-term, supplemental, one-carbon metabolism–related vitamin B use in relation to lung cancer risk in the vitamins and lifestyle (VITAL) cohort. J Clin Oncol. 2017;35(30):3440–8. https://doi.org/10.1200/JCO.2017.72.7735.
12. Carmeli E, Fogelman Y. Antioxidant effect of polyphenolic glabridin on LDL oxidation. Toxicol Ind Health. 2009;25(4–5):321–4. https://doi.org/10.1177/0748233709103034.
13. Chuang S-Y, Chiu THT, Lee C-Y, Liu T-T, Tsao CK, Hsiung CA, Chiu Y-F. Vegetarian diet reduces the risk of hypertension independent of abdominal obesity and inflammation: a prospective study. J Hypertens. 2016;34(11):2164–71. https://doi.org/10.1097/HJH.0000000000001068.
14. Craig WJ, Mangels AR, American Dietetic Association. Position of the American Dietetic association: vegetarian diets. J Am Diet Assoc. 2009a;109(7):1266–82. https://doi.org/10.1016/j.jada.2009.05.027.
15. Davey GK, Spencer EA, Appleby PN, Allen NE, Knox KH, Key TJ. EPIC–Oxford: lifestyle characteristics and nutrient intakes in a cohort of 33 883 meat-eaters and 31 546 non meat-eaters in the UK. Public Health Nutr. 2003;6(03). https://doi.org/10.1079/PHN2002430.
16. Di Pasquale MG. The essentials of essential fatty acids. J Diet Suppl. 2009;6(2):143–61. https://doi.org/10.1080/19390210902861841.
17. Donaldson MS. Metabolic vitamin B12 status on a mostly raw vegan diet with follow-up using tablets, nutritional yeast, or probiotic supplements. Ann Nutr Metab. 2000;44(5–6):229–34. https://doi.org/10.1159/000046689.
18. Epstein FH, Ross R. Atherosclerosis — an inflammatory disease. N Engl J Med. 1999;340(2):115–26. https://doi.org/10.1056/NEJM199901143400207.
19. Esselstyn CB. Resolving the coronary artery disease epidemic through plant-based nutrition. Prev Cardiol. 2001;4(4):171–7. https://doi.org/10.1111/j.1520-037X.2001.00538.x.
20. Estruch R, Ros E, Salas-Salvadó J, Covas M-I, Corella D, Arós F, Gómez-Gracia E, et al. Primary prevention of cardiovascular disease with a Mediterranean diet supplemented with extra-virgin olive oil or nuts. N Engl J Med. 2018;378(25):e34. https://doi.org/10.1056/NEJMoa1800389.
21. Feigin VL, Norrving B, Mensah GA. Global burden of stroke. Circ Res. 2017;120(3):439–48. https://doi.org/10.1161/CIRCRESAHA.116.308413.
22. Feskanich D, Willett WC, Colditz GA. Calcium, vitamin D, milk consumption, and hip fractures: a prospective study among postmenopausal women. Am J Clin Nutr. 2003;77(2):504–11. https://doi.org/10.1093/ajcn/77.2.504.
23. Forouzanfar MH, Liu P, Roth GA, Ng M, Biryukov S, Marczak L, Alexander L, et al. Global burden of hypertension and systolic blood pressure of at least 110 to 115 mm hg, 1990–2015. JAMA. 2017;317(2):165. https://doi.org/10.1001/jama.2016.19043.
24. Fraser GE. Vegetarian diets: what do we know of their effects on common chronic diseases? Am J Clin Nutr. 2009;89(5):1607S–12S. https://doi.org/10.3945/ajcn.2009.26736K.
25. Frémont L, Belguendouz L, Delpal S. Antioxidant activity of resveratrol and alcohol-free wine polyphenols related to LDL oxidation and polyunsaturated fatty acids. Life Sci. 1999;64(26):2511–21. https://doi.org/10.1016/S0024-3205(99)00209-X.
26. Fung TT, Rexrode KM, Mantzoros CS, Manson JAE, Willett WC, Hu FB. Mediterranean diet and incidence of and mortality from coronary heart disease and stroke in women. Circulation. 2009;119(8):1093–100. https://doi.org/10.1161/CIRCULATIONAHA.108.816736.
27. Gutiérrez OM, Muntner P, Rizk DV, McClellan WM, Warnock DG, Newby PK, Judd SE. Dietary patterns and risk of death and progression to ESRD in individuals with CKD: a cohort study. Am J Kidney Dis. 2014;64(2):204–13. https://doi.org/10.1053/j.ajkd.2014.02.013.
28. Haddad EH, Berk LS, Kettering JD, Hubbard RW, Peters WR. Dietary intake and biochemical, hematologic, and immune status of vegans compared with nonvegetarians. Am J Clin Nutr. 1999;70(3 Suppl):586S–93S.
29. Hertog MG, Sweetnam PM, Fehily AM, Elwood PC, Kromhout D. Antioxidant flavonols and ischemic heart disease in a welsh population of men: the Caerphilly Study. Am J Clin Nutr. 1997;65(5):1489–94.

30. Hu D, Huang J, Wang Y, Zhang D, Qu Y. Fruits and vegetables consumption and risk of stroke: a meta-analysis of prospective cohort studies. Stroke. 2014;45(6):1613–9. https://doi.org/10.1161/STROKEAHA.114.004836.

31. Hunt JR. Moving toward a plant-based diet: are iron and zinc at risk? Nutr Rev. 2002;60(5):127–34. https://doi.org/10.1301/00296640260093788.

32. Jenkins DJA. Effects of a dietary portfolio of cholesterol-lowering foods vs lovastatin on serum lipids and C-reactive protein. JAMA. 2003;290(4):502. https://doi.org/10.1001/jama.290.4.502.

33. Jian Z-H, Chiang Y-C, Lung C-C, Ho C-C, Ko P-C, Ndi Nfor O, Chang H-C, Liaw Y-C, Liang Y-C, Liaw Y-P. Vegetarian diet and cholesterol and TAG levels by gender. Public Health Nutr. 2015;18(04):721–6. https://doi.org/10.1017/S1368980014000883.

34. Jiang R, Manson JAE, Stampfer MJ, Liu S, Willett WC, Frank BH. Nut and peanut butter consumption and risk of type 2 diabetes in women. JAMA. 2002;288(20):2554–60.

35. John JH, Ziebland S, Yudkin P, Roe LS, Neil HAW, Oxford Fruit and Vegetable Study Group. Effects of fruit and vegetable consumption on plasma antioxidant concentrations and blood pressure: a randomised controlled trial. Lancet (London, England). 2002;359(9322):1969–74.

36. Joshi S, Shah S, Kalantar-Zadeh K. Adequacy of plant-based proteins in chronic kidney disease. J Ren Nutr, August. 2018; https://doi.org/10.1053/j.jrn.2018.06.006.

37. Kahleova H, Matoulek M, Malinska H, Oliyarnik O, Kazdova L, Neskudla T, Skoch A, et al. Vegetarian diet improves insulin resistance and oxidative stress markers more than conventional diet in subjects with type 2 diabetes. Diabet Med. 2011;28(5):549–59. https://doi.org/10.1111/j.1464-5491.2010.03209.x.

38. Kahleova H, Levin S, Barnard N. Cardio-metabolic benefits of plant-based diets. Nutrients. 2017;9(8):848. https://doi.org/10.3390/nu9080848.

39. Kahleova H, Levin S, Barnard ND. Vegetarian dietary patterns and cardiovascular disease. Prog Cardiovasc Dis. 2018;61(1):54–61. https://doi.org/10.1016/j.pcad.2018.05.002.

40. Khatri M, Moon YP, Scarmeas N, Gu Y, Gardener H, Cheung K, Wright CB, Sacco RL, Nickolas TL, Elkind MSV. The association between a Mediterranean-style diet and kidney function in the northern Manhattan study cohort. Clin J Am Soc Nephrol. 2014;9(11):1868–75. https://doi.org/10.2215/CJN.01080114.

41. Koeth RA, Wang Z, Levison BS, Buffa JA, Org E, Sheehy BT, Britt EB, et al. Intestinal microbiota metabolism of L-carnitine, a nutrient in red meat, promotes atherosclerosis. Nat Med. 2013;19(5):576–85. https://doi.org/10.1038/nm.3145.

42. Lanou AJ. Calcium, dairy products, and bone health in children and young adults: a reevaluation of the evidence. Pediatrics. 2005;115(3):736–43. https://doi.org/10.1542/peds.2004-0548.

43. Lin J, Fung TT, Hu FB, Curhan GC. Association of dietary patterns with albuminuria and kidney function decline in older White women: a subgroup analysis from the Nurses' Health Study. Am J Kidney Dis. 2011;57(2):245–54. https://doi.org/10.1053/j.ajkd.2010.09.027.

44. Marathe PH, Gao HX, Close KL. American Diabetes Association standards of medical care in diabetes 2017. J Diabetes. 2017;9(4):320–4. https://doi.org/10.1111/1753-0407.12524.

45. Meyer KA, Kushi LH, Jacobs DR, Slavin J, Sellers TA, Folsom AR. Carbohydrates, dietary fiber, and incident type 2 diabetes in older women. Am J Clin Nutr. 2000;71(4):921–30.

46. Moe SM, Zidehsarai MP, Chambers MA, Jackman LA, Radcliffe JS, Trevino LL, Donahue SE, Asplin JR. Vegetarian compared with meat dietary protein source and phosphorus homeostasis in chronic kidney disease. Clin J Am Soc Nephrol. 2011;6(2):257–64. https://doi.org/10.2215/CJN.05040610.

47. Mozaffarian D, Benjamin EJ, Go AS, Arnett DK, Blaha MJ, Cushman M, Das SR, et al. Heart disease and stroke statistics—2016 update. Circulation. 2016;133(4):e38–360. https://doi.org/10.1161/CIR.0000000000000350.

48. Mukamal KJ. Tea consumption and mortality after acute myocardial infarction. Circulation. 2002;105(21):2476–81. https://doi.org/10.1161/01.CIR.0000017201.88994.F7.

49. National Cholesterol Education Program, National Heart, Lung, and Blood Institute, National Institutes of Health. Third report of the National Cholesterol Education Program (NCEP) expert panel on detection, evaluation, and treatment of high blood cholesterol in adults (adult treatment panel III) final report. NIH Publication No. 02–5215. Circulation. 2002;106(25):3143–421.

50. Ornish D, Scherwitz LW, Billings JH, Brown SE, Gould KL, Merritt TA, Sparler S, et al. Intensive lifestyle changes for reversal of coronary heart disease. JAMA. 1998;280(23):2001–7.

51. Ornish D. Intensive lifestyle changes for reversal of coronary heart disease. JAMA. 1998;280(23):2001. https://doi.org/10.1001/jama.280.23.2001.

52. Pagenkemper J. Planning a vegetarian renal diet. J Ren Nutr. 1995;5(4):234–8. https://doi.org/10.1016/1051-2276(95)90009-8.

53. Prevention, Centers for Disease Control. Chronic kidney disease surveillance system—United States. 2018. https://nccd.cdc.gov/ckd/.

54. Rinaldi S, Campbell EE, Fournier J, O'Connor C, Madill J. A comprehensive review of the literature supporting recommendations from the Canadian Diabetes Association for the use of a plant-based diet for management of Type 2 diabetes. Can J Diabetes. 2016;40(5):471–7. https://doi.org/10.1016/j.jcjd.2016.02.011.

55. Satija A, Bhupathiraju SN, Spiegelman D, Chiuve SE, Manson JE, Willett W, Rexrode KM, Rimm EB, Hu FB. Healthful and unhealthful plant-based diets and the risk of coronary heart disease in U.S. Adults. J Am Coll 2017;70(4):411–22. https://www.ncbi.nlm.nih.gov/pmc/articles/PMC5555375/.

56. Scialla JJ, Appel LJ, Wolf M, Yang W, Zhang X, Sozio SM, Miller ER, et al. Plant protein intake is associated with fibroblast growth factor 23 and serum bicarbonate levels in patients with chronic kidney disease: the chronic renal insufficiency cohort study. J Ren Nutr. 2012;22(4):379–388.e1. https://doi.org/10.1053/j.jrn.2012.01.026.

57. Šebeková K, Boor P, Valachovičová M, Blažíček P, Parrák V, Babinská K, Heidland A, Krajčovičová-Kudláčková M. Association of metabolic syndrome risk factors with selected markers of oxidative status and microinflammation in healthy omnivores and vegetarians. Mol Nutr Food Res. 2006;50(9):858–68. https://doi.org/10.1002/mnfr.200500170.

58. Sonneville KR, Gordon CM, Kocher MS, Pierce LM, Ramappa A, Field AE. Vitamin D, calcium, and dairy intakes and stress fractures among female adolescents. Arch Pediatr Adolesc Med. 2012;166(7). https://doi.org/10.1001/archpediatrics.2012.5.

59. Stampfer MJ, Hu FB, Manson JE, Rimm EB, Willett WC. Primary prevention of coronary heart disease in women through diet and lifestyle. N Engl J Med. 2000;343(1):16–22. https://doi.org/10.1056/NEJM200007063430103.

60. Steffen LM, Kroenke CH, Xinhua Y, Pereira MA, Slattery ML, Van Horn L, Gross MD, Jacobs DR. Associations of plant food, dairy product, and meat intakes with 15-y incidence of elevated blood pressure in young black and White adults: the coronary artery risk development in young adults (CARDIA) study. Am J Clin Nutr. 2005;82(6):1169–77; quiz 1363-4.

61. Tang WHW, Wang Z, Levison BS, Koeth RA, Britt EB, Fu X, Wu Y, Hazen SL. Intestinal microbial metabolism of phosphatidylcholine and cardiovascular risk. N Engl J Med. 2013;368(17):1575–84. https://doi.org/10.1056/NEJMoa1109400.

62. Tonstad S, Stewart K, Oda K, Batech M, Herring RP, Fraser GE. Vegetarian diets and incidence of diabetes in the Adventist Health Study-2. Nutr Metab Cardiovasc Dis. 2013;23(4):292–9. https://doi.org/10.1016/j.numecd.2011.07.004.

63. Tonstad S, Butler T, Yan R, Fraser GE. Type of vegetarian diet, body weight, and prevalence of type 2 diabetes. Diabetes Care. 2009;32(5):791–6. https://doi.org/10.2337/dc08-1886.

64. Trang HM, Cole DE, Rubin LA, Pierratos A, Siu S, Vieth R. Evidence that vitamin D3 increases serum 25-hydroxyvitamin D more efficiently than does vitamin D2. Am J Clin Nutr. 1998;68(4):854–8.

65. Tuso PJ, Ismail MH, Ha BP, Bartolotto C. Nutritional update for physicians: plant-based diets. Perm J. 2013;17(2):61–6. https://doi.org/10.7812/TPP/12-085.

66. Vita JA. Polyphenols and cardiovascular disease: effects on endothelial and platelet function. Am J Clin Nutr. 2005;81(1 Suppl):292S–7S.

67. Wang F, Zheng J, Yang B, Jiang J, Fu Y, Li D. Effects of vegetarian diets on blood lipids: a systematic review and meta-analysis of randomized controlled trials. J Am Heart Assoc. 2015;4(10):e002408. https://doi.org/10.1161/JAHA.115.002408.

68. Wang Z, Klipfell E, Bennett BJ, Koeth R, Levison BS, DuGar B, Feldstein AE, et al. Gut flora metabolism of phosphatidylcholine promotes cardiovascular disease. Nature. 2011;472(7341):57–63. https://doi.org/10.1038/nature09922.

69. Wilson AK, Ball MJ. Nutrient intake and iron status of Australian male vegetarians. Eur J Clin Nutr. 1999;53(3):189–94.

70. Wilson JM, Nguyen AT, Schuyler AJ, Commins SP, Taylor AM, Platts-Mills TAE, McNamara CA. IgE to the mammalian oligosaccharide galactose-α-1,3-galactose is associated with increased atheroma volume and plaques with unstable characteristics—brief report. Arterioscler Thromb Vasc Biol. 2018;38(7):1665–9. https://doi.org/10.1161/ATVBAHA.118.311222.

71. Wolk A. Potential health hazards of eating red meat. J Intern Med. 2017;281(2):106–22. https://doi.org/10.1111/joim.12543.

72. Yang C, Pan L, Sun C, Xi Y, Wang L, Li D. Red meat consumption and the risk of stroke: a dose–response meta-analysis of prospective cohort studies. J Stroke Cerebrovasc Dis. 2016;25(5):1177–86. https://doi.org/10.1016/j.jstrokecerebrovasdis.2016.01.040.

73. Yang S-Y, Zhang H-J, Sun S-Y, Wang L-Y, Yan B, Liu C-Q, Zhang W, Li X-J. Relationship of carotid intima-media thickness and duration of vegetarian diet in Chinese male vegetarians. Nutr Metabol. 2011;8(1):63. https://doi.org/10.1186/1743-7075-8-63.

74. Yokoyama Y, Barnard ND, Levin SM, Watanabe M. Vegetarian diets and glycemic control in diabetes: a systematic review and meta-analysis. Cardiovasc Diagn Ther. 2014a;4(5):373–82. https://doi.org/10.3978/j.issn.2223-3652.2014.10.04.
75. Yokoyama Y, Levin SM, Barnard ND. Association between plant-based diets and plasma lipids: a systematic review and meta-analysis. Nutr Rev. 2017;75(9):683–98. https://doi.org/10.1093/nutrit/nux030.
76. Yokoyama Y, Nishimura K, Barnard ND, Takegami M, Watanabe M, Sekikawa A, Okamura T, Miyamoto Y. Vegetarian diets and blood pressure: a meta-analysis. JAMA Intern Med. 2014b;174(4):577–87. https://doi.org/10.1001/jamainternmed.2013.14547.
77. Young VR, Pellett PL. Plant proteins in relation to human protein and amino acid nutrition. Am J Clin Nutr. 1994;59(5 Suppl):1203S–12S.

Chapter 4
The Low AGE Diet

Jaime Uribarri

Keywords AGEs · Oxidative stress · Inflammation · Nutrition · Diabetes · Cardiovascular disease

Key Points
- AGEs are endogenous and exogenous biomarkers of microinflammation and oxidative stress.
- Exogenous AGEs are concentrated in animal proteins and fats, and food preparation has a dramatic effect increasing its levels.
- Cooking techniques to limit AGEs can be easily implemented.
- Most clinical trials of dietary AGE restriction have focused on biomarkers, but hard outcomes are lacking in the current literature.

Introduction

Compared to the third world, modern western living is associated with better overall survival but a significant increase in noninfectious chronic diseases such as type 2 diabetes and cardiovascular disease. Diet is an important factor in modern lifestyle and likely plays a significant role in these changes. Advanced glycation end products (AGEs) are a heterogeneous group of biological compounds with significant prooxidant and pro-inflammatory effects shown in vitro and in vivo in many animal models. AGEs, abundantly present in the usual western diet, have been shown to have same biological effects as their endogenous counterparts. Experimentally, a high dietary AGE in mice induces atherosclerosis, kidney disease, and diabetes, while a low AGE diet prevents and/or reverses these conditions. This experimental background has allowed the performance of several clinical trials to demonstrate the effect of a low AGE diet in humans, which will be the main emphasis in this chapter.

What Are AGEs

AGEs are a large and heterogenous group of highly reactive compounds that can form by several different pathways. Traditionally, AGEs have been considered to form through the spontaneous, nonenzymatic reaction of reducing sugars with free amino groups in amino acids. A series of intermediary

J. Uribarri (✉)
Division of Nephrology, Department of Medicine, Icahn School of Medicine at Mount Sinai, New York, NY, USA
e-mail: jaime.uribarri@mssm.edu

© Springer Nature Switzerland AG 2020
J. Uribarri, J. A. Vassalotti (eds.), *Nutrition, Fitness, and Mindfulness*, Nutrition and Health,
https://doi.org/10.1007/978-3-030-30892-6_4

reactions leads ultimately to the formation of irreversible compounds called AGEs. This is the classic Maillard reaction also known as browning reaction. AGEs can also form through many other reactions, including oxidation of sugars, lipids, and amino acids that create reactive aldehydes [1].

AGEs that form endogenously in these reactions can also form in any system in nature if the needed reagents are present. For example, AGEs form spontaneously in food, but cooking the food with direct heat markedly increases their formation [2]. A fraction of the AGEs contained in the ingested food gets absorbed and incorporates into the body AGE pool, where they are indistinguishable from their endogenous counterparts [3].

Numerous AGE compounds have been identified with pentosidine, carboxymethyllysine (CML), and methylglyoxal-derivatives such as MG-H1 among the better-characterized ones and often used as AGE biomarkers. There are many methods to measure AGEs. The simplest method is detection of their fluorescence capacity, but unfortunately it is nonspecific. More specific methods include immunoassays, HPLC, and mass spectrometry, each with advantages and disadvantages. Chemically and immunologically distinct AGEs can coexist on the same carrier proteins.

The biological effects of AGEs occur through two general mechanisms. AGEs can crosslink proteins directly modifying their structure and therefore their function [1]. As examples, glycation of collagen fibers in the skin and vessel wall changes the characteristics of these proteins leading to wrinkling under the skin and stiffness of arterial walls; direct glycation of the active site of a protein like albumin might modify albumin binding to certain drugs or, in the case of other proteins, modify their ability to bind to receptors.

Another important action of AGEs is their ability to activate several intracellular pathways leading to increased oxidative stress (OS) and inflammatory cytokines through receptors and non-receptor mechanisms. AGEs interact with different cell receptors. The interaction with receptors such as RAGE, EGFR, and TLR4 leads to stimulation of intracellular pathways that include NF-κB increasing formation of reactive oxygen species (ROS) and pro-inflammatory cytokines such as TNFα [4]. On the other hand, stimulation of receptors such as AGE receptor 1 (AGER1) increases AGE breakdown, activates sirtuin 1 (SIRT1), and decreases cellular pro-inflammatory activity [5]. AGER1 has been found to be directly associated with levels of circulating AGEs in healthy subjects, but its levels are very suppressed in subjects who are exposed to a chronic high OS state such as chronic kidney disease (CKD) and diabetes mellitus patients [6].

Steady-state levels of circulating AGEs at any particular point in time represent the balance between endogenous and exogenous sources and elimination via tissue degradation and kidneys. There are several potential mechanisms of AGE elimination. MGO, an AGE precursor, for example, is effectively catabolized by the enzymes glyoxalase I and glyoxalase II. Circulating proteins such as lysozyme bind AGEs increasing macrophage endocytosis and degradation of AGEs into smaller peptides facilitating their renal excretion. AGE peptides are filtered by the glomerulus and reabsorbed to a variable degree by proximal tubular cells [7]. A potential role for colonic degradation of AGEs has been postulated [8], but the relative contribution to balance of AGEs remains unproven.

What Are Dietary AGEs

As previously noted, AGEs form spontaneously in foods, during storage at room temperature, but their rate of formation markedly accelerates as temperature increases during direct heat cooking, particularly during browning of foods. Other factors that affect AGE generation in food include nutrient composition, water content, pH, presence of trace metals, and duration of cooking [2, 9]. Food scientists have learned to manipulate cooking techniques to generate AGEs and get the exact color, aroma, and taste of food they desire.

Table 4.1 AGE content of foods depending on cooking technique

Low AGE content items		High AGE content items	
Food item	AGE content	Food item	AGE content
Beef (stewed)	2199	Beef (broiled)	6731
Chicken (boiled)	1011	Chicken (fried)	6651
Salmon (poached)	1621	Salmon (broiled)	3012
Lamb leg (boiled)	1096	Lamb leg (broiled)	2188

Adapted from Uribarri et al. [9]
AGE content expressed in kilounits/serving

Databases of food CML content, a commonly measured AGE, have become available [2, 9, 10]. Using these databases investigators have been able to estimate daily dietary AGE intake based on food records as well as to design diets with variable AGE content. These databases show that foods rich in both animal protein and fat and cooked at high and dry heat, such as in broiling, grilling, frying, and roasting, tend to be the richest dietary sources of AGEs, whereas low-fat carbohydrate-rich foods tend to be relatively low in AGEs. This may reflect the fact that the AGEs in the diet are generated not just by the Maillard reaction but also by interactions between oxidized lipids and protein; such reactions are known to give rise to AGEs such as CML. Since these fat-rich foods are the ones commonly consumed in the Western diet, this population is ingesting a high AGE diet.

Knowledge of the effect of cooking temperature, duration of cooking, use of water, and pH of the solution in the generation of food AGEs is of great importance to develop culinary techniques, which allow reduction of food AGE content without necessarily changing the taste and quantity of foods consumed. The essential concept is that it is not only the actual nutrient composition of the food but also the way in which the food is cooked that determines its AGE content. Table 4.1 illustrates this concept by showing that AGE content of the same piece of chicken, expressed in arbitrary AGE kilounits/serving, changes from 1011 AGE kilounits when boiled to 6651 kilounits after broiled. Stewing or steaming of meat, which maintains food moisture during cooking, will generate much less AGE than broiling or frying. Marinating with lemon juice or vinegar will also have an AGE-reducing effect by maintaining the moisture and lowering the pH of food.

What Is the Low AGE Diet

As explained above, dietary AGE intake can be easily decreased by simply changing the cooking method from a high dry direct heat application to a low heat and high humidity, independent of its nutrient composition. Dry heat cooking methods, such as broiling, searing, and frying, significantly increase the AGE content of foods, compared to methods that use lower temperatures and higher moisture such as stewing, steaming, and boiling. Since the emphasis of the low AGE diet is on the cooking method, not the food being cooked, it can be broadly applied. The same principle will apply whether the patient is healthy, has diabetes, or has any other medical condition.

Studies have demonstrated that consumers can be educated about the use of low AGE-generating cooking methods such as poaching, steaming, stewing, and boiling. The generous application of herbs, condiments, and spices, some of which may have intrinsic antiglycation activity, could also make any food, however it is cooked, tastier. Although the highest AGE values are found in meats and meat-substitute food groups, pre-treatment of meats with lemon, vinegar, or with any acidic marinade prior to cooking may reduce the AGE content.

Whenever instructing patients on a low AGE diet, a multipronged strategy delineated in Table 4.2 is suggested. Only point 1, the AGE-restricted diet, however, has been tested clinically, and the table suggestions assume the simultaneous application of points 2–5 will have beneficial and synergistic effects. Avoidance of cigarette smoking, rich in AGEs, should also be a prominent part of an anti-AGE strategy [11].

Table 4.2 The low AGE diet

1. Decrease intake of foods rich in AGEs (by changing culinary methods based on existing databases)
2. Increase use of foods that have been shown to be associated with decreasing body AGEs, for example, brown rice and mushrooms
3. High intake of foods rich in antioxidants
4. Generous use of herbs, spices, and condiments that improve taste of food and also have antiglycation effect (curcumin, cinnamon, parsley, thyme, clove, and extracts from a variety of other culinary herbs and spices) (See also Chap. 6)

Table 4.3 Clinical trials with a Low AGE diet

Study (author/year)	Study population	Study design	Study outcomes
Vlassara et al. (2002) [19]	Diabetics (US)	Crossover	Decreased circulating AGEs and markers of OS/Infl
Uribarri et al. (2003) [22]	Nondiabetic ESRD (US)	Two parallel groups (high and low AGE diets)	Decreased circulating AGEs and markers of Infl
Vlassara et al. (2009) [12]	Healthy and nondiabetic CKD (US)	Two parallel groups (high and low AGE diets)	Decreased circulating AGEs and markers of OS/Infl
Uribarri et al. (2011) [6]	Type 2 diabetics (US)	Two parallel groups (high and low AGE diets)	Decreased circulating AGEs and markers of OS/Infl and decreased HOMA
Birlouez-Aragon et al. (2010) [14]	Healthy (France)	Two parallel groups (high and low AGE diets)	Decreased circulating AGEs and HOMA
Luevano-Contreras et al. (2013) [16]	Type 2 diabetics (Mexico)	Two parallel groups (high and low AGE diets)	Decreased circulating markers of OS/Infl
Mark et al. (2014) [17]	Overweight women (Denmark)	Two parallel groups (high and low AGE diets)	Decreased urinary AGEs and HOMA
Semba et al. (2014) [13]	Healthy (US)	Two parallel groups (high and low AGE diets)	Decreased circulating AGEs but no changes in markers OS/Infl
De Courten et al. (2016) [18]	Overweight healthy men and women (Denmark)	Two parallel groups (high and low AGE diets)	Decreased circulating AGEs and insulin resistance
Vlassara et al. (2016) [15]	Men and women with metabolic syndrome (US)	Two parallel groups (high and low AGE diets) × 1 year	Decreased circulating AGEs and markers of OS/Infl and decreased HOMA

Unfortunately, outside of the clinical trials arena, education of patients requires effort and time that many busy clinicians do not have. Moreover, a person who is used to cooking in a certain way needs a lot of support and encouragement to change habits. Another potential hurdle is that the patient is often only one of several members of a family, making it necessary to try to convince the enitre group and especially the person who cooks of the benefits of this diet.

Clinical Trials with a Low AGE Diet

There are many published clinical intervention trials of the low AGE diet (Table 4.3).

Low AGE Intervention in Healthy Subjects

A group of healthy subjects, equally divided among young and older ages, were randomly assigned to either their own usual high AGE diet or a low AGE diet for 4 months [12]. The design included balancing the control and AGE-restricted diets in caloric, nutrient, and micronutrient contents. Participants received detailed instructions on how to prepare food at home by a study dietitian who was in frequent telephone contact with them. Subjects were required to have a baseline high-normal dietary AGE intake as an entry criterion. After 4 months, significant reductions in serum AGE (both CML and MGO) levels were noted, with parallel reductions in plasma levels of 8-isoprostanes (OS biomarker), VCAM-1 (endothelial function biomarker), and peripheral mononuclear cell-derived TNFα (inflammation biomarker), below baseline values. There was no age difference in the response to the dietary intervention.

Another randomized, parallel-arm, controlled dietary intervention was conducted with 24 healthy adults, aged 50–69 years for 6 weeks. At the end of the study, the low AGE group had lower levels of serum and urinary CML, but no impact in any of the inflammatory markers measured [13].

In another randomized crossover study, the authors compared the effect of two diets, one based on mild steam cooking (low AGE) and the other one on high-temperature cooking (high AGE), each one followed for 1 month in 62 healthy volunteers in France. The low AGE diet significantly decreased circulating CML levels and improved insulin sensitivity as assessed by the HOMA index [14].

Low AGE Intervention in Obese Patients with the Metabolic Syndrome

A randomized 1-year trial was conducted in obese individuals with the metabolic syndrome divided in two parallel groups: low AGE diet vs a regular diet, high in AGEs. The low AGE diet significantly lowered serum AGEs, markers of OS, and inflammation and enhanced the protective factors sirtuin 1 (SIRT1), AGE receptor 1 (AGER1), and glyoxalase I as well as markedly decreased insulin resistance with just a modest decrease in body weight [15]. Three other trials have also explored the effects of a low AGE diet in overweight subjects and with similar results [16–18].

Low AGE Intervention in Diabetic Patients

The first randomized study on the effect of an AGE-restricted diet in diabetic patients was a crossover study between low and regular AGE diets for a period of 6 weeks. Meals were prepared in the clinical research unit kitchen, and patients picked them up twice a week during the duration of the study. Patients in the low AGE diet demonstrated decreased levels of circulating AGEs (both CML and MGO), VCAM-1, CRP, and TNFα [19]. Notably, circulating AGE levels decreased as much as 40%, despite same degree of diabetic control. High serum AGE levels in diabetic patients had previously been thought to result exclusively from endogenous overproduction due to hyperglycemia, and therefore this significant fall of their levels on the low AGE diet, while maintaining overall same glycemic control, was unexpected.

In another study, diabetic patients were randomized to follow either their regular AGE diet or a low AGE diet for 4 months [6]. A study dietitian followed the patients closely and instructed them how to prepare their own meals at home. At the end of the study, patients in the low AGE diet showed not only decreased circulating levels of AGEs, 8-isoprostane, RAGE, and TNFα but also decreased HOMA and increased AGER1 and SIRT1 [6].

The reduction of HOMA observed in diabetic patients and subjects with the metabolic syndrome implies improvement of insulin sensitivity in response to the low AGE diet. Hyperglycemia in diabetes can increase endogenous production of AGEs, but this study suggests that AGEs in turn have an important role in modifying insulin resistance and therefore diabetes itself. This concept that AGEs can induce diabetes in humans is supported by previous animal experiments showing that a high AGE diet can induce insulin resistance and in turn diabetes mellitus, while a low AGE diet is protective [20, 21].

This relationship between AGEs and insulin resistance needs to be further confirmed in additional clinical trials but is a potential opportunity for a safe, inexpensive, and effective dietary modulation to either prevent or improve diabetes control.

A group in Mexico has also shown that diabetic patients on a low AGE diet intervention showed lower circulating markers of inflammation and OS compared to those on a high AGE diet [16].

Low AGE Intervention in Chronic Kidney Disease (CKD) Patients

The impact of the intervention on subjects with impaired kidney function was tested in a small group of patients with established CKD not yet on dialysis exposed to an AGE-restricted diet for 4 months. The effects of the low AGE diet in these CKD patients mimicked those in healthy participants and in diabetic patients, namely, reduction in serum AGEs and in markers of inflammation and OS [12].

Low AGE Intervention in End-Stage Renal Disease (ESRD) Patients on Peritoneal Dialysis

An AGE-restricted diet has also been tested for 4 weeks in a group of nondiabetic ESRD patients on maintenance peritoneal dialysis. The results showed significant reduction of serum AGEs and hsCRP, a marker of inflammation [22].

Diabetic CKD Subjects on a Regular AGE Diet but Exposed to an Oral Medication that Binds AGEs in the GI Tract

Recently, 20 diabetic CKD patients were studied in a crossover design with one period of sevelamer carbonate (1600 mg with meals) and another one of calcium carbonate (1200 mg with meals) for 8 weeks each. Sevelamer therapy, in contrast to calcium carbonate, reproduced all the previous findings observed on the low dietary AGE intervention, namely, reduced circulating levels of AGEs, 8-isoprostane, and TNFα and increased AGER1 and SIRT1. Sevelamer, not calcium carbonate, was shown to bind AGEs quite effectively in vitro, and the presumption is that sevelamer trapped AGEs in the intestinal lumen of these patients [23]. A second study using sevelamer in a larger number of CKD patients confirmed previous results [24].

How Does the Low AGE Diet Differ from Other Popular Diets?

The essence of the low AGE diet is its simplicity: preferential use of some culinary techniques such as poaching, steaming, stewing, and boiling that generate less AGEs. No specific advice is given in terms of macronutrient intake; the only advice is in the way to cook. This is not a low-protein, or low-fat, or low-carbohydrate diet. Since cooking meats with less dry heat generates less aromas (such as the home cooking smell of barbecues) that people may be used to, experts advise generous use of spices and condiments to enhance flavor.

Plant-Derived Diet

The low AGE diet is not necessarily a plant-based nutrition, although vegetables/fruits are strongly advised because they are low in AGE and their high antioxidant effects could potentially antagonize the prooxidant effects of AGEs. The low AGE diet is much more flexible than a plant-based diet and therefore can be more broadly applied in practice.

DASH Diet

The low AGE diet is different from the DASH diet, although it also favors relatively low sodium and high potassium intake.

Raw Diet

Although the low AGE diet applies low heat and includes the use of fresh vegetables and fruits, it is quite different than the raw diet. Clearly, a raw diet is a very low AGE diet, but experts believe there are too many health risks related to its wide application.

Mediterranean Diet

The low AGE diet has many similarities with the Mediterranean diet, but they are not synonymous. In the low AGE diet, in contrast to the Mediterranean diet, every kind of food can be used provided it is cooked a certain way.

Paleo Diet

Paleo diet. The low AGE diet is different from the paleo diet that restricts intake of important foods such as grains, dairy, and legumes and plays excessive emphasis on meats.

Summary

The results from the clinical trials discussed above suggest a new paradigm for the pathogenesis of chronic diseases: chronic exposure to these exogenous prooxidant AGEs may help to gradually erode native defenses, setting the stage for abnormally high OS and inflammation, precursors of chronic diseases. Real-life dietary patterns are complex and include the simultaneous presence of many factors other than AGEs. Some of these dietary factors are pro-inflammatory such as fats and AGEs, while others are clearly anti-inflammatory such as polyphenols and a variety of antioxidants. The final biological effect of dietary patterns most likely reflects the combined influence of all these factors, each one of them acting in different directions and with different intensity. The combination of types of foods and their respective amounts over the day are overall more important rather than any specific food item AGE content. Detailed information on how to initiate and maintain a low AGE diet has been published. The restriction of dietary AGEs is a safe and feasible dietary intervention that effectively reverses increased inflammation and OS, both in health and in the chronic disease state. A final proof of a therapeutic role for the low AGE diet will require large, prospective, and randomized clinical trials, which indeed may never take place. In the meantime, however, a careful analysis of the currently available data makes it reasonable and prudent to advise limitation of dietary AGEs. This is particularly important since consumption of lower AGE foods and preparation methods can easily be integrated into meal patterns that are consistent with current recommendations designed to promote public health and prevent cardiovascular disease, cancer, diabetes, and obesity.

References

1. Uribarri J, Tuttle KR. Advanced glycation end products and nephrotoxicity of high-protein diets. Clin J Am Soc Nephrol. 2006;26:633–41.
2. Goldberg T, Cai W, Peppa M, Dardaine V, Baliga BS, Uribarri J, Vlassara H. Advanced glycoxidation end products in commonly consumed foods. J Am Diet Assoc. 2004;104:1287–91.
3. Koschinsky T, He C, Mitsuhashi T, Bucala R, Liu C, Buenting C, Heitmann K, Vlassara H. Orally absorbed reactive glycation products (glycotoxins): a potential risk factor in diabetic nephropathy. Proc Natl Acad Sci U S A. 1997;94:6474–9.
4. Yan SF, Ramsamy R, Schmidt AM. The RAGE axis: a fundamental mechanism signaling danger to the vulnerable vasculature. Circ Res. 2010;106:1040–51.
5. Cai W, He JC, Zhu L, Lu C, Vlassara H. Advanced glycation end product (AGE) receptor 1 suppresses cell oxidant stress and activation signaling via EGF receptor. Proc Natl Acad Sci U S A. 2006;103:13801–6.
6. Uribarri J, Cai W, Ramdas M, Goodman S, Pyzik R, Chen X, Zhu L, Striker GE, Vlassara H. Restriction of advanced glycation end products improves insulin resistance in human type 2 diabetes: potential role of AGER1 and SIRT1. Diabetes Care. 2011;34:1610–6.
7. Gugliucci A, Bendayan M. Renal fate of circulating advanced glycated end products (AGE): evidence for reabsorption and catabolism of AGE-peptides by renal proximal tubular cells. Diabetologia. 1996;39:149–60.
8. Yacoub R, Nugent M, Cai W, Nadkarni GN, Chaves LD, Abyad S, et al. Advanced glycation end products dietary restriction effects on bacterial gut microbiota in peritoneal dialysis patients; a randomized open label controlled trial. PLoS One. 2017;12(9):e0184789.
9. Uribarri J, Woodruff S, Goodman S, Cai W, Chen X, Pyzik R, Yong A, Striker GE, Vlassara H. Advanced glycation end products in foods and a practical guide to their reduction in the diet. J Am Diet Assoc. 2010;110:911–6.
10. Scheijen JLJM, Clevers E, Engelen L, et al. Analysis of advanced glycation endproducts in selected food items by ultra-performance liquid chromatography tandem mass spectrometry: presentation of a dietary AGE database. Food Chem. 2016;190:1145–50.
11. Cerami C, Founds H, Nicholl I, Mitsuhashi T, Giordano D, Vanpatten S, Lee A, Al-Abed Y, Vlassara H, Bucala R, Cerami A. Tobacco smoke is a source of toxic reactive glycation products. Proc Natl Acad Sci U S A. 1997;94:13915–20.
12. Vlassara H, Cai W, Goodman S, Pyzik R, Young A, Zhu L, Neade T, Beeri M, Silverman JM, Ferrucci L, Tansman L, Striker GE, Uribarri J. Protection against loss of innate defenses in adulthood by low AGE intake; role of a new anti-inflammatory AGE-receptor-1. J Clin Endocrinol Metab. 2009;94:4483–91.
13. Semba RD, et al. Dietary intake of advanced glycation end products did not affect endothelial function and inflammation in healthy adults in a randomized controlled trial. J Nutr. 2014;144:1037–42.
14. Birlouez-Aragon I, Saaveda G, Tessier FJ, Galinier A, Ait-Ameur L, Lacoste F, Niamba CN, Alt N, Somoza V, Lecerf JM. A diet based on high-heat-treated foods promotes risk factors for diabetes mellitus and cardiovascular disease. Am J Clin Nutr. 2010;91:1220–6.
15. Vlassara H, Cai W, Tripp E, Pyzik R, Yee K, Goldberg L, et al. Oral AGE restriction ameliorates insulin resistance in obese individuals with the metabolic syndrome: a randomised controlled trial. Diabetologia. 2016;59(10):2181–92.
16. Luevano-Contreras C, Garay-Sevilla ME, Wrobel K, Malacara JM, Wrobel K. Dietary advanced glycation end products restriction diminishes inflammation markers and oxidative stress in patients with type 2 diabetes mellitus. J Clin Biochem Nutr. 2013;52(1):22–6.
17. Mark AB, Poulsen MW, Andersen S, Andersen JM, Bak MJ, Ritz C, et al. Consumption of a diet low in advanced glycation end products for 4 weeks improves insulin sensitivity in overweight women. Diabetes Care. 2014;37:88–95.

18. De Courten B, de Courten MP, Soldats G, et al. Diet low in advanced glycation end products increases insulin sensitivity in healthy overweight individuals: a double-blind, randomized, crossover trial. Am J Clin Nutr. 2016;103:1426–33.
19. Vlassara H, Cai W, Crandall J, Goldberg T, Oberstein R, Dardaine V, et al. Inflammatory mediators are induced by dietary glycotoxins, a major risk factor for diabetic angiopathy. Proc Natl Acad Sci U S A. 2002;99(24):15596–601.
20. Hofmann SM, Dong HJ, Li Z, Cai W, Altomonte J, Thung SN, Zeng F, Fisher EA, Vlassara H. Improved insulin sensitivity is associated with restricted intake of dietary glycoxidation products in the db/db mouse. Diabetes. 2002;51:2082–9.
21. Sandu O, Song K, Cai W, Zheng F, Uribarri J, Vlassara H. Insulin resistance and type 2 diabetes in high-fat-fed mice are linked to high glycotoxin intake. Diabetes. 2005;54:2314–9.
22. Uribarri J, Peppa M, Cai W, Goldberg T, Lu M, He C, Vlassara H. Restriction of dietary glycotoxins reduces excessive advanced glycation end products in renal failure patients. J Am Soc Nephrol. 2003;14:728–31.
23. Vlassara H, Uribarri J, Cai W, Goodman S, Pyzik R, Post J, Grosjean F, Woodward M, Striker GE. Effects of sevelamer on HbA1c, inflammation, and advanced glycation end products in diabetic kidney disease. Clin J Am Soc Nephrol. 2012;7:934–42.
24. Yubero-Serrano EM, Woodward M, Poretsky L, Vlassara H, Striker GE, AGE-less Study Group. Effects of sevelamer carbonate on advanced glycation end products and antioxidant/pro-oxidant status in patients with diabetic kidney disease. Clin J Am Soc Nephrol. 2015;10(5):759–66.

Chapter 5
Healthy Drinks

Joseph A. Vassalotti

Keywords Health · Beverages · Water · Sugar · Calories

Key Points
- Beverages comprise approximately 20% of daily calories.
- Drinking plain water, tap or bottled, rather than high-caloric beverages, reduces dietary calorie consumption and may contribute to maintaining a healthy body weight.
- Sugar-sweetened beverages are associated with obesity, type-2 diabetes mellitus, cardiovascular disease, and chronic kidney disease.
- Sugar-sweetened beverages should be limited or avoided.
- Artificially sweetened beverages are probably safer than sugar-sweetened beverages, but the data are conflicting.

Introduction

The public consciousness of healthy eating conjures images of a balanced meal, including fruits, vegetables, whole grains, and lean protein sources, without considering drinks. Thus, drinks have been called hidden or empty calories for their potential to contribute a high-caloric content without significant nutritional value in an imperceptible fashion for the consumer. Beverage consumption comprises almost 20% of calorie intake. Importantly, the intake of all foods and beverages must be accounted for when striving for healthy eating patterns. The purpose of this chapter is to review the current literature to guide simple, practical healthy-drinking interventions for the busy clinician. The consumption of plain water as a widely available, inexpensive, non-caloric healthy drink is the main message that should be implemented by clinicians for their patients [17].

J. A. Vassalotti (✉)
Division of Nephrology, Department of Medicine, Icahn School of Medicine at Mount Sinai, New York, NY, USA

The National Kidney Foundation, Inc., New York, NY, USA
e-mail: joseph.vassalotti@mssm.edu

© Springer Nature Switzerland AG 2020
J. Uribarri, J. A. Vassalotti (eds.), *Nutrition, Fitness, and Mindfulness*, Nutrition and Health,
https://doi.org/10.1007/978-3-030-30892-6_5

Water as the Primary Drink

Drinking water is an effective way to promote adequate hydration without calories [11]. Drinking plain water, tap or bottled, rather than high-caloric beverages, reduces dietary calorie consumption and may contribute to maintaining a healthy body weight. Observational studies from national surveys reveal that plain water consumption is inversely proportional to calorie or energy intake. Two 24-hour dietary survey assessments of over 18 thousand adults in the US National Health and Nutrition Examination Survey (NHANES) 2005–2012 revealed every one percent increase in the proportion of daily plain water in total dietary water daily consumption was associated with a reduction in mean daily total calorie intake 8.58 (95% confidence interval [CI], 7.87–9.29) kcal, with a significant corresponding reduction in intakes from multiple other sources, including sugar-sweetened beverages (SSB) 1.43 (CI, 1.27–1.59) kcal, total fat intake 0.21 (CI, 0.17–0.25) g, saturated fat intake 0.07 (CI, 0.06–0.09) g, sugar intake 0.74 (CI, 0.67–0.82) g, sodium intake 9.80 (CI, 8.20–11.39) mg, and cholesterol intake 0.88 (CI, 0.64–1.13) g [1]. The effects of plain water intake on diet in this study were similar across race/ethnicity, education attainment, income level, and body mass index (BMI) [1].

Tap water is an inexpensive, widely available healthy drink with no calories and low in sodium. Although water consumption in the USA is predominantly from tap water, a significant percentage comes from bottled water. Many factors influence the decision to drink tap versus bottled water, including access, cost, convenience, taste, marketing, and perceptions of safety [25]. Several regional and national US surveys show that urban and particularly Hispanic and Black adults are more likely to consider bottled water as safer, and this perception has a negative effect on primarily consuming tap water [11, 25, 29]. Water filters are a practical intervention to address concerns about the safety of tap water [25]. Unfortunately, in parts of the world where safe drinking water is unavailable, bottled water may be a more convenient option than treating water with boiling and filtering or other measures.

Although adequate water intake can help avoid dehydration, acute electrolyte disorders, and hemodynamically mediated acute kidney injury, the precise optimal quantity of plain water intake is difficult to quantify, and thus recommendations should be generally be individualized.

The major health benefit of water is the replacement of other potentially deleterious high-calorie drinks. Moreover, plain water intake before or with meals may contribute to satiety, and in turn reduce calorie intake.

Aqua Therapy: High Volume Plain Water Intake Benefits and Risks

Patients with kidney stones as well as a subset of patients with CKD may benefit from increasing water intake above thirst [12, 30]. Poor quality evidence suggests increasing fluid intake to reduce arginine vasopressin (AVP) secretion may slow kidney cyst growth in CKD caused by autosomal dominant polycystic kidney disease (ADPKD). The PREVENT-ADPKD trial is an RCT of 1:1 allocation of increasing fluid intake to target urinary osmolarity <270 mOsmol/L versus usual care in patients with CKD stage G1-3 [30]. The primary endpoint of this ongoing trial will be total kidney volume.

The CKD WIT (Chronic Kidney Disease Water Intake Trial) enrolled CKD stage G3 or eGFR 30–60 mL/min/1.73 m^2 at 9 centers in Ontario, Canada, from 2013 to 2017 to increase water intake with coaching ($n = 316$) versus control ($n = 315$) [5]. Exclusion criteria were a 24-hour urine volume of 3 L or more, a history of kidney stones in the past 5 years, currently taking lithium or a high dose diuretic. The primary etiologies for CKD were similar in the hydration and control groups, respectively, with DM (38.0% and 33.3%), hypertension (40.2% and 27.8%), glomerulonephritis (4.7% and 8.3%), and ADPKD (2.9% and 2.8%). There was no difference in the primary outcome, change in kidney function (eGFR from baseline to 12 months), -2.2 mL/min/1.73 m^2 in the hydration group vs. -1.9 mL/min/1.73 m^2 in the control group (adjusted between-group difference, -0.3 mL/min/1.73 m^2 [CI, -1.8 to 1.2; p = 0.74]) [5]. The intervention implementation was successful as assessed by 1-year follow-up mean increase in 24-hour urine volume 0.6 L per day higher in the hydration group (95% CI, 0.5–0.7; p < 0.001). The authors concluded that for adults with CKD, coaching to increase water intake compared with control intake did not significantly slow the decline in kidney function after 1 year.

Individualizing fluid intake is important to emphasize. There is little data to support a uniform intake threshold to avoid volume depletion. Use of urinary osmolarity or specific gravity could guide decision-making in selected cases. One small study suggests a first morning voided urine-specific gravity of 1.013 or less may be desirable in healthy persons [22]. An easy rule of thumb to judge adequate hydration is the color of the urine; darker urine suggests concentration in response to reduced volume.

Avoid High Calorie Drinks

Between 1950 and 2000, the average US per capita annual consumption of SSB increased almost fivefold from 10.8 to 49.3 gallons, but consumption has declined in more recent years [3]. Sugary drinks are a major source of calories and the primary source of added sugar in the US diet, comprising 25% of total added sugar; see Fig. 5.1 [28]. These drinks generally contain sugar, high-fructose corn syrup, or fructose as single ingredients or in combination. These beverages are associated with obesity, type-2 diabetes mellitus (T2DM), cardiovascular disease (CVD), and chronic kidney disease (CKD) [3, 19, 20]. Putative mechanisms for SSB induction of chronic diseases include both increased caloric intake and inappropriate suppression of satiety [1, 3]. Fructose may play a role in visceral fat accumulation and in turn the development of non-alcoholic fatty liver disease by altering hepatic gene expression patterns, inhibiting satiety factors in the brain, and inducing leptin resistance [8].

Visceral versus peripheral fat has been associated with microinflammation, CVD, and CKD. A Framingham third generation cohort study of over one thousand adults showed significantly increased visceral adipose tissue in SSB drinkers compared to nondrinkers and diet soda consumers as assessed by CT scans approximately 6 years apart [19]. Visceral adipose tissue volume increased from 658 cm^3 (CI, 602–713) to 852 cm^3 (CI, 760–943) for non-consumers vs. daily SSB consumers [19]. A European Prospective Investigation into Cancer and Nutrition (EPIC)-Norfolk study of beverage consumption in over 25 thousand UK adults without DM (1993–1997) used 7-day food diaries to evaluate associations with respect to the 847 (3.3%) who developed incident T2DM over 10.8 years of mean follow-up [20]. The adjusted Cox regression analyses showed significant associations for SSB use and T2DM with hazard ratios for soft drinks at 1.21 (CI, 1.05–1.39) and for sweetened-milk beverages at 1.22 (CI, 1.05–1.43) [20]. There was a dose-response relationship with total SSB that was not attenuated after adjustment for baseline BMI. The authors estimated that substituting water for SSB would be associated with a 25% reduction in T2DM risk. If sweet beverage consumers reduced intake to below 2% energy, 15% of incident T2DM might be prevented [20]. A meta-analysis and survey analysis of 17 cohorts with over 38 thousand patients with over 10 million patient years showed higher consumption of SSB was associated with a greater incidence of T2DM by 18% (CI, 9–28%) per serving per day that was attenuated to 13% (CI, 6–21%) after adjustment for adiposity [16]. These findings support the implementation of clinician-level and population-based interventions to reduce SSB consumption and increase the consumption of suitable alternatives, particularly plain water.

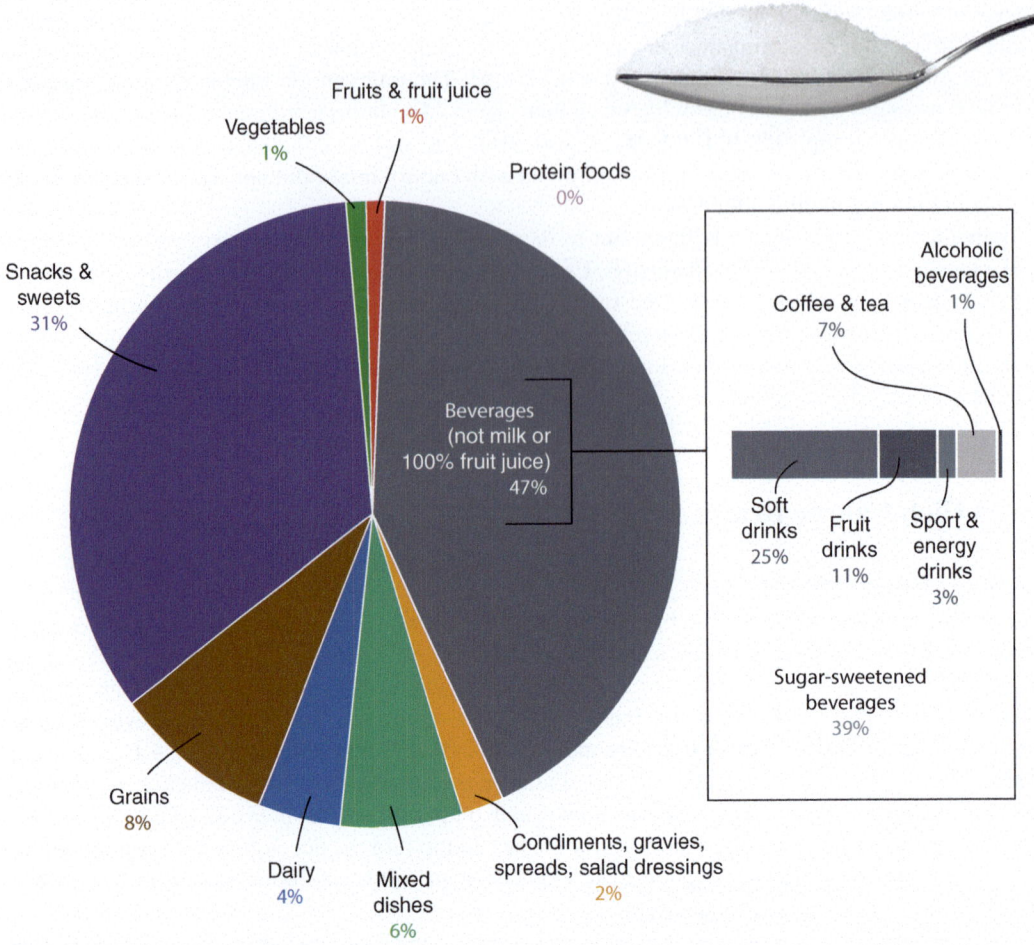

Fig. 5.1 Food category sources of added sugars in the US population ages 2 years and older. (Data source: What We Eat in America (WWEIA) Food Category analyses for the 2015 Dietary Guidelines Advisory Committee. Estimates based on day one dietary recalls from WWEIA, NHANES 2009–2010 [28])

Diet Drinks: Healthful or Harmful?

As the health hazards of SSB because widely known, health policies and public health programs to limit sugary drinks indirectly culminated in a surge in low-calorie beverage (LCB) use in the USA, containing any of the six FDA-approved artificial sweeteners. Artificially sweetened diet drinks and LCB are used interchangeably. Per capita consumption of diet beverages is higher in North America than any other region of the world [23] with LCB comprising 32% of drinks consumed by adults and 19% of beverages consumed by children from 2007 to 2010 [17]. Potential risks of LCB include increased waist circumference, metabolic syndrome, and T2DM. Whether LCB are detrimental to health remains controversial as observational studies are limited by residual confounding and reverse causality. The latter limitation reflects intake of diet drinks may be an epiphenomenon of these chronic conditions rather than cause them, because people with and at risk for T2DM may be more likely to consume LCB than others. Lastly, an American Heart Association science advisory concluded that there is dearth of evidence on the potential adverse effects of LCB relative to potential benefits [17].

A Woman's Health Initiative observational study of postmenopausal women showed self-reported T2DM developed among 4675 (7.2%) of 64,850 participants over a mean follow-up of 8.4 years with hazard ratios of 1.43 (CI 1.17–1.75) for SSB and 1.21 (CI 1.08–1.36) for LCB [15]. The authors inferred that the 21% increased risk of T2DM could be potentially be eliminated by substituting water for diet beverages. The previously described EPIC-Norfolk study showed an association of T2DM with LCB 1.22 (CI, 1.11–1.33), but not for sweetened tea/coffee 0.98 (CI, 0.94–1.02) or fruit juice 1.01 (CI, 0.88–1.15) [20]. Further adjustment for adiposity attenuated the association for LCB, HR 1.06 (CI, 0.93–1.20). Substituting LCB for any SSB did not reduce the T2DM incidence in analyses accounting for energy intake and adiposity. Substituting one serving/day of water or unsweetened tea/coffee for soft drinks and for sweetened-milk beverages reduced the incidence by 14–25%. The results of two food frequency questionnaires at baseline (1987–1989) and in follow-up (1993–1995) for over 15 thousand participants in the atherosclerosis risk in communities (ARIC) study showed a significant dose relationship between weekly diet soda intake and end stage kidney disease (ESKD) with corresponding hazard ratios <1 serving (reference), 1–4 servings 1.08 (CI, 0.75–1.55), 5–7 servings 1.33 (CI, 1.01–1.75), and >7 servings 1.83 (CI, 1.01–2.52) [24]. There were similar associations after adjustment for multiple potentially confounding variables, including physical activity and total caloric intake, among many others. The results were only significant for those who were overweight or obese at baseline [24]. In conclusion, based on the limited available data, the choice of LCB is likely a safer alternative to SSB in general, but plain water remains the optimal drink.

Moderate Alcohol Use

Whether or not light-to-moderate alcohol or ethanol use is preferable to abstaining for health benefits remains unclear, since the observational data are conflicting and controversial. Ethanol consumption may alter endothelial and smooth muscle cell function as well as microvascular function in a beneficial fashion. In contrast, heavy alcohol use is associated with hypertension, alcoholic cardiomyopathy, atrial fibrillation; fatal and nonfatal stroke; and fatal and nonfatal malignancies [6, 14]. Alcohol is not a component of the USDA Food Patterns, and recent guidelines advise if alcohol is consumed, it should be in moderation—up to one drink per day for women and up to two drinks per day for men. Obviously, consumption should only be by adults of legal drinking age. For those who choose to drink, moderate alcohol consumption can be incorporated into the calorie limits of most healthy eating patterns.

A meta-analysis of 34 prospective studies found mortality rate reductions of 17% in men and 18% in women with low levels of alcohol intake, with the lowest mortality rate at 6 g of alcohol (approximately one half drink) per day [9]. Most of the studies included in the analysis were performed in healthy cohorts, and data in patients with ischemic heart disease are limited [9]. A post-hoc analyses of the Baseline Double Exposure cohort study examined alcohol consumption and gender in association with 24-hour ambulatory BP monitoring (ABPM) in 248 Canadian participants, 54.4% of whom were women, with a mean age 50.8 ± 6.6 years and normal or elevated and untreated BP [27]. The main effects model, including BMI, multiple regression analysis with systolic ABPM as the dependent variable found that alcohol consumption more than 10 drinks/week was associated with a 4.4 mmHg increase for men (p = 0.033) and an 8.4 mmHg increase for women (p = 0.007) [27].

An analysis that evaluated the relationship between light-to-moderate alcohol consumption and outcomes in patients with ischemic or non-ischemic LV dysfunction used the Studies Of Left Ventricular Dysfunction (SOLVD) data, which enrolled patients with an left ventricular (LV) ejection fraction ≤0.35 [6]. In the context of baseline characteristics versus subsequent event rates of participants who consumed 1–14 alcoholic drinks per week (light-to-moderate drinkers, n = 2594) were compared with those who reported no alcohol consumption (nondrinkers, n = 3719) [6]. Mortality rates were lower among light-to-moderate drinkers than among nondrinkers (7.2 vs. 9.4 deaths/100 person-years, p < 0.001). Among patients with ischemic LV dysfunction, light-to-moderate alcohol consumption was independently associated with a reduced relative risk (RR) 0.85, p = 0.01, particularly for death from myocardial infarction (MI) 0.55, p < 0.001. The relative risks of heart failure hospitalization, cardiovascular death, death from heart failure, and dysrhythmia death were similar for light-to-moderate drinkers and nondrinkers. Among patients with non-ischemic LV dysfunction, light-to-moderate alcohol consumption had no significant effect on mortality RR 0.93, p = 0.5. Light-to-moderate alcohol consumption was not associated with an adverse prognosis in patients with LV systolic dysfunction, and it may reduce the risk of fatal myocardial infarction in patients with ischemic LV dysfunction. A modest anticoagulant effect could be speculated in the causal pathway for this observation. The authors advised caution regarding recommending alcohol intake to nondrinkers with ischemic LV dysfunction patients on the basis of this study but recommended that continued light-to-moderate alcohol intake could be continued in this context.

Red Wine

Some researchers have suggested that the potential health benefits of alcohol may be particularly due to red wine, as part of the so-called "French Paradox" [9]. For example, a meta-analysis showed a significant inverse association between light-to-moderate wine consumption and vascular risk RR 0.68 (95% CI, 0.59–0.77) relative to nondrinkers [9] and a similar but smaller RR 0.78 (95% CI, 0.70 –0.86) for beer consumption [9]. Others are examining the potential benefits of components in red wine such as flavonoids, resveratrol, and other antioxidants in reducing heart disease risk. These studies may be confounded by healthy lifestyle factors rather than alcohol, including increased physical activity, and a diet high in fruits and vegetables and lower in saturated fats. No direct comparison trials have been done to determine the specific effect of wine or other alcohol on the risk of developing heart disease or stroke. The American Heart Association does not recommend drinking wine or any other form of alcohol to gain these potential benefits.

Drinks as Complementary Medicine

Hibiscus and Green Tea

Hibiscus sabdariffa is used in herbal teas that may also treat hypertension, yet the evidence from randomized controlled trials (RCTs) has been mixed. The most promising study selected five RCTs comprising 390 participants, of whom 225 were allocated to the *Hibiscus sabdariffa* group and 165 to the control group [26]. The fixed-effect meta-regression analysis indicated a significant effect of *Hibiscus sabdariffa* supplementation in lowering both SBP weighed mean difference −7.58 mmHg (CI, −9.69 to −5.46, p < 0.00001) and DBP weighed mean difference −3.53 mmHg (CI, −5.16 to −1.89, p < 0.0001) [26]. Thus, this meta-analysis of RCTs showed a significant effect of *Hibiscus sabdariffa* in lowering both SBP and DBP. The authors recommended that additional well-designed trials are necessary to validate these results. A Meta-analysis of ten trials including both green and black tea in 834 participants with hypertension or elevated BP showed statistically significant reductions in SBP −2.36 mmHg (95% CI, −4.20 to −0.52) and DBP −1.77 mmHg (CI, −3.03 to −0.52) [31]. These teas may be offered as a low-risk adjunctive therapy for hypertension, but should not be used as a substitute for drugs.

Coffee

One of the world's most widely consumed beverages is coffee, which is a major source of caffeine, metabolized by the polymorphic cytochrome P450 1A2 enzyme [7]. About 75% of Americans drink coffee with 50% as daily drinkers. There are no important large-scale prospective trials to assess the impact of coffee on important outcomes. Thus, the relationship between coffee consumption and cardiovascular disease remains controversial, since the results from observational studies and case-control studies are mixed. Starting with the risks of coffee consumption, a case-crossover design study of 503 nonfatal acute MI between 1994 and 1998 in Costa Rica revealed the relative risk (RR) for heart attack in the first hour after coffee consumption was 1.49 (CI = 1.17–1.89) overall [2]. The relative risk was inversely proportional to the chronic coffee consumption by occasional ($\leq$1 cup/day, n = 103) 4.14 (CI, 2.03–8.42), moderate (2–3 cups/day, n = 280) 1.60 (CI, 1.16–2.21), and heavy ($\geq$4 cups/d, n = 120) 1.06 (CI, 0.69–1.63; p = 0.006) [2]. As expected, more than three cardiovascular risk factors or sedentary lifestyle significantly increased the relative risk of acute MI vs. attenuated relative risk in those without three risk factors or an active lifestyle. Coffee may trigger an acute MI, particularly in the first hour after consumption for light drinkers. A case-control study from the same group of over 2 thousand patients with nonfatal MI versus a similar number of population-based controls in Costa Rica between 1994 and 2004 revealed intake of coffee was associated with an increased risk of nonfatal MI only among individuals with slow caffeine metabolism, suggesting that caffeine plays a role in this association [7].

Perhaps the most compelling data to support the potential health benefits of coffee drinking is the National Institutes of Health–AARP Diet and Health Study of over 400,000 subjects who were 50–71 years of age at baseline with 5,148,760 person-years of subsequent follow-up between 1995 and 2008 for cause-specific and all-cause mortality [13]. Participants with cancer, heart disease, and stroke were excluded. Coffee consumption was assessed once at baseline. In age-adjusted models, the risk of death was increased among coffee drinkers. However, coffee drinkers were also more likely to smoke, and, after adjustment for tobacco-smoking status and other potential confounders, there was a significant inverse association between coffee consumption and mortality. Adjusted hazard ratios for death among men by daily coffee intake as compared with those who did not were as follows: 0.99 (CI, 0.95–1.04) for less than 1 cup per day, 0.94 (CI, 0.90–0.99) for 1 cup, 0.90 (CI, 0.86–0.93) for 2 or 3 cups, 0.88 (CI, 0.84–0.93) for 4 or 5 cups, and 0.90 (CI, 0.85–0.96) for 6 or more cups of coffee per day (p < 0.001 for trend); the respective hazard ratios among women were 1.01 (CI, 0.96–1.07), 0.95 (CI, 0.90–1.01), 0.87 (CI, 0.83–0.92), 0.84 (CI, 0.79–0.90), and 0.85 (CI, 0.78–0.93) (p < 0.001) [13]. Results were similar in other subgroups. The authors concluded that coffee consumption was inversely associated with total and cause-specific mortality, but weather this relationship is a causal or an associational finding cannot be determined from the available data.

A meta-analysis of the dose response of coffee drinking and cardiovascular disease revealed thirty-six studies with 1,279,804 participants and 36,352 CVD cases. A significant nonlinear relationship of coffee consumption with CVD risk was identified. Compared with the lowest category of coffee consumption (median, 0 cups per day), the relative risk of CVD was 0.95 (CI, 0.87–1.03) for the highest category (median, 5 cups per day), 0.85 (CI, 0.80–0.90) for the second highest category (median, 3.5 cups per day), and 0.89 (CI, 0.84–0.94) for the third highest category (median, 1.5 cups per day) [10]. Increased physical activity associated with coffee consumption has been suggested as the confounding explanation for lower mortality [18]. Lastly, any recommendation about coffee intake should account for how the coffee is consumed, since black coffee with 4 sugar packets is essentially transformed into a SSB with the deleterious risks noted above. In summary, the available evidence suggests that coffee consumption benefits seem to outweigh the risks, although associated increase in physical activity may contribute to the mechanism.

Evaluating Drinks

As previously noted, beverages are a major source of dietary added sugars, accounting for about half of daily intake (Fig. 5.1) [28]. A simple way to limit added sugars from drinks is to drink plain water. Water can be flavored with juices from lemons or limes to add flavor. For those who prefer other drinks, nutrition labels are informational tools with the potential for encouraging healthy choices. The nutrition facts label, present on most beverages in the USA, is a tool for making daily informed drink choices [4]. Unfortunately, the underutilization of the nutrition facts panel is common and is associated with low levels of both education and health literacy [4, 21]. The amount of sugar and calories can vary considerably in drinks so the focus on these elements is important to avoid or limit SSB drinking. For example, review of the nutrition facts label for products such as sports drinks, which may be marketed as healthful beverages, but may be especially important to emphasize as these are often SSB, see Fig. 5.1. Sugars have no percent Daily Value (%DV), thus the amount in grams (g) on the label should be reviewed. The Dietary Guidelines for Americans 2015–2020 recommend consuming less than 10% of calories per day from added sugars. Since each g of sugar comprises 4 calories, patients on 2000 calorie a day intake should target sugar intake of less than 50 g sugar/day corresponding to 200 calories/day. Patients could also be educated to look for added sugars on the ingredient list on a beverage package with examples including corn sweetener, corn syrup, dextrose, fructose sweetener, fruit juice concentrates, glucose, high-fructose corn syrup, malt syrup, maple syrup, molasses, pancake syrup, sucrose, and sugar. These ingredients are listed in descending order by weight, so that the closer they are to the beginning of the list, the more of that ingredient is in the drink. Lastly, nutrition labels obviously do not account for sugar packets and other sweeteners or dairy products subsequently added to a beverage.

Conclusion

The typical US diet includes almost 20% of calories from beverages. Thus, the substitution of plain water as the primary drink is a simple, scalable, inexpensive way to reduce mean calorie intake by up to 400 calories per day, assuming 2000 calorie intake. Observational data support that increasing plain water intake is associated with reduced calorie consumption. Sugar-sweetened beverages should be limited or avoided because of strong associations with increased abdominal obesity and T2DM. Artificially sweetened beverages are probably safer than SSB, but less desirable than plain water.

References

1. An R, McCaffrey J. Plain water consumption in relation to energy intake and diet quality among US adults, 2005–2012. J Hum Nutr Diet. 2016;29:624–32.
2. Baylin A, Hernandez-Diaz S, Kabagambe EK, et al. Transient exposure to coffee as a trigger of a first nonfatal myocardial infarction. Epidemiology. 2006;17(5):506–11.
3. Bray GA, Popkin BM. Dietary sugar and body weight: have we reached a crisis in the epidemic of obesity and diabetes?: health be damned! Pour on the sugar. Diabetes Care. 2014;37(4):950–6.
4. Christoph MJ, Larson N, Laska MN, et al. Nutrition facts panels: who uses them, what do they use, and how does use relate to dietary intake? J Acad Nutr Diet. 2018;118(2):217–28.
5. Clark WF, Sontrop JM, Huang SH, et al. Effect of coaching to increase water intake on kidney function decline in adults with chronic kidney disease: the CKD WIT randomized clinical trial. JAMA. 2018;319(18):1870–9.
6. Cooper HA, Exner DV, Domanski MJ. Light-to-moderate alcohol consumption and prognosis in patients with left ventricular systolic dysfunction. J Am Coll Cardiol. 2000;35(7):1753–9.

7. Cornelis MC, El-Sohemy A, Kabagambe EK, et al. Coffee, CYP1A2 genotype, and risk of myocardial infarction Campos H. JAMA. 2006;295(10):1135–41.
8. Dekker MF, Su Q, Baker C, Rugtledge AC, Adeli K. Fructose: a highly lipogenic nutrient implicated in insulin resistance, hepatic steatosis, and the metabolic syndrome. Am J Physiol Endocrinol Metab. 2010;299(5):E685–94.
9. Di Castelnuovo A, Rotondo S, Iacoviello L, et al. Meta-analysis of wine and beer consumption in relation to vascular risk. Circulation. 2002;105:2836–44.
10. Ding M, Bhupathiraju SN, Satija A, et al. Long-term coffee consumption and risk of cardiovascular disease: a systematic review and a dose-response meta-analysis of prospective cohort studies. Circulation. 2014;129(6):643–59.
11. Drewnowski A, Rehm C, Constant F. Water and beverage consumption among adults in the United States: cross-sectional study using data from NHANES 2005–2010. BMC Public Health. 2013;13(1):1068.
12. Feehally J, Khosravi M. Effect of acute and chronic hydration on kidney health and function. Nutr Rev. 2015;73(Suppl 2):110–9.
13. Freedman ND, Park Y, Abnet CC, et al. Association of coffee drinking with total and cause-specific mortality. N Engl J Med. 2012;366:1891–904.
14. Goldberg RJ, Burchfiel CM, Reed DM, et al. A prospective study of the health effects of alcohol consumption in middle-aged and elderly men. The Honolulu Heart Program. Circulation. 1994;89(2):651–9.
15. Huang M, Quddus A, Stinson L, et al. Artificially sweetened beverages, sugar-sweetened beverages, plain water, and incident diabetes mellitus in postmenopausal women: the prospective Women's Health Initiative observational study. Am J Clin Nutr. 2017;106(2):614–22.
16. Imamura F, Mukamal KJ, Meigs JB, et al. Risk factors for type 2 diabetes mellitus preceded by β-cell dysfunction, insulin resistance, or both in older adults: the Cardiovascular Health Study. Am J Epidemiol. 2013;177(12):1418–29.
17. Johnson RK, Lichtenstein AH, Anderson CAM, et al. Low-calorie sweetened beverages and cardiometabolic health: a science advisory from the American Heart Association. Circulation. 2018;138:e126–40.
18. Lewis SF, Hennekens CH. Energy expenditure may explain why coffee drinkers have lower mortality. J Cardiovasc Pharmacol Ther. 2018;23(3):270–2.
19. Ma J, McKeown NM, Hwang S, et al. Sugar-sweetened beverage consumption is associated with change of visceral adipose tissue over 6 years of follow-up. Circulation. 2016;133:370–7.
20. O'Connor L, Inamura F, Lentiges MA, et al. Prospective associations and population impact of sweet beverage intake and type 2 diabetes, and effects of substitutions with alternative beverages. Diabetologia. 2015;58(7):1474–83.
21. Persoskie A, Hennessy E, Nelson WL. US consumers' understanding of nutrition labels in 2013: the importance of health literacy. Prev Chronic Dis. 2017;14:E86.
22. Perrier ET, Bottin JH, Vecchio M, et al. Criterion values for urine-specific gravity and urine color representing adequate water intake in healthy adults. Eur J Clin Nutr. 2017;71(4):561–3.
23. Popkin BM, Hawkes C. Sweetening of the global diet, particularly beverages: patterns, trends, and policy responses. Lancet Diabetes Endocrinol. 2016;4(2):174–86.
24. Rebholz CM, Grams ME, Steffen LM, et al. Diet soda consumption and risk of incident end stage renal disease. Clin J Am Soc Nephrol. 2017;12:79–86.
25. Rosinger AY, Herrick K, Wutich A, et al. Disparities in plain, tap and bottled water consumption among US adults: National Health and Nutrition Examination Survey (NHANES) 2007–2014. Public Health Nutr. 2018;21(8):1455–64.
26. Serban C, Sahebkar A, Ursoniu S, et al. Effect of sour tea (Hibiscus sabdariffa L.) on arterial hypertension: a systematic review and meta-analysis of randomized controlled trials. J Hypertens. 2015;33(6):1119–27.
27. Tobe SW, Soberman H, Kiss A, et al. The effect of alcohol and gender on ambulatory blood pressure: results from the Baseline Double Exposure study. Am J Hypertens. 2006;19(2):136–9.
28. U.S. Department of Health and Human Services and U.S. Department of Agriculture. 2015–2020 dietary guidelines for Americans. 8th ed. 2015. Available at: https://health.gov/dietaryguidelines/2015/guidelines/.
29. van Erp B, Webber WL, Stoddard P, et al. Demographic factors associated with perceptions about water safety and tap water consumption among adults in Santa Clara County, California, 2011. Prev Chronic Dis. 2014;11:130437.
30. Wong ATY, Mannix C, Grantham JJ, et al. Randomised controlled trial to determine the efficacy and safety of prescribed water intake to prevent kidney failure due to autosomal dominant polycystic kidney disease (PREVENT-ADPKD). BMJ Open. 2018;8(1):e018794.
31. Yarmolinsky J, Gon G, Edwards P. Effect of tea on blood pressure for secondary prevention of cardiovascular disease: a systematic review and meta-analysis of randomized controlled trials. Nutr Rev. 2015;73(4):236–46.

Chapter 6
Beneficial Herbs and Spices

Teresa Herrera, Amaia Iriondo-DeHond, Jaime Uribarri, and María Dolores del Castillo

Keywords Chronic diseases · Food applications · Functional food · Health claims · Herbs · Spices Therapeutic properties

Abbreviations

8-OHdG	8-hydroxy-2'-deoxyguanosine
BHT	Butylated hydroxytoluene
CAT	Catalase
CCSCH	Codex Committee on Spices and Culinary Herbs
CVDs	Cardiovascular diseases
DSLD	Dietary Supplement Label Database
EFSA	European Food Safety Authority
EU	European Union
FDA	Food and Drug Administration
$GABA_A$	γ-aminobutyric acid
GAE	Gallic acid equivalent
GMP	Good Manufacturing Practices
GPx	Glutathione peroxidase
GT	Green tea
HbA1c	Glycosylated hemoglobin
HDL	High-density lipoprotein
LDL	Low-density lipoprotein
LPO	Lipid peroxidation
MPO	Myeloperoxidase
SOD	Superoxide dismutase
T2DM	Type 2 diabetes mellitus
US	United States
VLDL	Very-low-density lipoprotein

T. Herrera · A. Iriondo-DeHond · M. D. del Castillo (✉)
Department of Bioactivity and Food Analysis, Instituto de Investigación en Ciencias de la Alimentación (CIAL) (CSIC-UAM), Madrid, Spain
e-mail: teresa.herrera@csic.es; amaia.iriondo@csic.es; mdolores.delcastillo@csic.es

J. Uribarri
Division of Nephrology, Department of Medicine, Icahn School of Medicine at Mount Sinai, New York, NY, USA
e-mail: jaime.uribarri@mountsinai.org

© Springer Nature Switzerland AG 2020
J. Uribarri, J. A. Vassalotti (eds.), *Nutrition, Fitness, and Mindfulness*, Nutrition and Health, https://doi.org/10.1007/978-3-030-30892-6_6

Key Points
- Herbs and spices have been widely used from ancient times for both food and medicinal purposes.
- Some of the health claims for herbs and spices may not have been fully demonstrated, and more regulations are needed to regulate these claims.
- Trial evidence for the use of herbs and spices has uniformly demonstrated safety, but the efficacy data are limited by small subject size and short duration trials.
- Efficacy evidence is most robust for the herb green tea and the turmeric spice.

Introduction

Diet and nutrition are important elements in the promotion and maintenance of good health [96]. The World Health Organization recommends regular consumption of fruits and vegetables, including herbs and spices, because of their potential to decrease the incidence of several chronic diseases [98]. The Codex Committee on Spices and Culinary Herbs (CCSCH) is responsible for establishing worldwide standards for spices and culinary herbs in their dried and dehydrated state in whole, ground, and cracked or crushed form and consulting, as necessary, with other international organizations in the standard development process to avoid duplication. According to CODEX [22], herbs come from plant leaves or flowering parts either fresh or dried, and spices come from other parts of the plant such as roots, stem, bark, seeds, and bulb [94]. They are also usually dried before used. In some cases, herbs and spices may come from the same plant but from different parts. Herbs and spices have been widely used for both food and medicinal purposes (Fig. 6.1). In culinary practices, they are employed as preservatives (antioxidants or antimicrobials), flavor enhancers, colorants, and ingredient substitution of salt and sugar. Efforts to assess dietary intake of spices and herbs are complicated because their use is varied and they are consumed in trace amounts together with other foods.

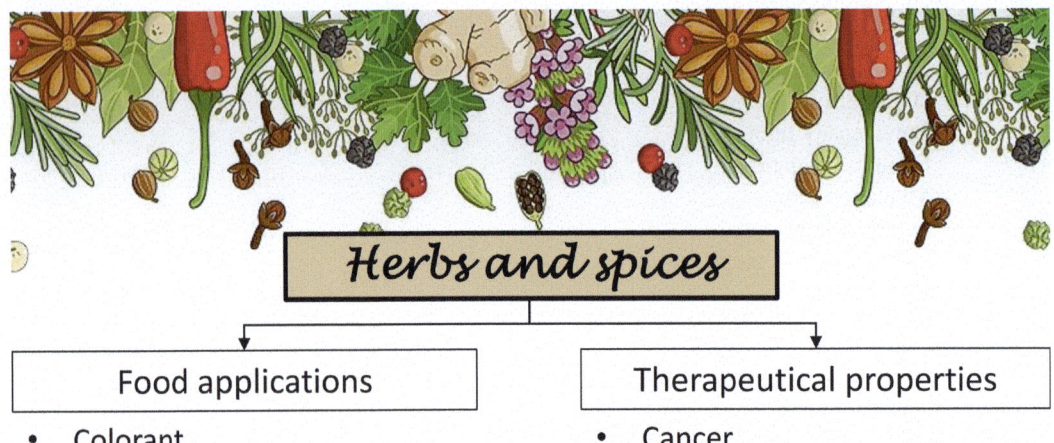

Fig. 6.1 Food applications and therapeutic uses of herbs and spices

Concentrations of herbs and spices in finished foods frequently fall within the range of 0.5–1% [49]. In medicine, they are used to reduce the risk or treat noncommunicable chronic diseases associated with oxidative stress and inflammation [76]. Herbs and spices are rich sources of bioactive phytochemicals such as phenolic compounds, carotenoids, sterols, terpenes, alkaloids, glucosinolates, and other sulfur-containing compounds, the majority of which have powerful antioxidant capacity. These phytochemicals seem to be responsible for the therapeutic effect of herbs and spices, and they provide a variety of health benefits [73] such as anticancer [49], anti-inflammatory [12], antibacterial [87], antiviral [47], and antioxidant effects [94]. The above statement accounts for the increasing interest in the health-promoting and protective properties of culinary herbs and spices.

The use of plant ingredients in food products is well established as vegetables and fruits, herbs and spices, herbal teas and infusions, beverages, and plant food supplements and has steadily increased in the last decade [17]. Health claims are increasingly appearing on our food, but the food industry is not allowed to make medicinal claims about food. In the European Union (EU), the discrepancy between the assessment of medical claims and health claims regarding the use of traditional data made the Commission of the European Food Safety Authority (EFSA) in September 2010 decide not to continue with the assessment of health claims for plant and herbal substances, the so-called "botanical" substances. The Scientific Committee decided alternatively to focus its work first on the safety assessment of botanicals and botanical preparations used as ingredients in food supplements. Since the Commission and member countries need more time to decide how to assess safety, evaluation of health claims was deferred. However, there are a few authoritative recommendations regarding the intake of herbs and spices in existing national dietary guidelines.

Research has begun to identify not only culinary uses but also other potential benefits of spices and herbs in human health according to that described in Fig. 6.2. Authorized health claims in food labeling are claims that have been reviewed by the Food and Drug Administration (FDA) or EFSA

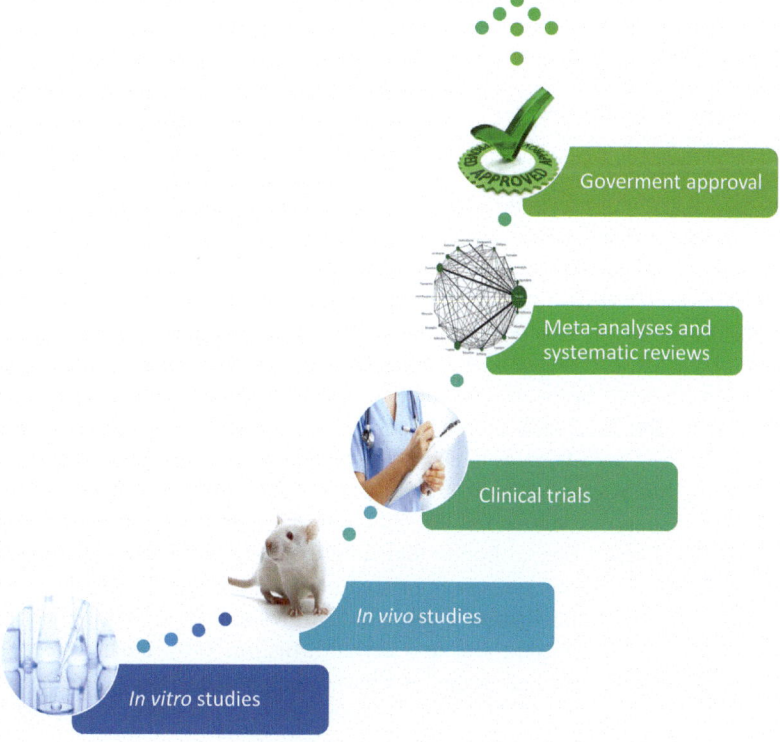

Fig. 6.2 Research steps for the approval of a health claim of herbs or spices

and are allowed on food products or dietary supplements to show that a food or food component may reduce the risk of a disease or a health-related condition. Health claims are truthful, clear, reliable, and useful to the consumer. Permitted health claims must provide scientific evidence on the relationship existing between a food category, a food or one of its constituents, and health benefit.

In the past decade, the number of clinical trials involving spices and herbs has increased sixfold [27]. Clinical trials aim to evaluate a medical intervention in human populations. Before the clinical trial, in vitro laboratory tests and in vivo studies in animals to test potential therapy's safety and efficacy are performed. After the success of a clinical trial, the FDA or EFSA may approve the drug for clinical use and continues to monitor its effects [70]. If a health claim is rejected, further research and an appeal for resubmission should be conducted. In addition, if a cause-effect relationship cannot be demonstrated, in some cases a nutrition claim can be included in the label. Nutrition claims state that a food has particular beneficial nutritional properties in terms of energy amount, nutrients, or other substances, for instance, "reduced salt" or "high in fiber." If neither a health nor a nutrition claim is approved, the herb or spice can still be used as a food ingredient or additive, but it would not have the corresponding claim indicated on its label. The declaration of the ingredient on its food label will depend on the legislation in the country in which the product will be commercialized.

In order to increase our understanding on the mechanisms of action of the potential health-promoting properties, phytochemicals, their bioactivity, and impact in human health and disease, the use of the term "phytochemomics" has been proposed as an advanced analytical approach. This multidisciplinary research field is essential for establishing a cause-effect relationship and authorizing or rejecting nutrition and health claims made on foods, herbs, and botanicals enriched in phytochemicals [15]. Therefore, the aim of the present chapter is to review the most significant findings related to the food applications and therapeutic properties of herbs and spices, focusing on the beneficial effects reported in clinical trials.

Herbs

Herbs may be defined as the dried leaves of aromatic plants used to impart flavor and odor to foods with, sometimes, the addition of color [74]. Table 6.1 shows the information regarding the food applications and therapeutic properties of the 25 most commonly consumed herbs.

Herbs can be consumed in different forms as a condiment in cooking, as beverages, or as essential oils due to their characteristic chemical composition. Beverages composed from herbs can be separated into tea or herbal infusions. The common tea is made from leaves of the plant *Camellia sinensis*, and four types are produced: white tea, green tea (both unfermented), Oolong tea (semifermented), and black tea (fermented) [42]. Nevertheless, the term herbal infusion usually refers to infusions made with other herbs, for instance, boldo, feverfew, linden, lemon verbena, lovage, senna, St. John's wort, hibiscus, and thyme. Other difference between these beverages is the temperature of water; in the case of tea, it is usually prepared with boiling water, while herbal infusions are made with hot water (without reaching boiling point). In general, herbal beverages constitute an important part of the food culture in countries where traditional medicines are widely used such as some Asian countries, although their interest and consumption have increased exponentially in nontraditional regions, such as in many European countries. Due to the potential beneficial health effects related to tea drinking, there are studies that have determined and compared the chemical composition of different teas and herbal infusions [40]. Furthermore, herbs can be used fresh, where their highly delicate aromatic character is best preserved, but the vast majority of the trade is based on dried herbs. In this sense, herbs are used as natural preservatives (antioxidant or antimicrobial), colorants, and flavorings in the food industry.

Table 6.1 Food applications and therapeutic properties of the most consumed herbs

Herbs	Scientific name	Family	Tissue	Food applications	Therapeutic properties	Registered clinical trials (n)
Basil	*Ocimum basilicum* L.	Lamiaceae	Leaves	Flavoring, antimicrobial	Cancer[a], metabolic disorders[b]	2
Bay	*Laurus nobilis*	Lauraceae	Leaves	Flavoring, colorant	Metabolic disorders[a, b]	1
Boldo	*Peumus boldus molina*	Monimiaceae	Leaves	Beverage	–	0
Borage	*Borago officinalis* L.	Boraginaceae	Leaves	Antioxidant	Cardiovascular diseases[b], metabolic disorders[b]	10
Calendula	*Calendula officinalis* L.	Asteraceae	Flowers	Flavoring, Colorant	Cardiovascular diseases[b], neurodegeneratives disorders[b]	8
Chamomile	*Matricaria chamomilla* L.	Asteraceae	Flowers	Colorant	Cardiovascular diseases[b]	23
Chervil	*Anthriscus cerefolium*	Apiaceae	Leaves	Flavoring	–	0
Chives	*Allium schoenosprasum*	Amaryllidaceae	Leaves	Flavoring	–	0
Feverfew	*Tanacetum parthenium* L.	Asteraceae	Leaves	Beverage	Migraine[b]	1
Lemon balm	*Melissa officinalis* L.	Lamiaceae	Leaves	Flavoring, Antioxidant	Neurodegeneratives disorders[a, b], metabolic disorders[a, b], cancer[b], cardiovascular diseases[b]	2
Lemon grass	*Cymbopogon citratus*	Poaceae	Leaves	Flavoring, beverage	Cancer[a]	0
Lemon verbena	*Aloysia citrodora*	Verbenaceae	Leaves	Beverage	Neuromuscular diseases[b]	1
Linden	*Tilia americana* L.	Malvaceae	Leaves	Beverage	Neurodegeneratives disorders[b]	1
Lovage	*Levisticum officinale*	Apiaceae	Leaves	Beverage	Urologic diseases[b]	1
Marjoram	*Origanum majorana*	Lamiaceae	Leaves	Flavoring, antioxidant	Respiratory disorders[b]	1
Oregano	*Origanum vulgare*	Lamiaceae	Leaves	Flavoring, antioxidant, antimicrobial	Metabolic disorders[a, b], cardiovascular diseases[b], sleep desorders[b], respiratory disorders[b]	10
Parsley	*Petroselinum crispum*	Apiaceae	Leaves	Flavoring	Metabolic disorders[b], urinary disorders[b]	5
Pennyroyal	*Mentha pulegium* L.	Lamiaceae	Leaves	Flavoring, beverage		0
Rosemary	*Rosmarinus officinalis*	Lamiaceae	Leaves	Flavoring, antioxidant, antimicrobial	Cancer[a], metobolic disorders[a, b], cardiovascular diseases[b], respiratory disorders[b], urinary disorders[b]	26

(continued)

Table 6.1 (continued)

Herbs	Scientific name	Family	Tissue	Food applications	Therapeutic properties	Registered clinical trials (n)
Sage	*Salvia officinalis*	Lamiaceae	Leaves	Flavoring, antioxidant, antimicrobial	Metabolic disorders[a, b], cardiovascular diseases[b]	10
Senna plant	*Cassia angustifolia*	Fabaceae	Leaves, flowers	Beverage		0
St. John's wort	*Hypericum perforatum* L.	Clusiaceae	Flowers	Beverage	Cancer[b], metobolic disorders[b], cardiovascular diseases[b], anxiety disroders[b]	38
Tea	*Camellia sinensis* L.	Theaceae	Leaves	Antioxidant, beverage	Metabolic disorders[a, b], cancer[a, b], cardiovascular diseases[b], neurodegenerative diseases[b], urinary disorders[b]	396
Thyme	*Thymus vulgaris*	Lamiaceae	Leaves	Antioxidant, antimicrobial	Metabolic disorders[b], respiratory disorders[b]	13

Number of clinical trials registered in ClinicalTrials.gov in November 2018
[a]Published human studies of the therapeutic properties of herbs
[b]Currently ongoing clinical trials studying therapeutic properties herbs

Food Applications

Flavorings

A culinary herb is an edible plant that when consumed in small quantities, provides substantial flavor and aroma. Fresh or dried leaves from different types of herbs (Table 6.1) can be often used as a food ingredient in many dishes such as salads, pasta, sausages, soups, marinades, meat, egg, vinegar, even in desserts, biscuits, and some alcoholic beverages such as liqueurs and wine [13, 94]. Aromatic compounds in herbs are either phenolic or terpene-based compounds. Some important chemical compounds for the flavoring potential of herbs are carvacrol, thymol (in oregano and thyme), and linalool (in sage and rosemary) [74].

Colorants

Colorants are food additives that add or restore color in foods [71]. They are used to improve the appearance of foods and to maintain their natural color during processing and storage [60]. Plant-derived pigments are divided in four groups: green chlorophylls, yellow-orange-red carotenoids, red-blue-purple anthocyanins, and red betanin. Nowadays, there is increasing interest in the development of colorants from natural sources, especially in food industries. Color and freshness are the main criteria favored essentially by the social trend toward the consumption of natural products instead of synthetic ones because of their side effects, toxicity, and allergic reactions [85]. In herbs, the principal compounds responsible for color are flavonoids which dye in colors from pale yellow (isoflavones) through deep yellow (chalcones, flavones, flavonols, aurones), orange (aurones) to reds and blues (anthocyanins) [74].

Some herbs have been described as natural colorants. Bay leaf has been employed as a food colorant due to the presence of anthocyanins [61]. The flower of *Calendula* is normally used as a food colorant to bring a yellow color due to the presence of carotenoids. The stability of these compounds during commercial shelf life is very important if the final products have to be attractive and acceptable [82]. In addition, essential oils obtained from fresh or dried flower heads of chamomile have coloring properties [28]. However, spices are more commonly used as a source of natural colorants than herbs.

Preservatives: Antioxidants

The Codex General Standard for Food Additives defines antioxidants as food additives that prolong the shelf life of foods by protecting against deterioration caused by oxidation [35]. Several studies have proven the excellent preservative capacity of different plant extracts in different food matrices. Antioxidants, even in low amounts, significantly delay or prevent oxidation reactions of susceptible ingredients such as lipids [34]. Many herbs are excellent sources of natural antioxidants, and their antioxidant properties are associated to flavones, isoflavones, flavonoids, anthocyanins, coumarins, lignans, catechins, and isocatechins [5].

Rosemary, oregano, sage, marjoram, thyme, borage, balm, and tea, among others, are natural sources of antioxidants (Table 6.1) and are considered as free radical scavengers [30]. Kumar et al. reviewed the use of herbs in meat and meat products [56]. In this sense, rosemary and oregano extracts were used in raw pork batters to identify the main antioxidant compounds and their effect on color and oxidation. Results showed that rosemary extracts had a high antioxidant activity, even more than the phenol compounds separately. These extracts also showed the highest antioxidant capacity, possibly due to the presence of high concentrations of carnosic acid and carnosol, among other compounds. However, ethanol oregano extracts containing high concentrations of phenols, mainly rosmarinic acid, efficiently prevented color deterioration [38]. Borage has also been added as an antioxidant in fermented sausages [20] and balm in meat products [21]. Sage was effective in controlling lipid and cholesterol oxidation, minimizing the prooxidant effects of salt, cooking, and storage in chicken meat [63]. Green tea extract has also been used to protect Turkish dry-fermented sausage (sucuk) against oxidation during the ripening periods, and it showed more effectiveness than butylated hydroxytoluene (BHT). Green tea extract has shown capacity to scavenge oxygen radicals and to chelate metal ions [14].

Rosemary extract (E-392) has been classified as a food additive in the EU and in the USA, and it is the only herb commercially available for its use as an antioxidant. Carnosic acid and its derivative carnosol are also used and regulated as key antioxidant compounds in rosemary extracts by the European Commission [10, 32]. Rosemary leaf extract antioxidant is prepared by solvent extraction (ethanol, acetone, or ethanol followed by hexane) or supercritical carbon dioxide extraction, which are then deodorized, decolorized, and standardized. According to the EU regulation, only deodorized rosemary extracts containing carnosic acid and carnosol are considered additives. Application areas are food matrices, including oils, animal fats, sauces, and bakery wares, and meat and fish products [10]. Rosemary is known to be a superoxide radical scavenger, lipid antioxidant, and metal chelator [30].

Preservatives: Antimicrobials

There is increasing interest in the antimicrobial properties of herbs and their products to reduce the occurrence of microbial (bacteria, yeast, fungi) contamination in foods caused by undesirable pathogenic microorganisms such as *Listeria monocytogenes*, *Escherichia coli* O157:H7, *Salmonella typhimurium*, *Bacillus cereus*, and *Staphylococcus aureus*. Antimicrobial compounds and extracts improve shelf life of foods and generally minimize pathogens and toxins produced by microorganisms. However, these compounds or their extracts act as antimicrobials in vitro, and to achieve the same effect in foods, a greater concentration is needed. Only a few food preservatives possessing antioxidant and antimicrobial properties containing essential oils from rosemary, sage, thyme, oregano, and basil are already commercially available. They have been used successfully alone or in combination with other preservation methods. Rosemary hydroalcoholic extract has been effective against *Streptococcus mitis*, *Streptococcus sanguinis*, *Streptococcus mutans*, *Streptococcus sobrinus*, and *Lactobacillus casei* standard strains, and its antimicrobial activity has been proved in all tests, except against *Streptococcus mitis* [89]. Costa et al. [23] have studied the antibacterial activity of essential oils from oregano against multiresistant bacteria (including *Escherichia coli*, *Listeria monocytogenes*, *Bacillus cereus*, *Staphylococcus aureus*, *Enterococcus faecalis*, and *Saccharomyces cerevisiae*) [23]. Essential oils from oregano, thyme, marjoram, and basil were also active against strains of *Listeria monocytogenes* and *Salmonella enteritidis* in meat products but were more active against gram-positive bacteria [90].

Therapeutic Properties

In order to overcome the difficulties of applying the pharmaceutical regulation to herbal medicinal products in a uniform manner, specific provisions for traditional herbal medicinal products have been introduced in the EU relating to medicinal products for human use (Directive 2001/83/EC). Bibliographical or expert evidence to the effect that the medicinal product in question has been in medicinal use throughout a period of at least 30 years preceding the date of the application, including at least 15 years within the community, is required for assessing the safety of the medicinal product [33]. The following section reviews all the clinical trials studying the health-promoting properties of herbs in metabolic disorders, cardiovascular diseases, cancer, and neurodegenerative disorders.

Metabolic Disorders

Several in vitro studies show antidiabetic properties of herbs, but only a few clinical trials investigating the effect of herbs on metabolic disorders have been conducted. In a parallel randomized double-blind clinical trial with 82 patients with borderline hyperlipidemia, the consumption of 3 g of lemon balm leaf powder per day for 2 months was associated with a significant decrease in mean serum LDL cholesterol [46].

The effect of bay leaf ingestion for 30 days in men and women over the age of 40 showed reduced fasting serum glucose, total cholesterol, LDL, and triglycerides compared to the placebo group [53]. Similarly, males and females over 40 years old with controlled type I diabetes consuming 3 g of bay leaf per day for 4 weeks had reduced serum total cholesterol, LDL, triglycerides and fasting glucose and had greater serum HDL compared to baseline [3]. These results suggest that bay leaf consumption may help manage hyperlipidemia.

The potential hypolipidemic effect of consuming oregano extract has also been studied in humans. Forty-five non-smoking men were divided in three groups: placebo group (mango-orange juice, $n = 15$); low phenolic group (mango-orange juice enriched with oregano extract, in which daily dosage of total phenolic compounds from the extract was 300 mg gallic acid equivalent (GAE), $n = 15$); and high phenolic group (mango-orange juice enriched with oregano extract, in which daily dosage of total phenolic compounds from the extract was 600 mg GAE, $n = 15$). Results after 90 min of juice ingestion showed a significant reduction in LDL oxidation in the low phenolic group [72].

Sage extract also has beneficial effects on blood lipid profile in humans. In a randomized double-blind placebo-controlled clinical study, newly diagnosed primary hyperlipidemia patients consumed a capsule containing 500 mg of sage extract every 8 hours for 2 months. At the end of the study, subjects had lower serum total cholesterol, triglycerides, LDL, and VLDL and increased HDL compared to both baseline and placebo groups [54]. In another study on healthy female subjects between the ages of 40 and 50, consumption of sage aqueous infusion twice a day for 2 weeks was associated with lower plasma LDL, total cholesterol, and greater plasma HDL [83]. In a double-blind, placebo-controlled trial, 56 obese, hypertensive subjects were randomized to receive a daily supplement of 1 capsule that contained either 379 mg of green tea extract or a matching placebo, for 3 months. Results showed that a daily supplementation with 379 mg of green tea extract favorably influences blood pressure, insulin resistance, inflammation, oxidative stress, and lipid profile in patients with obesity-related hypertension [11].

Cardiovascular Diseases

Herbs have been used in patients with congestive heart failure, systolic hypertension, angina pectoris, atherosclerosis, cerebral insufficiency, venous insufficiency, and arrhythmia [81]. A study regarding the effect of lemon balm infusion drunk twice a day for 30 days in 55 radiology staff showed that the activity of superoxide dismutase (SOD), catalase (CAT), and guttation peroxidase (GPx) increased significantly, but the level of lipid peroxidation (LPO), 8-hydroxy-2'-deoxyguanosine (8-OHdG), and the activity of myeloperoxidase (MPO) significantly decreased. Hence, it decreases radiation-induced oxidative stress biomarkers, and since oxidative stress is related to cardiovascular diseases (CVDs), lemon balm may have potential in the prevention or treatment of these diseases [103]. The antioxidant potential of lemon balm infusion may be due to its phenolic compounds, especially phenolic acids (rosmarinic acid, gallic acid, and ferulic acid), flavonoids (luteolin 7-O-glucoside, quercetin 3-rutinoside, and quercetin 3-O galactoside), and their antioxidant capacity [55]. In another clinical trial, participants with hypercholesterolemia who consumed 140 mg of lemon grass oil daily experienced a significant drop in mean cholesterol concentrations up to 38 mg/dL, but this trial had no control group [29]. Hawthorn is an herb used for improving blood flow. The leaves, fruit, and flowers of hawthorn are widely used in Europe for improving the pumping capacity of the heart and for treating angina. The major activity of hawthorn is thought to be mediated by various flavonoids. Patients with congestive heart failure (NY Heart Association class II) who were given 600 mg/day of a hawthorn extract had significantly lower blood pressure, heart rates, and less shortness of breath when exercising compared with subjects not receiving hawthorn [86]. Studies have suggested that green tea may lower blood cholesterol concentrations and blood pressure and may be effective for the treatment of hypertension and hyperlipidemia in both patients on medications and healthy subjects [68]. A double-blind, randomized, placebo-controlled, parallel-group trial studied the effect of daily intake of a capsule containing 75 mg theaflavin, 150 mg of green tea catechins, and 150 mg of other tea polyphenols for 12 weeks on subjects with mild-to-moderate hypercholesterolemia already consuming a low-fat diet. Results showed that the extract decreased mean serum total cholesterol and LDL by 11.3% and 16.4%, respectively, in treated volunteers compared to the placebo group [64]. Similar results were recently described in a randomized, double-blind trial with 115 women with central obesity. A high-dose of green tea extract with epigallocatechin gallate (EGCG) at a daily dosage of 856.8 mg resulted in significant weight loss, reduced waist circumference, and a consistent decrease in total cholesterol and LDL plasma levels without any side effects [18].

Hibiscus tea has demonstrated antihypertensive properties in several clinical trials studies. Anthocyanin compounds (delphinidin-3-sambubioside and cyanidin-3-sambubioside) were involved in these effects [41]. Previous studies conducted in hypertensive patients used a higher dose of hibiscus tea to compare its effects with that of either black tea, for instance, in a sequential randomized controlled clinical trial, 60 diabetic patients with mild hypertension were randomly allocated in 2 groups, hibiscus tea and black tea. In each group, they consumed their corresponding infusion two times per day for one month. Results showed a significant decrease from 134.4 to 112.7 mm Hg for hibiscus tea consumers group, and so consuming hibiscus tea had positive effects on blood pressure in type 2 diabetic (T2DM) patients with mild hypertension [69]. In addition, the first reported placebo-controlled clinical trial in order to examine the effect of hibiscus tea on blood pressure was described by McKey et al. [66]. In a randomized study, double-blind, placebo-controlled clinical trial, 65 pre- and mildly hypertensive adults were distributed in 2 groups, hibiscus tea and placebo group. For 6 weeks, participants consumed daily a bag of hibiscus tea or placebo (which contain artificial hibiscus flavor). Results showed at 6 weeks of treatment, hibiscus tea lowered systolic (-7.2 ± 11.4 mm Hg) and diastolic (-3.1 ± 7.0 mm Hg) blood pressure compared with placebo, although in the last case this change did not differ from placebo group. Results suggest daily consumption of hibiscus tea, in an amount readily incorporated into the diet, lowers blood pressure in pre- and mildly hypertensive adults and may be an effective component of the dietary changes recommended for people with these conditions [66].

Chamomile, rosemary, sage, and thyme have high flavonoid contents, and therefore they have an important role in dietary flavonoid intake, but there is little evidence to support a direct cardiovascular health benefit from these herbs apart from some epidemiological studies [94].

Cancer

Worldwide, more than 3000 plants have been reported to have anticancer properties. There are several in vitro studies and rodent in vivo studies suggesting that certain herbs may have a chemopreventive effect against the early initiating stages of cancer. Herbs containing known anticarcinogenic effects in animal models of cancer include basil, rosemary, mint, and lemon grass [94]. Nevertheless, limited data are available concerning the effectiveness of herbal extracts as anticarcinogenic agents in humans [4]. Experimentally, several medicinal plants and herbal ingredients have been reported to have anticancer effects. Herbs may be able to inhibit carcinogen bioactivation, decrease free radical formation, suppress cell division, and promote apoptosis in cancerous cells [50].

Green tea is the only herb that has shown clinical evidence for supporting its anticancer effects [43]. A double-blind placebo-controlled study showed that green tea catechins were safe and effective for treating premalignant prostate cancer [8]. In contrast, other studies showed that green tea has minimal clinical activity against prostate cancer [19, 48]. Catechins (phenolic compounds) have been identified as the main active constituents responsible for most of the biological properties of green tea.

Bioactive compounds present in herbs with cancer-preventive properties include terpenes (basil, marjoram, mint, rosemary, oregano, sage, and thyme), polyphenols, mainly flavonoids compounds (basil, marjoram, mint, rosemary, oregano, sage, parsley and thyme), and epigallocatechin gallate and other catechins (green tea) [7, 44, 100, 101].

Neurodegenerative Disorders

Lemon balm has been used traditionally for the treatment of dementia and amnesia, two disorders that are closely associated with Alzheimer's disease. A clinical trial of 42 patients during 16 weeks demonstrated reduction of agitation and improvement in cognitive and behavioral functions after administration of hydroalcoholic extract of lemon balm (60 drops/day) standardized to contain 500 μg citral/mL (terpenoid compound) [1]. Based on limited data, a proposed mechanism for the memory-enhancing effects of lemon balm may be attributed to the inhibition of acetylcholinesterase activity, the stimulation of acetylcholine (nicotinic and muscarinic receptors), and γ-aminobutyric acid (GABA$_A$) receptors, as well as the inhibition of matrix metalloproteinase-2 (MMP-2).

Spices

According to the FDA, spices are defined as "aromatic vegetable substances, in the whole, broken, or ground form, whose significant function in food is seasoning rather than nutrition." Table 6.2 shows the food applications and therapeutic properties of the most consumed spices.

Table 6.2 Food applications and therapeutic properties of the most consumed spices

Spices	Scientific name	Family	Tissue	Food applications	Therapeutical properties	Registered clinical trials (n)
Anise	*Pimpinella anisum*	Apiaceae	Fruit	Flavoring	Metabolic disorders[a, b]	6
Caraway	*Carum carvi*	Apiaceae	Fruit	Antioxidant	Metabolic disorders[b], back pain[b]	12
Cardamom	*Elettaria cardamomum*	Zingiberaceae	Fruit	Flavoring, antioxidant	Cancer[b], cardiovascular disease[b]	5
Celery	*Apium graveolens*	Apiaceae	Fruit	Flavoring	Cardiovascular disease[b], neurodegenerative disorders[b]	10
Cinnamon	*Cinnamomum zeylanicum*	Lauraceae	Bark	Flavoring, antioxidant, antimicrobial	Cardiovascular disease[a, b], metabolic disorders[a, b], neurodegenerative disorders[b], dental caries[b]	58
Cloves	*Eugenia aromaticum*	Myrtaceae	Flower bud	Flavoring, antioxidant, antimicrobial	Cardiovascular disease[a], metabolic disorders[a], cancer[b], dental caries[b]	15
Coriander	*Coriandrum sativum*	Apiaceae	Fruit	Flavoring, antioxidant	Cardiovascular disease[b], metabolic disorders[a]	7
Cumin	*Cuminum cyminum*	Apiaceae	Fruit	Flavoring, antioxidant, antimicrobial	Metabolic disorders[a, b], fungal infection[b]	20
Dill	*Anethum graveolens*	Apiaceae	Fruit	Flavoring	Cancer[b], kidney injury[b]	16
Fennel	*Foeniculum vulgare*	Apiaceae	Fruit	Flavoring, antioxidant	Chronic constipation[b]	4
Fenugreek	*Trigonella foenum-graecum*	Fabaceae	Fruit	Flavoring	Metabolic disorders[a, b], hypogonadism[b]	19
Garlic	*Allium sativum*	Liliaceae	Bulb	Flavoring	Cancer[a, b], cardiovascular disease[a, b], metabolic disorders[a, b]	54
Ginger	*Zingiber officinale*	Zingiberaceae	Rhizome	Flavoring, antioxidant	Cardiovascular disease[a], metabolic disorders[a, b], anxiety[b], psoriasis[b]	144
Horseradish	*Armoracia lapathifolia*	Brassicaceae	Root	Flavoring	Metabolic disorders[b]	10

(continued)

Table 6.2 (continued)

Spices	Scientific name	Family	Tissue	Food applications	Therapeutical properties	Registered clinical trials (n)
Mustard seed	*Brassica nigra, Brassica juncea, Brassica hirta*	Brassicaceae	Seed	Flavoring, antimicrobial	Cancer[b], metabolic disorders[b]	5
Nutmeg	*Myristica fragrans*	Myristicaceae	Kernel of the seed	Flavoring, antioxidant	–	0
Onion	*Allium cepa*	Liliaceae	Bulb	Flavoring	Cardiovascular disease[b], metabolic disorders[a, b]	29
Paprika	*Capsicum annum*	Solanaceae	Fruit	Flavoring, colorant	Cardiovascular disease[a], headache[b]	2
Pepper, black/white	*Piper nigrum*	Piperaceae	Fruit	Flavoring, antioxidant	Cardiovascular disease[a, b], metabolic disorders[b]	119
Pepper, red	*Capsicum frutescens*	Piperaceae	Fruit	Flavoring	Metabolic disorders[b], neurodegenerative disorders[b]	41
Saffron	*Crocus sativus*	Iridaceae	Stigma	Colorant	Metabolic disorders[b], macular degeneration[b]	4
Star anise	*Illicium verum*	Illiciaceae	Fruit	Antioxidant	–	0
Turmeric	*Curcuma longa*	Zingiberaceae	Rhizome	Colorant, antimicrobial	Cancer[a, b], cardiovascular disease[a, b], neurodegenerative disorders[a, b], metabolic disorders[a, b] skin inflammation[b], osteoarthritis[b]	117
Vanilla	*Vanilla tahitensis*	Orchidaceae	Fruit	Flavoring	Metabolic disorders[b], osteoporosis[b]	57

Number of clinical trials registered in ClinicalTrials.gov in November 2018
[a]Published human studies of the therapeutic properties of spices
[b]Currently ongoing clinical trials studying therapeutic properties spices

Food Applications

Flavorings

Flavoring food is one of the most common uses of spices. There is a conventional classification of spices based on the degree of taste [74]:

- Hot spices: Black, red, and white pepper, ginger, and mustard
- Mild spices: Paprika and coriander
- Aromatic spices: Allspice, cardamom, celery, cinnamon, clove, cumin, dill, fennel, fenugreek, onion, garlic, and nutmeg

The most important flavor compounds found in culinary spices are eugenol (allspice, cinnamon, and clove), piperine (black pepper), gingerol (ginger), myristicin (nutmeg), and turmerone (turmeric) [74].

Colorants

Paprika (E160c) and curcumin (E100) are the two natural colorants obtained from spices allowed as food additives in the EU and in the USA [31, 58]. Paprika extract (E160c) is a natural dark red dye obtained by solvent extraction from the ground fruit pods, with or without seeds, of *Capsicum annuum*, and it contains capsanthin and capsorubin as the principle coloring compounds [32]. In both the EU and the USA, paprika extract (E 160c) is permitted *quantum satis*, which means that no maximum numerical level is specified and it shall be used in accordance with good manufacturing practice, at a level not higher than is necessary to achieve the intended purpose and provided the consumer is not misled [31]. However, for meat preparations and processed meat, there is an established limit by the European Commission of 10 mg/kg product [58]. Curcumin (E100) is obtained by solvent extraction of turmeric, the ground rhizomes of *Curcuma longa*. Curcumin, which represents about 2–8% of most turmeric preparations, gives turmeric its distinct color and flavor. A concentrated curcumin powder is obtained by crystallization. The orange-yellow powder consists essentially of curcumins, the coloring principle (1,7-bis(4-hydroxy-3-methoxyphenyl)hepta-1,6-dien-3,5-dione), and its two desmethoxy derivatives in varying proportions [32]. The EU has established an acceptable daily intake of curcumin of 3 mg/kg; however, the USA limits the amount of turmeric used in foods by the good manufacturing practices (GMP) where manufacturers use only the amount of an additive necessary to achieve the desired result [58].

Preservatives: Antioxidants

Different spices have been studied to preserve different food matrixes. For instance, coriander has been proven to be efficient as an antioxidant in the control of lipid oxidation in white hake fish meatballs during frozen storage [84]. Dwivedi et al. [26] have studied Chinese five-spice ingredients composed of cinnamon, cloves, fennel, pepper, and star anise alone and in combination in cooked ground beef. Results showed that all spices and blends reduced rancid odor/flavor in cooked ground beef. However, the spices did not mask rancid off-flavors but had antioxidant effects [26]. Cooked ground beef has also been used as a food matrix to study the antioxidant effect and sensory attributes of individual ingredients (black pepper, caraway, cardamom, chili powder, cinnamon, cloves, coriander, cumin, fennel, ginger, nutmeg, salt, star anise) of an Indian spice blend (garam masala). All individual spices of garam masala were effective in maintaining low rancidity levels in cooked beef during refrigeration in addition to significant reduction of perception of rancid odor and rancid flavor [97]. The antioxidant properties of spices are due to their chemical composition, especially to phenolic compounds. In fact, there is a linear relationship between the phenolic and flavonoid content and the antioxidant capacity of a spice [99]. Most of the antioxidants from spices act by reacting with free radicals created during the initiation stage of autoxidation or by forming complexes with metal ions [30].

Preservatives: Antimicrobials

The use of spices as preservatives has been assessed in multiple foods such as meat, fish, dairy products, vegetables, rice, fruit, and animal food. Spices can exert antimicrobial activity in two ways: by preventing the growth of spoilage microorganisms (food preservation) and by inhibiting the growth of those pathogenic (food safety) [36]. Many extracts obtained from spices possess antimicrobial activity against a wide range of bacteria, yeast, molds, and viruses due to the presence of high levels of phenolic compounds. Cumin and clove essential oils inhibited the growth of total bacteria on meat samples for 15 days at 2 °C [39]. In addition, treatment of raw chicken meat with extracts of clove, oregano, cinnamon, and black mustard was effective against microbial growth [78]. The addition of turmeric extract (1.5%) to whole gutted rainbow trout can also retard microbial growth, delay the chemical changes, maintain sensory attributes (texture, odor, color, and overall acceptance), and extend the shelf life during refrigerated storage [75]. Although the antimicrobial effects of spices and their derivatives have been tested against a wide range of microorganisms over the years, their mode of action is still not completely understood. In fact, spices and their essential oils can contain many different bioactive compounds present in variable amounts.

Bioactive compounds of spices such as terpenes, terpenoids (thymol and carvacrol), and phenylpropenes (eugenol and cinnamaldehyde) are responsible for their antimicrobial activity. Terpenes possess lesser antimicrobial activity than the other compounds. Terpenoids exert their antimicrobial activity by their functional groups (hydroxyl groups and delocalized electrons) affecting the permeability or disrupting important energy-generating processes leading to cell death. The antimicrobial activity of eugenol is performed at membrane and protein level and reacts and cross-links with DNA and proteins. Overall, antimicrobial activity of spices is a synergistic effect of the combination of all the bioactive compounds present in them [36]. The main limitation of spices as antimicrobial agents is the need of high amounts of natural compounds that comprise the organoleptic profile of foods. Therefore, combinations of spices or their pure natural compounds and additional technologies represent a promising alternative to reduce the amount of spices used and solve this problem.

Therapeutic Properties

Numerous studies have shown that nutraceuticals derived from spices such as clove, coriander, garlic, ginger, onion, pepper, and turmeric prevent various chronic diseases by targeting inflammatory pathways [57]. Nutraceuticals are natural, bioactive chemical compounds that have health-promoting, disease-preventing, or general medicinal properties [16].

A recent cross-sectional study carried out in adults living in Midwestern USA concluded that the majority of participants currently used one or more spices on a daily basis but were unaware of their potential health benefits [45]. This study also concluded that most participants shared interest in learning about the health benefits of spices. Therefore, since limited clinical studies have examined the therapeutic effects of spice-derived nutraceuticals in humans, the aim of this section is to gather and review all the beneficial effects of spices on human health supported by clinical studies. Table 6.2 shows the most commonly used spices according to the FDA, their proved health-promoting properties (published clinical trials and currently on going), and the number of registered clinical trials [95].

Metabolic Disorders

Many spices have antioxidant and anti-inflammatory properties and could also have potential therapeutic properties in diabetes [2]. Only few spices have demonstrated to reduce the glycemic response in animals and human clinical trials. Cumin, cinnamon, garlic, ginger, onion, and turmeric have shown antidiabetic properties in human studies [6]. The antidiabetic properties of these spices involve improving insulin sensitivity, stimulating insulin secretion, decreasing carbohydrate absorption, increasing peripheral glucose uptake, inhibiting hepatic glycogenolysis, exerting antioxidant effects, inhibiting hepatic glycogenolysis, and potentiating endogenous incretins [6].

Cinnamon has the potential to lower blood glucose in animal models and humans. To date, several randomized controlled studies have studied the effect of cinnamon on T2DM in adults. These studies have evaluated the effect of cinnamon on glycosylated hemoglobin, fasting plasma glucose, total cholesterol, LDL cholesterol, and triglycerides [67]. However, the short duration of studies is flawed; design has made the available evidence difficult to interpret.

The first randomized double-blind placebo-controlled clinical trial to evaluate the effects of cinnamon on individuals with T2DM was conducted in 2003. Sixty diabetic patients (30 men and 30 women) received either placebo or 3 different doses of cinnamon powder (1, 3, 6 g/day, respectively) for 40 days. Cinnamon was found to reduce fasting blood glucose, triglycerides, LDL cholesterol, and total cholesterol levels [52]. Other clinical study has reported that cinnamon decreased glycosylated hemoglobin (HbA1c) in 109 patients with T2DM [24].

Fenugreek seeds have been found to diminish hyperglycemia in normal individuals and those with diabetes in several different clinical trials carried out in the past few years [91]. Fasting blood glucose, 24-h urinary sugar excretion, serum cholesterol, and triglyceride levels were significantly reduced in diabetic patients. Clinical symptoms like polyuria, polyphagia, and polydipsia were also improved. These effects of fenugreek seeds seem to be due to the gum fiber present in them. Inclusion of fenugreek in amounts of 25–50 g in the daily diet can be an effective supportive therapy in the management of diabetes. Fenugreek is reported to be absolutely safe for consumption based on a long-term animal study [91].

Ginger supplementation might be considered as a beneficial natural remedy for regulating triglycerides and LDL cholesterol. The lowering effect of ≤ 2 g/day ginger was greater on triglycerides and total cholesterol [77]. Ginger is a safe, non-expensive, and available traditional remedy with negligible side effects at usual dosages. However, further long-term studies are needed to confirm these results.

Turmeric is another important spice claimed to possess beneficial hypoglycemic effects and to improve glucose tolerance in a limited number of clinical studies. Moreover, it has been demonstrated that turmeric had a synergistic effect with metformin in T2DM in lowering fasting blood glucose. When T2DM patients received turmeric supplementation with metformin, both fasting blood glucose and HbA1c levels were significantly reduced as compared to controls treated metformin alone [62].

Cumin supplementation has been found to be more effective than glibenclamide in the treatment of T2DM. The antihyperglycemic effect of cumin may be due to the protection of surviving pancreatic β-cells, the increase in insulin secretion, and glycogen storage [9].

The antidiabetic, hypolipidemic, and antioxidant properties of coriander and anise have been assessed in vivo by the administration of coriander seed powder (5 g/day) to diabetic patients for 60 days. It was found that coriander and anise decreased blood sugar, decreased serum lipids and lipoproteins, improved HDL, and controlled lipid peroxidation [80].

Clove extracts also improved the function of insulin and lower glucose, total cholesterol, LDL, and triglycerides in people with diabetes. Thirty-six people with T2DM were given capsules containing 0, 1, 2, or 3 g of cloves per day for 30 days followed by a 10-day washout period. At the end of the 30 days, the diabetic patients who had been taking some level of clove supplementation showed a decrease in serum glucose, triglycerides, serum total cholesterol, and LDL [51].

Cardiovascular Diseases

Although very few clinical studies regarding the use of spices and cardiovascular diseases have been performed, Harvard Medical School recommends the use of spices instead of salt and butter in order to prevent high blood pressure and heart disease. A salty diet may raise blood pressure, increasing the risk of heart attack and stroke. It has been found that people who enjoy spicy foods (especially chili peppers) eat less salt and have lower blood pressure than people who prefer less spicy foods. These findings suggest that gradually adding small amounts of spice to your food may help reduce use of salt and, therefore, lower blood pressure [37].

A randomized crossover study has shown that the post meal triglyceride response can be reduced by the inclusion of a culinary spice blend (black pepper, cinnamon, cloves, garlic, ginger, oregano, paprika, rosemary, and turmeric) in a high-fat meal by the inhibition of enzymes responsible for lipid digestion in the small intestine [65]. Post-meal triglycerides are an important indicator of cardiovascular risk and a potential target for therapeutic intervention. These data suggest that the regular inclusion of spices in the diet may help attenuate the effect of large fat loads on cardiovascular risk.

Cancer

There are several spices such as turmeric, garlic, ginger, and black cumin with proven anticarcinogenic effects in animal models of cancer. These spices have shown chemopreventive effects against different types of cancers – skin, stomach, pancreas, liver, colon, and oral – in experimental models. Zheng et al. [104] have reviewed recent studies on some spices for the prevention and treatment of cancers paying special attention to bioactive components and mechanisms of action. These authors suggest the potential therapeutic strategy of using spices to prevent or treat cancers [104]. However, cancer-preventive effects have not been conclusively proven in humans. Bioactive compounds composing these spices reduce oxidative stress inhibit cell division, promote apoptosis in cancerous cells, and regulate inflammation contributing to cancer prevention [92].

One of the most studied spices for the application in cancer treatment is turmeric. Curcumin obtained from turmeric shows antioxidant, anti-inflammatory, and antitumor properties demonstrated in preclinical and clinical trials. Antitumor activity is proposed to be due to the activation of apoptosis and inhibition of inflammation, angiogenesis, and metastasis in the tumor microenvironment [25]. There are numerous clinical trials being carried out to allow corroborating the in vitro antitumor activity of curcumin and its effectiveness as a therapeutic agent in different types of tumors such as: colon, gastric, cervical, endometrial, breast, pancreatic, prostate, lung, and lymphoma [25]. Consequently, numerous patents have been developed in connection with the administration and use of curcumin against different types of cancer.

Garlic has also been studied in a few clinical trials to examine its potential anticancer effects. Different randomized clinical trials have evaluated the effect of garlic intake on gastric cancer risk. In one study, patients who received garlic extract had a reduction of risk for all tumors combined by 33% and the risk for stomach cancer by 52% in comparison with the placebo group [59]. In contrast, findings from another randomized trial involving individuals with precancerous stomach lesions found that garlic supplementation (800 mg garlic extract plus 4 mg steam-distilled garlic oil daily) did not improve the prevalence of precancerous gastric lesions or reduced the incidence of gastric cancer [102]. A randomized study in Japan compared the effects of daily high-dose and low-dose intakes of garlic extract on individuals with colorectal adenomas, and after 12 months, 67% of the low-intake group developed new adenomas compared with 47% in the high-intake group [93]. Diallyl disulfide and diallyl trisulfide may be the main contributors of the anticancer action of garlic. Garlic compounds may work by multiple mechanisms, including mutagenesis inhibition, induction of phase II detoxification enzymes, inhibition of DNA adduct formation, affecting the intrinsic pathway for apoptotic cell death, and cell cycle machinery that may cumulatively contribute to their anticancer activities [92]. Future research is needed in the clinical assessment of these compounds for the prevention or treatment of cancers in humans.

Neurodegenerative Disorders

Recently, numerous spices, medicinal plants, fruits, and vegetables possessing high antioxidant activity have received much attention as food supplements to slow the loss of cognitive function with aging and to protect against Alzheimer's disease. A 6-month trial examined curcumin's safety and its effects on biochemical and cognitive measures on Alzheimer's disease. Thirty-three patients were randomly assigned to receive 1–4 g of curcumin as capsule or powder. A rise of amyloid β_{40} levels in serum and a slower disease progression was observed in patients treated with curcumin. This finding indicated that curcumin disaggregates amyloid β_{40} deposits in the brain, releasing amyloid β_{40} for circulation and disposal. In addition, this study found no side effects from curcumin [88]. Not all studies have demonstrated benefits, although a 12-month randomized, placebo-controlled, double-blind study of 1500 mg/d BiocurcumaxTM showed that most of the benefit was attributed to a significant decline in the placebo arm at 6 months as assessed by the Montreal Cognitive Assessment [79].

Most of the literature about nutraceuticals derived from spices discusses only curcumin, given that this spice may have potential against neurodegenerative diseases, owing to its strong anti-inflammatory and antioxidant properties. However, the potential of many other spices needs also to be explored. Therefore, more preclinical and clinical studies are urgently needed to fully explore the potential of spice-derived nutraceuticals as neuroprotective agents.

Conclusion

Herbs and spices have been traditionally used in culinary practices and in traditional medicine for centuries. Among all the herbs reviewed in this chapter, green tea is the one with the most compelling evidence for health benefits in humans. Turmeric is the spice with more scientific evidence from human studies with potential health-promoting properties in cancer, cardiovascular diseases, neurodegenerative disorders, and metabolic disorders. Despite the numerous studies regarding the health properties of green tea and turmeric, they still have not received neither the FDA nor the EFSA approval to prevent or treat disease. Daily intake of herbs and spices has the potential to contribute to a better health. However, there is a need for an increase in research in the mechanism of action ("phytochemomics") and clinical trials, to improve the evidence-based regarding the efficacy of most herbs and spices.

Acknowledgments The SUSCOFFEE (AGL 2014-57239-R) and ALIBIRD-CM (S2013/ABI-2728) projects funded this work. A. Iriondo-DeHond is a fellow of the FPI predoctoral program of MINECO (BES-2015-072191).

References

1. Akhondzadeh S, et al. *Melissa officinalis* extract in the treatment of patients with mild to moderate Alzheimer's disease: a double blind, randomised, placebo controlled trial. J Neurol Neurosurg Psychiatry. 2003;74(7):863–6. https://doi.org/10.1136/JNNP.74.7.863.
2. Al-Waili N, et al. Natural antioxidants in the treatment and prevention of diabetic nephropathy; a potential approach that warrants clinical trials. Redox Rep. 2017;22(3):99–118. https://doi.org/10.1080/13510002.2017.12 97885.
3. Aljamal A. Effects of bay leaves on blood glucose and lipid profiles on the patients with type 1 diabetes. World Acad Sci Eng Technol. 2010;4(9):409–12.
4. Alonso-Castro AJ, et al. Mexican medicinal plants used for cancer treatment: pharmacological, phytochemical and ethnobotanical studies. J Ethnopharmacol. 2011;133(3):945–72. https://doi.org/10.1016/J.JEP.2010.11.055.
5. Aqil F, Ahmad I, Mehmood Z. Antioxidant and free radical scavenging properties of twelve traditionally used Indian medicinal plants. Turk J Biol. 2006;30(3):177–83. https://doi.org/10.1207/S15326950DP3102_03.
6. Beidokhti MN, Jäger AK. Review of antidiabetic fruits, vegetables, beverages, oils and spices commonly consumed in the diet. J Ethnopharmacol. 2017;201:26–41. https://doi.org/10.1016/j.jep.2017.02.031.
7. Berrington D, Lall N. Anticancer activity of certain herbs and spices on the cervical epithelial carcinoma (HeLa) cell line. Evid Based Complement Alternat Med. 2012;2012:11. https://doi.org/10.1155/2012/564927.
8. Bettuzzi S, et al. Chemoprevention of human prostate cancer by oral administration of green tea catechins in volunteers with high-grade prostate intraepithelial neoplasia: a preliminary report from a one-year proof-of-principle study. Cancer Res. 2006;66(2):1234–40. https://doi.org/10.1158/0008-5472.CAN-05-1145.

9. Bi X, Lim J, Henry CJ. Spices in the management of diabetes mellitus. Food Chem. 2017;217:281–93. https://doi. org/10.1016/j.foodchem.2016.08.111.

10. Birtić S, et al. Carnosic acid. Phytochemistry. 2015;115:9–19. https://doi.org/10.1016/J.PHYTOCHEM.2014.12.026.

11. Bogdanski P, et al. Green tea extract reduces blood pressure, inflammatory biomarkers, and oxidative stress and improves parameters associated with insulin resistance in obese, hypertensive patients. Nutr Res. 2012;32(6):421–7. https://doi.org/10.1016/j.nutres.2012.05.007.

12. Bower A, Marquez S, de Mejia EG. The health benefits of selected culinary herbs and spices found in the traditional mediterranean diet. Crit Rev Food Sci Nutr. 2016;56(16):2728–46. https://doi.org/10.1080/10408398.2013.805713.

13. Bown D. New encyclopedia of herbs and their uses: the definitive guide to the identification, cultivation and uses of herbs. New York: Dorling Ki; 2001.

14. Bozkurt H. Utilization of natural antioxidants: green tea extract and Thymbra spicata oil in Turkish dry-fermented sausage. Meat Sci. 2006;73(3):442–50. https://doi.org/10.1016/J.MEATSCI.2006.01.005.

15. del Castillo MD, et al. Phytochemomics and other omics for permitting health claims made on foods. Food Res Int. 2013;54(1):1237–49. https://doi.org/10.1016/j.foodres.2013.05.014.

16. del Castillo MD, Iriondo-DeHond A, Martirosyan DM. Are functional foods essential for sustainable health? Ann Nutr Food Sci. 2018;2(1):1015.

17. CBI. Through what channels can you get spices and herbs onto the European market? Centre for the promotion of imports from developing countries. 2018.

18. Chen IJ, et al. Therapeutic effect of high-dose green tea extract on weight reduction: a randomized, double-blind, placebo-controlled clinical trial. Clin Nutr. 2016;35(3):592–9. https://doi.org/10.1016/j.clnu.2015.05.003.

19. Choan E, et al. A prospective clinical trial of green tea for hormone refractory prostate cancer: an evaluation of the complementary/alternative therapy approach. Urol Oncol. 2005;23(2):108–13. https://doi.org/10.1016/j. urolonc.2004.10.008.

20. Ciriano MG, et al. Use of natural antioxidants from lyophilized water extracts of *Borago officinalis* in dry fermented sausages enriched in ω-3 PUFA. Meat Sci. 2009;83(2):271–7. https://doi.org/10.1016/J. MEATSCI.2009.05.009.

21. de Ciriano MG-I, et al. Effect of lyophilized water extracts of *Melissa officinalis* on the stability of algae and linseed oil-in-water emulsion to be used as a functional ingredient in meat products. Meat Sci. 2010;85(2):373–7. https://doi.org/10.1016/j.meatsci.2010.01.007.

22. Food and Agriculture Organization of the United Nations (FAO) Revision of The Classification of Food and Feed: Class A: Primary Food Commodities of Plant Origin Type 05: Herbs and Spices (Codex (Cx/Pr 18/50/7)); China. 2017;1–23.

23. Costa A, et al. Antibacterial activity of the essential oil of *Origanum vulgare* L.(Lamiaceae) against bacterial mul-tiresistant strains isolated from nosocomial patients. Rev Bras. 2009;19(1B):236–41.

24. Crawford P. Effectiveness of cinnamon for lowering hemoglobin A1C in patients with type 2 diabetes: a random-ized, controlled trial. J Am Board Fam Med. 2009;22(5):507–12. https://doi.org/10.3122/jabfm.2009.05.080093.

25. Doello K, et al. Latest in vitro and in vivo assay, clinical trials and patents in cancer treatment using curcumin: a literature review. Nutr Cancer. 2018;70(4):569–78. https://doi.org/10.1080/01635581.2018.1464347.

26. Dwivedi S, Vasavada MN, Cornforth D. Evaluation of antioxidant effects and sensory attributes of Chinese 5-spice ingredients in cooked ground beef. J Food Sci. 2006;71(1):C12–7. https://doi.org/10.1111/j.1365-2621.2006. tb12381.x.

27. Dwyer JT. The potential of spices and herbs to improve the health of the public through the combination of food science and nutrition. Nutr Today. 2014;49:S3–4. https://doi.org/10.1097/01.NT.0000453843.06840.2d.

28. El-Agbar ZA, et al. Comparative antioxidant activity of some edible plants. Turk J Biol. 2007;32:193–6.

29. Elson CE, et al. Impact of lemongrass oil, an essential oil, on serum cholesterol. Lipids. 1989;24(8):677–9. https:// doi.org/10.1007/BF02535203.

30. Embuscado ME. Spices and herbs: natural sources of antioxidants – a mini review. J Funct Foods. 2015;18:811–9. https://doi.org/10.1016/j.jff.2015.03.005.

31. European Commission. Regulation (Ec) No 1333/2008 of the European Parliament and of the Council of 16 December 2008 on food additives. Off J Eur Communities. 2008:1–342. https://doi.org/2004R0726-v.7. of 05.06.2013.

32. European Commission. Annex II Commission Regulation (EU) No 231/2012 of 9 March 2012 laying down specifications for food additives listed in Annexes II and III to Regulation (EC) No 1333/2008 of the European Parliament and of the Council. Off J Eur Union. 2012:1–295. https://doi.org/10.1201/9781315152752.

33. European Parliament. DIRECTIVE 2001/83/EC of the European Parliament and of the Council of 6 November 2001 on the Community code relating to medicinal products for human use. 2003; 8784(211011). https://doi. org/2004R0726-v.7. of 05.06.2013.

34. Farzaneh V, Carvalho IS. A review of the health benefit potentials of herbal plant infusions and their mechanism of actions. Ind Crop Prod. 2015;65:247–58. https://doi.org/10.1016/j.indcrop.2014.10.057.

35. Food and Agriculture Organization of the United Nations. Codex Alimentarius General Standard for Food Additives CODEX STAN 192-1995. 2018.
36. Gottardi D, et al. Beneficial effects of spices in food preservation and safety. Front Microbiol. 2016;7:1–20. https://doi.org/10.3389/fmicb.2016.01394.
37. Harvard Heart Letter. To eat less salt, enjoy the spice of life; 2018. https://www.health.harvard.edu/heart-health/to-eat-less-salt-enjoy-the-spice-of-life.
38. Hernández-Hernández E, et al. Antioxidant effect rosemary (*Rosmarinus officinalis* L.) and oregano (*Origanum vulgare* L.) extracts on TBARS and colour of model raw pork batters. Meat Sci. 2009;81(2):410–7. https://doi.org/10.1016/J.MEATSCI.2008.09.004.
39. Hernández-Ochoa L, et al. Use of essential oils and extracts from spices in meat protection. J Food Sci Technol. 2014;51(5):957–63. https://doi.org/10.1007/s13197-011-0598-3.
40. Herrera T, et al. Teas and herbal infusions as sources of melatonin and other bioactive non-nutrient components. LWT Food Sci Technol. 2018;89:65–73. https://doi.org/10.1016/j.lwt.2017.10.031.
41. Herrera-Arellano A, et al. Effectiveness and tolerability of a standardized extract from *Hibiscus sabdariffa* in patients with mild to moderate hypertension: a controlled and randomized clinical trial. Phytomedicine. 2004;11(5):375–82. https://doi.org/10.1016/j.phymed.2004.04.001.
42. Horžić D, et al. The composition of polyphenols and methylxanthines in teas and herbal infusions. Food Chem. 2009;115(2):441–8. https://doi.org/10.1016/J.FOODCHEM.2008.12.022.
43. Hosseini A, Ghorbani A. Cancer therapy with phytochemicals: evidence from clinical studies. Avicenna J Phytomed. 2015;5(2):84–97.
44. Huang W-Y, Cai Y-Z, Zhang Y. Natural phenolic compounds from medicinal herbs and dietary plants: potential use for cancer prevention. Nutr Cancer. 2009;62(1):1–20. https://doi.org/10.1080/01635580903191585.
45. Isbill J, Kandiah J, Khubchandani J. Use of ethnic spices by adults in the United States: an exploratory study. Health Promot Perspect. 2018;8(1):33–40. https://doi.org/10.15171/hpp.2018.04.
46. Jandaghi P, et al. Lemon balm: a promising herbal therapy for patients with borderline hyperlipidemia—a randomized double-blind placebo-controlled clinical trial. Complement Ther Med. 2016;26:136–40. https://doi.org/10.1016/j.ctim.2016.03.012.
47. Jassim SAA, Naji MA. Novel antiviral agents: a medicinal plant perspective. J Appl Microbiol. 2003;95(3):412–27. https://doi.org/10.1046/j.1365-2672.2003.02026.x.
48. Jatoi A, et al. A Phase II trial of green tea in the treatment of patients with androgen independent metastatic prostate carcinoma. Cancer. 2003;97(6):1442–6. https://doi.org/10.1002/cncr.11200.
49. Kaefer CM, Milner JA. The role of herbs and spices in cancer prevention. J Nutr Biochem. 2008;19(6):347–61. https://doi.org/10.1016/J.JNUTBIO.2007.11.003.
50. Kaefer CM, Milner JA. Herbs and spices in cancer prevention and treatment, herbal medicine: biomolecular and clinical aspects. Boca Raton, Florida, USA: CRC Press/Taylor & Francis; 2011.
51. Kahn SE, Hull RL, Utzschneider KM. Mechanisms linking obesity to insulin resistance and type 2 diabetes. Nature. 2006;444:840–6.
52. Khan A, et al. Cinnamon improves glucose and lipids of people with type 2 diabetes. Diabetes Care. 2003;26(12):3215–8.
53. Khan A, Zaman G, Anderson RA. Bay leaves improve glucose and lipid profile of people with type 2 diabetes. J Clin Biochem Nutr. 2009;44(1):52–6. https://doi.org/10.3164/jcbn.08-188.
54. Kianbakht S, et al. Antihyperlipidemic effects of *Salvia officinalis* L. Leaf extract in patients with hyperlipidemia: a randomized double-blind placebo-controlled clinical trial. Phytother Res. 2011;25(12):1849–53. https://doi.org/10.1002/ptr.3506.
55. Kulisic-Bilusic T, et al. Antioxidant and acetylcholinesterase inhibiting activity of several aqueous tea infusions *in vitro*. Food Technol Biotechnol. 2008;46(4):368–75.
56. Kumar Y, et al. Recent trends in the use of natural antioxidants for meat and meat products. Compr Rev Food Sci Food Saf. 2015;14(6):796–812. https://doi.org/10.1111/1541-4337.12156.
57. Kunnumakkara AB, et al. Chronic diseases, inflammation, and spices: how are they linked? J Transl Med. 2018;16(1):1–25. https://doi.org/10.1186/s12967-018-1381-2.
58. Lehto S, et al. Comparison of food colour regulations in the EU and the US: a review of current provisions. Food Addit Contam Part A Chem Anal Control Expo Risk Assess. 2017;34(3):335–55. https://doi.org/10.1080/19440049.2016.1274431.
59. Li H, et al. An intervention study to prevent gastric cancer by micro-selenium and large dose of allitridum. Chin Med J. 2004;117(8):1155–60. https://doi.org/10.1046/j.1528-1157.2003.32702.x.
60. Llamas NE, et al. Second order advantage in the determination of amaranth, sunset yellow FCF and tartrazine by UV–vis and multivariate curve resolution-alternating least squares. Anal Chim Acta. 2009;655(1–2):38–42. https://doi.org/10.1016/J.ACA.2009.10.001.
61. Longo L, Vasapollo G. Anthocyanins from Bay (*Laurus nobilis* L.) Berries. J Agric Food Chem. 2005;53(20):8063–7. https://doi.org/10.1021/jf051400e.

62. Maithili Karpaga Selvi N, et al. Efficacy of turmeric as adjuvant therapy in type 2 diabetic patients. Indian J Clin Biochem. 2015;30(2):180–6. https://doi.org/10.1007/s12291-014-0436-2.

63. Mariutti LRB, Nogueira GC, Bragagnolo N. Lipid and cholesterol oxidation in chicken meat are inhibited by sage but not by garlic. J Food Sci. 2011;76(6):C909–15. https://doi.org/10.1111/j.1750-3841.2011.02274.x.

64. Maron DJ, et al. Cholesterol-lowering effect of a theaflavin-enriched green tea extract. Arch Intern Med. 2003;163(12):1448. https://doi.org/10.1001/archinte.163.12.1448.

65. McCrea CE, et al. Effects of culinary spices and psychological stress on postprandial lipemia and lipase activity: results of a randomized crossover study and in vitro experiments. J Transl Med. 2015;13(1):1–12. https://doi.org/10.1186/s12967-014-0360-5.

66. McKay DL, et al. *Hibiscus Sabdariffa* L. tea (tisane) lowers blood pressure in prehypertensive and mildly hypertensive adults. J Nutr. 2009;140(2):298–303. https://doi.org/10.3945/jn.109.115097.

67. Medagama AB. The glycaemic outcomes of cinnamon, a review of the experimental evidence and clinical trials. Nutr J. 2015;14(1):1–12. https://doi.org/10.1186/s12937-015-0098-9.

68. Momose Y, Maeda-Yamamoto M, Nabetani H. Systematic review of green tea epigallocatechin gallate in reducing low-density lipoprotein cholesterol levels of humans. Int J Food Sci Nutr. 2016;67(6):606–13. https://doi.org/10.1080/09637486.2016.1196655.

69. Mozaffari-Khosravi H, et al. The effects of sour tea (*Hibiscus sabdariffa*) on hypertension in patients with type II diabetes. J Hum Hypertens. 2009;23(1):48–54. https://doi.org/10.1038/jhh.2008.100.

70. National Institute of Aging. What are clinical trials and studies? 2017. Available at: https://www.nia.nih.gov/health/what-are-clinical-trials-and-studies.

71. Nations, F. and A. O. of the U. Codex Alimentarius: general standard for food additives. In: Codex Alimentarius: general standard for food additives. Rome: Food and Agriculture Organization of the United Nations (FAO); 2017.

72. Nurmi A, et al. Consumption of juice fortified with oregano extract markedly increases excretion of phenolic acids but lacks short- and long-term effects on lipid peroxidation in healthy nonsmoking men. J Agric Food Chem. 2006;54(16):5790–6. https://doi.org/10.1021/jf0608928.

73. Opara EI, Chohan M. Culinary herbs and spices: their bioactive properties, the contribution of polyphenols and the challenges in deducing their true health benefits. Int J Mol Sci. 2014;15(10):19183–202. https://doi.org/10.3390/ijms151019183.

74. Peter KV, Shylaja MR. Introduction to herbs and spices: definitions, trade and applications. In: Peter KV, editor. Handbook of Herbs and Spices. Cambridge: Woodhead Publishing; 2012. p. 1–24.

75. Pezeshk S, Rezaei M, Hosseini H. Effects of turmeric, shallot extracts, and their combination on quality characteristics of vacuum-packaged rainbow trout stored at 4 ± 1°C. J Food Sci. 2011;76(6):387–91. https://doi.org/10.1111/j.1750-3841.2011.02242.x.

76. Pistollato F, Battino M. Role of plant-based diets in the prevention and regression of metabolic syndrome and neurodegenerative diseases. Trends Food Sci Technol. 2014;40:62–81. https://doi.org/10.1016/j.tifs.2014.07.012.

77. Pourmasoumi M, et al. The effect of ginger supplementation on lipid profile: a systematic review and meta-analysis of clinical trials. Phytomedicine. 2018;43:28–36. https://doi.org/10.1016/j.phymed.2018.03.043.

78. Radha Krishnan K, et al. Antimicrobial and antioxidant effects of spice extracts on the shelf life extension of raw chicken meat. Int J Food Microbiol. 2014;171:32–40. https://doi.org/10.1016/j.ijfoodmicro.2013.11.011.

79. Rainey-Smith S, Brown B, Sohrabi H, Shah T, Goozee K, Gupta V, Martins R. Curcumin and cognition: a randomised, placebo-controlled, double-blind study of community-dwelling older adults. Br J Nutr. 2016;115(12):2106–13. https://doi.org/10.1017/S0007114516001203.

80. Rajeshwari U, Shobba I, Andallu B. Comparison of aniseeds and coriander seeds for antidiabetic, hypolipidemic and antioxidant activities. Spatulla DD. 2011;1:9–16.

81. Rastogi S, Pandey MM, Rawat AKS. Traditional herbs: a remedy for cardiovascular disorders. Phytomedicine. 2016;23(11):1082–9. https://doi.org/10.1016/J.PHYMED.2015.10.012.

82. Rjzk EM, El-Gharably AM, Tolba KH. Carotenoid pigments composition of Calendula flower and its potential uses as antioxidant and natural colorant in manufacturing of hard candy. Arab Univ J Agric Sci. 2008;16(2):407–17.

83. Sá C, et al. Sage tea drinking improves lipid profile and antioxidant defences in humans. Int J Mol Sci. 2009;10(9):3937–50. https://doi.org/10.3390/ijms10093937.

84. Sancho RAS, et al. Effect of annatto seed and coriander leaves as natural antioxidants in fish meatballs during frozen storage. J Food Sci. 2011;76(6):C838–45. https://doi.org/10.1111/j.1750-3841.2011.02224.x.

85. Santos-Buelga C, Mateus N, De Freitas V. Anthocyanins. Plant pigments and beyond. J Agric Food Chem. 2014;62(29):6879–84. https://doi.org/10.1021/jf501950s.

86. Schmidt U, et al. Efficacy of the Hawthorn (*Crataegus*) preparation LI 132 in 78 patients with chronic congestive heart failure defined as NYHA functional class II. Phytomedicine. 1994;1(1):17–24. https://doi.org/10.1016/S0944-7113(11)80018-8.

87. Shan B, et al. The *in vitro* antibacterial activity of dietary spice and medicinal herb extracts. Int J Food Microbiol. 2007;117(1):112–9. https://doi.org/10.1016/J.IJFOODMICRO.2007.03.003.

88. Shim GS, et al. Six-month randomized, placebo-controlled, double-blind, pilot clinical trial of curcumin in patients with alzheimer disease. J Clin Psychopharmacol. 2008;28(1):110–3.

89. Silva IF, et al. Antimicrobial screening of some medicinal plants from Mato Grosso Cerrado. Braz J Pharmacogn. 2009;19(1 B):242–8. https://doi.org/10.1590/S0102-695X2009000200011.

90. Silva N, Fernandes Júnior A. Biological properties of medicinal plants: a review of their antimicrobial activity. J Venom Anim Toxins Incl Trop Dis. 2010;16(3):402–13. https://doi.org/10.1590/S1678-91992010000300006.

91. Srinivasan K. Plant foods in the management of diabetes mellitus: spices as beneficial antidiabetic food adjuncts. Int J Food Sci Nutr. 2005;56(6):399–414. https://doi.org/10.1080/09637480500512872.

92. Srinivasan K. Antimutagenic and cancer preventive potential of culinary spices and their bioactive compounds. PharmaNutrition. 2017;5(3):89–102. https://doi.org/10.1016/j.phanu.2017.06.001.

93. Tanaka S, et al. Aged garlic extract has potential suppressive effect on colorectal adenomas in humans. Hiroshima J Med Sci. 2004;53(3–4):39–45. https://doi.org/10.1093/jn/136.3.810S. [pii].

94. Tapsell LC, Scientific TC, Sullivan DR. Health benefits of herbs and spices: the past, the present, the future. Med J Aust. 2006;185(4 Suppl):S4–24.

95. U.S. Food and Drug Administration (FDA). CPG Sec. 525.750 spices – definitions. 2015. Available at: https://www.fda.gov/iceci/compliancemanuals/compliancepolicyguidancemanual/ucm074468.htm.

96. U.S. Department of Agriculture. Scientific Report of the 2015 Dietary Guidelines Advisory Committee. 2015. Available at: https://health.gov/dietaryguidelines/2015-scientific-report/pdfs/scientific-report-of-the-2015-dietary-guidelines-advisory-committee.pdf. Accessed 11 Oct 2016.

97. Vasavada MN, Dwivedi S, Cornforth D. Evaluation of garam masala spices and phosphates as antioxidants in cooked ground beef. J Food Sci. 2006;71(5):292–7. https://doi.org/10.1007/s00191-013-0315-7.

98. WHO. Diet, nutrition and the prevention of chronic diseases. World Health Organization Technical Report Series, 916. 2003, p. i–viii-1-149-backcover. ISBN 92 4 120916 X ISSN 0512-3054 (NLM classification: QU 145).

99. Wojdyło A, Oszmiański J, Czemerys R. Antioxidant activity and phenolic compounds in 32 selected herbs. Food Chem. 2007;105(3):940–9. https://doi.org/10.1016/j.foodchem.2007.04.038.

100. Yashin A, et al. Antioxidant activity of spices and their impact on human health: a review. Antioxidants. 2017;6(3):70. https://doi.org/10.3390/antiox6030070.

101. Yi W, Wetzstein HY. Anti-tumorigenic activity of five culinary and medicinal herbs grown under greenhouse conditions and their combination effects. J Sci Food Agric. 2011;91(10):1849–54. https://doi.org/10.1002/jsfa.4394.

102. You WC, et al. Randomized double-blind factorial trial of three treatments to reduce the prevalence of precancerous gastric lesions. J Natl Cancer Inst. 2006;98(14):974–83. https://doi.org/10.1093/jnci/djj264.

103. Zeraatpishe A, et al. Effects of *Melissa officinalis* L. on oxidative status and DNA damage in subjects exposed to long-term low-dose ionizing radiation. Toxicol Ind Health. 2011;27(3):205–12. https://doi.org/10.1177/0748233710383889.

104. Zheng J, et al. Spices for prevention and treatment of cancers. Nutrients. 2016;8(8):495. https://doi.org/10.5194/acpd-11-10449-2011.

Chapter 7
Integrating Healthy Eating and Drinking into Daily Life

Jerrilynn D. Burrowes and Josephine Wright

Keywords Healthy eating · Healthy beverage choices · *Dietary Guidelines for Americans* · Mobile health

Key Points
- Chronic diseases such as obesity, diabetes, hypertension, and cardiovascular disease are among the most prevalent health conditions in the US that can be prevented with a healthy eating and drinking lifestyle.
- In order to prevent the public from being deceived and receiving misinformation about food and nutrition, they should consult with a registered dietitian.
- The *Dietary Guidelines* aim to promote health, prevent chronic disease, and help people reach and maintain a healthy weight.
- The right mix of what we eat and drink today can help us be healthier in the future, since everything we eat and drink matters in the long term.
- More than two thirds of all Americans use a computer or smartphone to find health information for themselves or someone else, but choosing a mobile app can be challenging because the scientific evidence is limited for commercially available apps.

Introduction

Chronic diseases such as obesity, diabetes, hypertension, and cardiovascular disease are among the most prevalent and preventable health conditions in the US. Nearly half of all Americans suffer from at least one chronic disease, and the number is steadily increasing [1]. A history of poor-quality eating and drinking patterns and physical inactivity has a cumulative effect and has contributed to significant nutrition and physical activity-related health challenges that affect the US population. Individuals need to understand that the food and beverage choices they make every day, and over a lifetime, matters. This is one reason the US Department of Health and Human Services (USDHHS) and the US Department of Agriculture (USDA) have worked jointly every 5 years for the past 35 years to develop the *Dietary Guidelines for Americans*. One purpose of the guidelines is to provide scientific, evidence-based food and beverage recommendations for people 2 years of age and older. The guidelines are a

J. D. Burrowes (✉) · J. Wright
Department of Nutrition, School of Health Professions and Nursing, Brookeville, NY, USA
e-mail: jerrilynn.burrowes@liu.edu; josephine.wright@liu.edu

© Springer Nature Switzerland AG 2020
J. Uribarri, J. A. Vassalotti (eds.), *Nutrition, Fitness, and Mindfulness*, Nutrition and Health,
https://doi.org/10.1007/978-3-030-30892-6_7

tool for health professionals such as registered dietitians (RDs) to educate Americans on how to make healthy choices in their daily lives that will become good dietary habits. It is the goal that these habits will eventually promote overall health and reduce the risk of chronic disease across the life-span—all with a focus on disease prevention [2].

This chapter will first describe the qualifications that support the RD as the food and nutrition expert and explain how the RD can assist individuals in integrating healthy eating and drinking practices into their lifestyle using the recommendations from the *2015–2020 Dietary Guidelines for Americans* (hereafter referred to as the *Dietary Guidelines*). Strategies for healthy eating using evidence-based dietary practices such as volumetrics, mindful eating, and intuitive eating will be discussed. This chapter will also provide information about credible food, nutrition, and health resources that individuals can use to increase their knowledge. The last section of this chapter includes information on using mobile health such as the Internet, social media, apps, and blogs to implement healthy dietary and fitness practices.

The Food and Nutrition Expert

What Is the Difference Between a Nutritionist and a Registered Dietitian (RD)?

The short answer is that RDs (also referred to as registered dietitian/nutritionists [RDNs]) are nutritionists, but not all nutritionists are RDs. In many states, anyone can use the title "nutritionist" because there is no legal definition of a "nutritionist." As a result, people with little or no formal education, supervised training, or work experience may practice as nutritionists, but they are not required to obtain continuing education to maintain professional competence. On the other hand, some states have licensure for RDs that prevent people from practicing as nutritionists. While there may be some good nutritionists, the RD credential ensures that the individual has a well-defined, science-based, standardized education and is required to complete mandatory continuing education to keep abreast of the latest developments in the field. In order to prevent the public from being deceived and receiving misinformation about food and nutrition, they should consult with a RD.

When and How Is a RD Helpful in Promoting Healthy Eating and Drinking into Daily Life?

It is often difficult and challenging for some people to know what to believe about food, nutrition, and health since they are often bombarded with information from different sources such as the Internet, the media, social websites, and blogs—much of which may not be factual. The RD is a trusted source of credible food, nutrition, and health information who can dispel the myths and provide factual information. He/she can provide personalized service to individuals who want to improve their health by adopting a healthy eating and drinking lifestyle. With the assistance of the client, the RD can develop an eating plan using the *Dietary Guidelines* that are realistic and tailored to the client's needs and goals that are easy to follow and adhere to. He/she can also assist in meal planning and organize supermarket tours to make food shopping a fun, positive experience to teach the client how to identify a variety of healthful food and beverage options and how to read nutrition fact labels and ingredient lists. RDs can also develop educational materials using the *Dietary Guidelines* to promote healthy eating and drinking in a manner that is compelling, inspiring, empowering, and actionable for individuals and groups.

Integrating Healthy Eating into Daily Life

Strategies for Healthy Eating

Volumetrics

The basic principle of volumetrics is to eat a satisfying volume of food while controlling calories and meeting nutrient requirements [3]. This low-calorie, high-volume eating plan includes foods with a lot of water and fiber (e.g., fruits and vegetables), since both increase a sense of fullness. No food is banned in the volumetrics eating plan, and calorie-packed foods can be enjoyed as long as the recommended calorie intake is met [3].

Mindful Eating/Intuitive Eating

Choosing when, where, and how much to eat may be an arduous task for some people; it may become less stressful as one transitions away from diet-influenced, habitual ways of thinking about eating to more thoughtful approaches. Both mindful and intuitive eating are good dietary practices to improve one's relationship with food and build healthier, long-term eating habits [4].

Mindful Eating

Mindful eating is not the same as intuitive eating, and the terms should not be used interchangeably. Eating mindfully is about awareness and intention (i.e., paying attention to our food, on purpose, moment by moment, without judgment) [4–6]. It is an approach to food that focuses on an individuals' sensual awareness and experience with food. Mindful eating has little to do with calories, carbohydrates, fat, or protein. *The basic core principle of mindful eating is to slow down while eating and to be fully aware of each plate or bite of food by examining all the tastes and textures of the food.* It begins with the first thought about food and lasts until the final bite is swallowed, and the consequence of the food episode is experienced [4–6]. (See Table 7.1 for some helpful tips for practicing mindful eating.)

Table 7.1 Helpful tips for practicing mindful eating

Minimize distractions by turning off or silencing your devices and eating away from the television or computer or eating in the car
Become aware of the body's hunger and fullness cues, and utilize these cues to guide the decision to begin and end eating as opposed to following a regimented diet plan
Take a moment to clear your head and appreciate the food that's in front of you
Use all five of your senses to note the appearance, aroma, textures, flavors, and sounds of your food
As you eat your meal or snack, consider the five basic tastes that you are experiencing (i.e., umami, bitter, sweet, salty, and sour)
Notice the texture (i.e., is it crunchy or creamy, dry, or moist)
Set down the fork in between bites to slow down your pace (e.g., taking breaks during bites, chewing more slowly, taking a break to breathe and assess fullness)

Modified from: Food Insight. International Food Information Council (IFIC) Foundation [4]

Table 7.2 Ten principles of intuitive eating

1. *Reject the diet mentality:* Throw out the diets that offer false hope of losing weight quickly, easily, and permanently
2. *Honor your hunger:* Provide nutrition for your body before any feelings of excessive hunger manifest—intentions of moderation are irrelevant at this point
3. *Make peace with food:* Call a truce, stop the food fight! Provide unconditional permission to eat; can't or shouldn't foods lead to bingeing
4. *Challenge the food police:* Scream a loud "NO" to thoughts in your head that declare you're "good" for eating minimal calories or you're "bad" because you ate a piece of chocolate cake
5. *Respect your fullness:* Listen for the body signals that tell you that you are no longer hungry Observe the signs that show that you're comfortably full. Pause in the middle of a meal or food, and ask yourself how the food tastes and what is your current fullness level
6. *Discover the satisfaction factor:* Find pleasure and satisfaction in the eating experience. When you eat what you really want, in an environment that is inviting and conducive, you will find that it takes much less food to decide you've had "enough"
7. *Honor your feelings without using food:* Find ways to comfort, nurture, distract, and resolve your issues without using food. Anxiety, loneliness, boredom, and anger are emotions that have their own triggers that food won't fix. Eating for an emotional hunger will only make you feel worse in the long run. You'll ultimately have to deal with the source of the emotion, as well as the discomfort of overeating
8. *Respect your body:* Accept your genetic blueprint so you can feel better about who you are. It's hard to reject the diet mentality if you are unrealistic and overly critical about your body shape
9. *Exercise—feel the difference:* Get active and feel the difference. Shift the focus on how it feels to move your body, rather than the calorie burning effect of exercise
10. *Honor your health:* Make food choices that honor your health and taste buds while making you feel well. It's what you eat consistently over time that matters

Modified from: Intuitive Eating [47]

Intuitive Eating

The major principle underlying intuitive eating is to reject the diet mentality, adopting an "all foods fit mantra" and focusing on hunger cues (i.e., use instincts to decide when and how much food to eat) [4, 7]. The more we get "in tune" with our hunger cues, the better we become at choosing foods that are both nourishing and satisfying. Intuitive eating helps individuals find a balance between honoring their health with appropriate food choices, with being kind to themselves if they overeat or eat indulgent foods. It operates on the idea that we, as individuals, know what foods will make us feel best—typically those are the same nutritious foods the *Dietary Guidelines* advise us to eat. (See Table 7.2 for the principles of intuitive eating.)

Resources for Healthy Eating

Healthy Eating Guides

2015–2020 Dietary Guidelines for Americans

The *Dietary Guidelines* provide evidence-based food and beverage recommendations for Americans 2 years of age and older [2]. These recommendations aim to promote health, prevent chronic disease, and help people reach and maintain a healthy weight. Table 7.3 presents five recommendations from the *Dietary Guidelines* that should be applied in their entirety, given the interconnected relationship that each component has with the others to promote healthy eating

Table 7.3 Five guidelines from the 2015–2020 *Dietary Guidelines for Americans* that encourage healthy eating patterns

1. *Follow a healthy eating pattern across the life-span:* All food and beverage choices matter. Choose a healthy eating pattern at an appropriate calorie level to help achieve and maintain a healthy body weight, support adequate nutrient, and reduce the risk of chronic disease A healthy eating pattern includes: • A variety of vegetables from all of the subgroups—dark green, red, and orange, legumes (beans and peas), starchy, and other • Fruits, especially whole fruits • Grains, at least half of which are whole grains • Fat-free or low-fat dairy, including milk, yogurt, cheese, and/or fortified soy beverages • A variety of protein foods, including seafood, lean meats and poultry, eggs, legumes (beans and peas), nuts, seeds, and soy products • Oils
2. *Focus on variety, nutrient density, and amount:* To meet nutrient needs within calorie limits, choose a variety of nutrient-dense foods across and within all food groups in recommended amounts
3. *Limit calories from added sugars and saturated fats and reduce sodium intake:* Consume an eating pattern low in added sugars, saturated and *trans* fats, and sodium. Cut back on foods and beverages higher in these components to amounts that fit within healthy eating patterns • Consume less than 10% of calories per day from added sugars • Consume less than 10% of calories per day from saturated fats • Consume less than 2300 milligrams (mg) per day of sodium • If alcohol is consumed, it should be consumed in moderation—up to one drink per day for women and up to two drinks per day for men—and only by adults of legal drinking age
4. *Shift to healthier food and beverage choices:* Choose nutrient-dense foods and beverages across and within all food groups in place of less healthy choices. Consider cultural and personal preferences to make these shifts easier to accomplish and maintain
5. *Support healthy eating patterns from all*: Everyone has a role in helping to create and support healthy eating patterns in multiple settings nationwide, from home to school to work to communities

From: Office of Disease Prevention and Health Promotion [48]

patterns. A number of resources are available to assist individuals in implementing the *Dietary Guidelines*. These include information on cutting down on added sugars [8], saturated fats [9], and sodium [10]; how to build a healthy eating pattern [11]; and how to shift to healthier food and beverage choices [12].

MyPlate.Gov

MyPlate was developed to assist health professionals in promoting and implementing the *Dietary Guidelines* for the public so that individuals, families, and communities can become more aware of and educated about making healthy food and beverage choices over time [13]. MyPlate provides information about each of the target food groups (fruit [14], vegetables [15], grains [16], protein foods [17], and dairy [18]). It was created to be used in various settings and to be adaptable to the needs of specific population groups. This tool brings together the key elements of healthy eating patterns, translating the *Dietary Guidelines* into key consumer messages that can be used in educational materials for the public.

MyPlate is a reminder that individuals should find a healthy eating style and build it throughout their life-span. Eating healthy is a journey shaped by many factors, including stage of life, food preferences, budget, access to food, culture, traditions, and personal decisions made over time. The right mix of what you eat and drink today can help you be healthier in the future, since everything you eat and drink matters in the long term.

MyPlate Plan and MyPlate Tip Sheet

The MyPlate Plan [19] and MyPlate Tip Sheets [20] are resources available for the consumer to aid in using MyPlate. The MyPlate Plan, which is available in English and Spanish, is a personalized food plan that is based on the individual's age, sex, height, weight, and level of physical activity. It provides a guide for what and how much to eat within the individual's calorie allowance for each food group.

MyPlate Tip Sheets are for consumers to build a healthy eating style and maintain it for a lifetime; they are available in 19 different languages [20]. A MyPlate Tip Sheet that focuses on nutrients for healthy vegetarian eating is also available [21]. Individuals should choose foods and beverages from each MyPlate food group that is limited in sodium, saturated fat, and added sugars. The recommendations suggest starting with small changes to make healthier choices you can enjoy. (See Table 7.4 for ten tips to implementing MyPlate.)

Healthy Eating Patterns

Eating patterns, what we eat and drink on a daily basis, are at the core of the *Dietary Guidelines*. The USDA has developed three different food patterns (Healthy US-Style Eating Pattern, Mediterranean-Style Eating Pattern, and a Healthy Vegetarian Eating Pattern) to help individuals carry out the *Dietary Guidelines;* the latter two plans are adapted from the Healthy US-Style Eating Pattern. All eating patterns include 12 calorie levels (from 1000 to 3200) to meet the needs of individuals across the life-span [22].

The Healthy US-Style Pattern is based on the types and proportions of foods Americans typically consume but in nutrient-dense forms and appropriate amounts. The Healthy Mediterranean-Style Pattern modifies amounts recommended from some food groups (e.g., more fruits and seafood and less dairy) to more closely reflect eating patterns that have been associated with additional positive

Table 7.4 Ten tips: Choose MyPlate

1. *Find your healthy eating style*: Creating a healthy style means regularly eating a variety of foods to get the nutrients and calories you need. MyPlate's tips help you create your own healthy eating solutions—"MyWins"
2. *Make half your plate fruits and vegetables*: Eating colorful fruits and vegetables is important because they provide vitamins and minerals and most are low in calories
3. *Focus on whole fruits*: Choose whole fruits—fresh, frozen, dried, or canned in 100% juice. Enjoy fruit with meals, as snacks or as a dessert
4. *Vary your veggies*: Try adding fresh, frozen, or canned vegetables to salads, sides, and main dishes. Choose a variety of colorful vegetables prepared in healthful ways: steamed, sautéed, roasted, or raw
5. *Make half your grains whole grains*: Look for whole grains listed first or second on the ingredients list—try oatmeal, popcorn, whole-grain bread, and brown rice. Limit grain-based desserts and snacks, such as cakes, cookies, and pastries
6. *Move to low-fat or fat-free milk or yogurt*: Choose low-fat or fat-free milk, yogurt, and soy beverages (soymilk) to cut back on saturated fat. Replace sour cream, cream, and regular cheese with low-fat yogurt, milk, and cheese
7. *Vary your protein routine*: Mix up your protein foods to include seafood, beans and peas, unsalted nuts and seeds, soy products, eggs, and lean meats and poultry. Try main dishes made with beans or seafood like tuna salad or bean chili
8. *Drink and eat beverages and food with less sodium, saturated fat, and added sugars*: Use the Nutrition Facts label and ingredients list to limit items high in sodium, saturated fat, and added sugars. Choose vegetable oils instead of butter and oil-based sauces and dips instead of ones with butter, cream, or cheese
9. *Drink water instead of sugary drinks*: Water is calorie-free. Non-diet soda, energy or sports drinks, and other sugar-sweetened drinks contain a lot of calories from added sugars and have few nutrients
10. *Everything you eat and drink matters*: The right mix of foods can help you be healthier now and into the future. Turn small changes into your "MyPlate, MyWins"

From: US Department of Agriculture [49]

health outcomes. The Healthy Vegetarian Pattern modifies amounts recommended from some food groups to more closely reflect eating patterns reported by self-identified vegetarians in the National Health and Nutrition Examination Survey (NHANES). This eating pattern can be vegan if all dairy choices are comprised of fortified soy beverages (soymilk) or other plant-based dairy substitutes [22].

Additional Food, Nutrition, and Health Resources

Eight Healthy Eating Goals

The President's Council on Sports, Fitness, and Nutrition (PCSFN) has identified small dietary changes that will make a big difference in overall health. They suggest incorporating one new healthy eating goal each week for 6 weeks into your diet (see Table 7.5) [23].

The Nutrition Facts Label

The Nutrition Facts Label is required by the US Food and Drug Administration (FDA) on most packaged foods and beverages [24, 25]. The label provides detailed information about a food's nutrient content, such as the amount of fat, sugar, sodium, and fiber it contains. As of January 1, 2020, the Nutrition Facts Label will be more informative; it will include updated information and a refreshed label design to make it easier for consumers to identify food choices that support a healthful diet. (See Table 7.6 for a quick guide to reading the new Nutrition Facts Label.)

Table 7.5 Eight healthy eating goals

1. *Make half your plate fruits and vegetables*: Choose red, orange, and dark-green vegetables like tomatoes, sweet potatoes, and broccoli, along with other vegetables for your meals. Add fruit to meals as part of main or side dishes or as dessert. The more colorful you make your plate, the more likely you are to get the vitamins, minerals, and fiber your body needs to be healthy
2. *Make half the grains you eat whole grains*: An easy way to eat more whole grains is to switch from a refined-grain food to a whole-grain food. For example, eat whole-wheat bread instead of white bread. Read the ingredients list and choose products that list a whole-grain ingredients first. Look for things like "whole wheat," "brown rice," "bulgur," "buckwheat," "oatmeal," "rolled oats," "quinoa," or "wild rice"
3. *Switch to fat-free or low-fat (1%) milk*: Both have the same amount of calcium and other essential nutrients as whole milk but fewer calories and less saturated fat
4. *Choose a variety of lean protein foods*: Meat, poultry, seafood, dry beans or peas, eggs, nuts, and seeds are considered part of the protein foods group. Select leaner cuts of ground beef (where the label says 90% lean or higher), turkey breast, or chicken breast
5. *Compare sodium in foods*: Use the Nutrition Facts label to choose lower sodium versions of foods like soup, bread, and frozen meals. Select canned foods labeled "low sodium," "reduced sodium," or "no salt added"
6. *Drink water instead of sugary drinks*: Cut calories by drinking water or unsweetened beverages. Soda, energy drinks, and sports drinks are a major source of added sugar and calories in American diets. Try adding a slice of lemon, lime, or watermelon or a splash of 100% juice to your glass of water if you want some flavor
7. *Eat some seafood*: Seafood includes fish (such as salmon, tuna, and trout) and shellfish (such as crab, mussels, and oysters). Seafood has protein, minerals, and omega-3 fatty acids (heart-healthy fat). Adults should try to eat at least eight ounces a week of a variety of seafood. Children can eat smaller amounts of seafood, too
8. *Cut back on solid fats*: Eat fewer foods that contain solid fats. The major sources for Americans are cakes, cookies, and other desserts (often made with butter, margarine, or shortening); pizza; processed and fatty meats (e.g., sausages, hot dogs, bacon, ribs); and ice cream

From: US Department of Health and Human Services, President's Council on Sports, Fitness, and Nutrition [23]

Table 7.6 Quick guide to reading the Nutrition Facts Label

Nutrition Facts	
8 servings per container	
Serving size	2/3 cup (55g)
Amount per serving	
Calories	**230**
	% Daily Value*
Total Fat 8g	10%
Saturated Fat 1g	5%
Trans Fat 0g	
Cholesterol 0mg	0%
Sodium 160 mg	7%
Total Carbohydrate 37g	13%
Dietary Fiber 4g	14%
Total Sugars 12g	
Includes 10g Added Sugars	20%
Protein 3g	
Vitamin D 2mcg	10%
Calcium 260mg	20%
Iron 8mg	45%
Potassium 235mg	6%

* The % Daily Value (DV) tells you how much a nutrient in a serving of good contributes to a daily diet. 2,000 calories a day is used for general nutrition advice.

1	*Serving size*: The number of servings will be more prominent with a larger and bolder font. Additionally, serving size will also be modified to better represent the portion consumed by most Americans. For instance, a single serving of ice cream will be modified from 1/2 cup to 2/3 cup. The label also includes the number of servings per container to help you calculate the calories and nutrients in the entire package. The serving sizes are not meant to tell people how much to eat
2	*Calories*: This is the most obvious change you will see. The calorie count of a single serving will now be the most prominent information on the label. You can use this information to compare similar products
3	*Nutrients and daily values*: The label must list the amounts of total fat, saturated fat, trans fat, cholesterol, sodium, total carbohydrate, dietary fiber, sugars, protein, vitamin D, calcium, iron, and potassium that are in one serving. "Added sugars" was added as a new category under "total sugars." The daily value (DV) percent tells you how close you are to meeting your daily requirements for each nutrient based on a typical 2000-calorie-a-day diet. The DV can help you track whether you're getting enough, or too much, of all the nutrients you need in a day. Daily values for nutrients such as sodium, dietary fiber, and vitamin D are being updated based on the research that was used to develop the 2015–2020 *Dietary Guidelines for Americans*
4	*Nutrients to increase*: The typical American diet is low in fiber, vitamin D, calcium, iron, and potassium. They're listed on the label to encourage Americans to include more of these important nutrients in their diet. In addition to the percentage of the daily value, manufacturers will be required to list the actual milligrams or micrograms contained within the serving

Adapted from: US Department of Agriculture [24, 25]

Food and Nutrition Information Center (FNIC)

The Food and Nutrition Information Center (FNIC) is a leader in online global nutrition information. Located at the National Agricultural Library (NAL) of the USDA, the FNIC website contains over 2500 links to current and reliable information about food and human nutrition. The FNIC strives to serve the professional community (including educators, health professionals, and researchers) by providing access to a wide range of trustworthy food and nutrition resources from both government and non-government sources [26].

International Food Information Council (IFIC) Foundation

The mission of the International Food Information Council (IFIC) Foundation is dedicated to effectively communicating science-based information on health, nutrition, and food safety for the public good. The Foundation serves as a nutrition and food safety resource for consumers, health professionals, journalists, educators, government officials, and students. It provides important, timely, and consumer-friendly resources on a variety of topics such as weight management, diet (food) and health, food safety, food production, international food issues, and science communications [4].

Integrating Healthy Beverages into Daily Life

Beverage choices are important for good health and nutrition. There are a lot of beverage choices available today, which makes it difficult for the average consumer to decide which one(s) to choose. The amount of sugar, calories, and nutrients in these products can vary considerably.

When it comes to quenching your thirst with a healthy, zero-calorie, low-cost, and easily accessible beverage (for most people), plain tap water is undoubtedly the winner. Water is the most commonly consumed beverage, and drinking enough water every day is good for overall health. Water provides everything the body needs to restore fluids lost through metabolism, breathing, and sweating, especially during exercise, and for removing wastes from the body. Water also helps to prevent dehydration. Although there is no general recommendation for how much plain water adults and youth should drink daily, the Dietary Reference Intake for total water (from all beverages and foods) for women is about 2.7 L (about 11 cups) each day and for men about 3.7 L (about 15 cups) each day. This is not a daily target, but a general guide [27].

After water, tea and coffee are the other two most commonly consumed beverages. Plain tea and coffee are calorie-free beverages that are loaded with antioxidants, flavonoids, and other biologically active substances that may be beneficial for good health [28, 29]. The addition of cream, sugar, whipped cream, and/or flavorings can turn coffee or tea from a healthful beverage into one that is not so healthful. For example, a 16-ounce Cinnamon Roll Frappuccino Blended Coffee with dolce syrup, white chocolate mocha sauce, and vanilla bean, topped with whipped cream and a cinnamon dolce sprinkle, contains 500 calories, 16 grams of saturated fat, and 83 grams of sugar—the equivalent of 21 teaspoons of sugar [30], which is about three times the daily recommended intake of added sugars [31].

Sugar-sweetened beverages such as soda, energy drinks, sports drinks, fruit drinks, sweetened coffee and tea, and flavored waters with added sugar have calories and sugar, but little or no nutritional value. Sports drinks were originally developed for athletes to provide them with carbs, electrolytes (particularly sodium and potassium), and fluid during high-intensity workouts or playing hard or exercising for an hour or more on hot days. However, for the average individual, sports drinks are just another source of sugar and calories [32].

Consumers are seeking alternatives to sugar-sweetened beverages and looking for healthy beverage options. Homemade plain flavored water is a healthy alternative to bottled beverages. They can be infused with fruits and vegetables such as lemons, oranges, berries, and cucumbers. Plant-based waters, also referred to as alternative waters, are also increasing in popularity. These include coconut, aloe vera, cactus, maple, and birch water [33]. However, depending on the plant type, water can

Table 7.7 Better beverage choices made easy

Now that you know how much difference a drink can make, here are some ways to make smart beverage choices:
Drink water instead of sugar-sweetened beverages. Regular soda, energy or sports drinks, and other sweet drinks usually contain a lot of added sugar, which provides more calories than needed. Diet or low-calorie beverages instead of sugar-sweetened beverages are also an option
For a quick, easy, and inexpensive thirst-quencher, carry a water bottle and refill it throughout the day
Don't "stock the fridge" with sugar-sweetened beverages. Instead, keep a jug or bottles of cold water in the fridge
Drink water with and between meals. Adults and children take in about 400 calories per day as beverages; drinking water can help you manage your calories
Make water more exciting by adding slices of lemon, lime, cucumber, or watermelon, or drink sparkling water
Add a splash of 100% juice to plain sparkling water for a refreshing, low-calorie drink
When you choose milk or milk alternatives, select low-fat or fat-free milk or fortified soymilk. Each type of milk offers the same key nutrients such as calcium, vitamin D, and potassium, but the number of calories are very different
When you do opt for a sugar-sweetened beverage, go for the small size. Remember to check the serving size and the number of servings in the can, bottle, or container to stay within calorie needs. Select smaller cans, cups, or glasses instead of large or supersized options
Be a role model for your friends and family by choosing healthy, low-calorie beverages

Adapted from: Centers for Disease Control and Prevention [50]

be extracted or processed in many different ways. There is no standard definition for plant waters, and, depending on how the product is labeled, it may or may not be regulated by the FDA on nutrients and required labeling. These alternative waters have some nutritional value, but they also have calories [34].

Energy drinks are marketed to improve energy, stamina, athletic performance, and concentration. Most energy drinks contain similar ingredients including water, sugar, caffeine, nonnutritive stimulants (e.g., guarana, ginseng, yerba mate, taurine, l-carnitine, d-glucuronolactone, and inositol), and certain vitamins and minerals. The amount of sugar contained in one can (500 mL or 16.9 oz) of an energy drink is typically about 54 g [35]. In addition, some of these beverages may contain more than 500 mg of caffeine per 8-ounce serving [36], an amount equivalent to about 14 cans of cola. As a result, energy drinks can have serious health risks for children and adolescents, including increased heart rate and blood pressure, disrupted sleep, increased anxiety, irregular heart rhythms, seizures, and even death [37].

Diet sodas and other diet drinks are sweetened with calorie-free sugar substitutes such as aspartame (Equal®, NutraSweet®), saccharin (Sweet'N Low®), sucralose (Splenda®), or stevia. These diet drinks are a better choice than sugar-sweetened soft drinks because they are lower in calories [34]. (See Table 7.7 for a list of better beverage choices.)

Using the Internet and Social Media to Implement Healthy Dietary Patterns

Mobile health (mHealth) "is the use of mobile and wireless devices to improve health outcomes, healthcare services and health research" [38]. The use of mHealth includes short message service (SMS) known as text messages, mobile applications (apps), wearable devices, social media, and the Internet. Today, nearly 90% of all US adults use the Internet, an increase in 30% since early 2000 when the Pew Research Center started tracking Internet use by Americans [39]. Additionally, 77% of US adults own a smartphone [40]. In the most recent Health Information National Trends Survey (HINTS 2017) collected by the National Cancer Institute, 67.3% and 54.2% of Americans reported using a computer or smartphone to find health information for themselves or someone else, respectively [41].

Apps

In 2016, 3.2 billion mHealth apps were downloaded worldwide [42]. Nutrition apps are included in the mHealth market. A variety of nutrition apps are available with features that allow users to set goals and track daily food intake. Self-monitoring is associated with weight loss in behavior-based programs. In younger women, apps were more acceptable compared to paper-based food logs; therefore, they may increase adherence [43]. The use of mHealth apps in college-age students may also have a positive effect on eating behavior, particularly when more than one app is used [44]. Many of the mHealth apps provide dietary information about macro- and micronutrients, and users are able to find recipes and create grocery lists and meal plans. Scientific evidence is usually available for apps that are created primarily for research. Therefore, choosing an app can be challenging because the scientific evidence is limited for commercially available apps.

Tracking Dietary Intake

Dietary tracking apps allow users to set a profile and calorie goals based on a formula using height, weight, gender, age, activity, and goals for weight loss, maintenance, or gain. Some allow users to change these values or have the flexibility to adjust the macronutrients in the diet plan. Most allow users to enter foods into the logs by searching for the food in the database or by bar scan. These apps provide the user with nutrient information in the form of calories, macronutrients, and some micronutrients. Most apps today have a community for users to connect to and share progress or get help. The following are the most popular apps that track dietary intake with their unique features.

MyFitnessPal

Platform: Apple, Android
    Free or paid subscription ($9.99/month or $49.99/year)
    MyFitnessPal is an app that has a large food database with the ability to import recipes and log restaurant menu items. It also has a blog that is released daily to inspire and motivate users.
    Special features:

- Easy to change calorie levels if working with a nutrition professional or doctor
- Sharing diary with users who have a "key"
- Sync with fitness devices
- Set goals by calorie, weight, or nutrient (e.g., sodium)
- Track progress
- Includes challenges for those who are inspired by competition

    Paid features:

- Set specific macronutrient goals (e.g., fat, carb, protein).
- Export files
- Get information about eating behaviors

Lifesum

Platform: Apple, Android
    Free or paid subscription ($21.99/3 months, $34.99/6 months, or $44.99/year)

Lifesum is clean and user-friendly with tracking tools and recipes; the app also delivers extra tips and reminders to motivate users. The app allows users to integrate with social media to connect with friends for added motivation and inspiration.

Special features:

- Provides a classic diet plan (50% carbohydrate, 20% protein, and 30% fat) that cannot be changed in the free app

Paid features:

- Sync with fitness devices
- Specialized diets
- Detailed nutrition information
- Photo tracking—snap a picture of food and get nutritional details
- Weekly tips
- Individualized meal plan

Lose It

Platform: Apple, Android
    Free and paid subscription ($39.99/year)
    Lose It is a user-friendly app that allows users to set goals for weight and keep track of their daily intake.
    Special features:

- Easy to change calorie levels if working with a nutrition professional or doctor
- Pie chart visual for macronutrients
- Inspiration provided with badges
- Snap It photo capture technology—search database by photograph

    Paid features:

- Sync with fitness devices
- Track carbs
- Learn about calories and macronutrients
- View calorie and macronutrient trends
- Includes challenges for those who are inspired by competition

Fooducate

Platform: Apple, Android
    Free and paid subscription ($9.99/month, $49.99/year, $99.99/lifetime).
    Fooducate has a health tracker, food finder, community, healthy recipes, and diet tips. A summary of solid versus liquid calories, water consumption, real foods, macronutrients, sugars, and added sugars is provided. The app has sections on the community, recipes, and diet tips. The diet tips section is a blog where nutrition information is provided for users regarding healthy eating.
    Special features:

- Easy to change calorie levels if working with a nutrition professional or doctor.
- Uses a foodpoint system whereby foods with lower foodpoints are considered healthier.
- Foods in the database are given grades of "A" through "D"; this grading system was developed by nutrition scientists and RDs.
- An alternative tab is available for each food showing ten similar foods with better grades.

Paid features:

- Special diet plans are available such as gluten free and diets for those with food allergies.
- Tracking for more nutrients and also blood pressure, serum cholesterol, triglycerides, and other measures.
- Export data.
- "Learn from the experts" tab.
- Dietary help for the family pet.

Watches

Electronic wearable fitness devices or watches are activity monitors that track health-related metrics such as heart rate and distance traveled, but some also allow users to monitor calorie consumption. In 2017, consumer surveys found that 30% of US respondents owned an electronic wearable device and 44% used it daily [45]. As of 2016, the most popular electronic wearable device was Fitbit, which has 47% of the market [46].

Fitbit

The Fitbit is a small black band that measures movement. However, for dietary intake, the user needs to use the Fitbit app. Users do not need to have a Fitbit to use the app, but having a Fitbit allows the user to sync their Fitbit to the app so that calories and activity are automatically tracked. The website allows users to check compatibility of devices such as Android or Apple (https://www.fitbit.com/devices). The app dashboard shows the user the number of steps, floors, miles, calories, and minutes of activity for the day. There are buttons to track exercise, sleep, female health, weight, water intake, and log food intake.

Special features:

- Dashboard can be modified so the user can have the most used features on top.
- Diet tracker shows "calories in" versus "calories out" in graphical format.
- Macronutrient data is provided in chart form.

iWatch

The iWatch is a smartwatch that lets users take phone calls, text messages, listen to music, get e-mails, and track activity. Although users cannot directly track calories on the device, this minicomputer allows users to access apps on the screen. Many apps will sync to the iWatch, and some apps will connect through Apple's Health app, which can sync with iWatch.

Blogs

Blogs provide information that can be created by reputable sources or, in some cases, by people just sharing experiences. The Pew Research Center found that as of 2018, 98% of 18–49-year-olds are using the Internet and 87% of 50–64-year-olds are online. However, the age group over 65 uses the Internet the least at 66%, but this value has been increasing each year the survey has been administered [39]. In the 2017 HINTS data, approximately half of the respondents stated that they used the Internet to search for diet, weight, or physical activity information [41]. The blogs listed here are reliable sources of nutrition information.

President's Council on Sports, Fitness, and Nutrition

The USDHHS maintains the PCSFN website and blog at https://www.hhs.gov/fitness/index.html. Because this chapter focuses on nutrition and not physical activity, the "Eat Healthy" section of the website will be discussed. In this section there are four subsections: (1) Importance of Good Nutrition, (2) How to Eat Healthy, (3) School Breakfast Program, and (4) Dietary Guidelines for Americans. The blog, which can be accessed by the link in the navigation on the left, has an archive and search function. Users can search the tags including childhood obesity, fitness and nutrition, MyPlate, National Nutrition Month, and nutrition.

USDA: Food and Nutrition Blog

The USDA has a large blog that covers many topics. One of the topic areas is food and nutrition, which can be accessed at https://www.usda.gov/media/blog/category/food-and-nutrition. In this blog, readers will find information about various topics including child nutrition programs, dietary health, food security, and nutritional policies and programs. In the health and safety topic area of the blog, which can be accessed at https://www.usda.gov/media/blog/archive/category/health-and-safety, readers can find information about preventing food-borne illness. Archives are available and readers can search by topic or by month.

Summary and Conclusion

With nearly half of all Americans suffering from at least one chronic disease [1], this chapter described the qualifications of the RD as the nutrition expert and how the RD can assist individuals in integrating healthy eating and drinking practices into their lifestyle using recommendations from the *Dietary Guidelines*. Additionally, strategies for healthy eating using evidenced-based practices were introduced along with information about credible food, nutrition, and health resources, and mHealth technologies such as apps for dietary tracking, watches, and blogs. Using the resources to choose the right mix of food and beverages can help individuals live a healthier life.

References

1. Raghupathi W, Raghupathi V. An empirical study of chronic diseases in the United States: a visual analytics approach to public health. Int J Environ Res Public Health [Internet]. 2018 [cited 2018 Aug 12];15(3):431. Available from: https://doi.org/10.3390/ijerph15030431.
2. U.S. Department of Health and Human Services and U.S. Department of agriculture. 2015–2020 dietary guidelines for Americans. 8th ed. [Internet]; 2015 [cited 2018 Aug 12]. Available from: https://health.gov/dietaryguidelines/2015/guidelines/.
3. Rolls B, Barnett RA. The volumetrics weight control plan. New York: HarperCollins Publishers; 2000.
4. Food Insight. International Food Information Council (IFIC) Foundation. Mindful and intuitive eating: the perfect pair. [Internet]. 2018 [cited 2018 Aug 11]. Available from: https://www.foodinsight.org/mindful-intuitive-eating-differences-eating-pattern.

5. Fletcher M. What is mindful eating? [Internet]. 2016 [cited 2018 Aug 11]. Available from: https://www.mindful. org/what-is-mindful-eating/.

6. Nelson JB. Mindful eating: the art of presence while you eat. Diabetes Spectr. 2017;30(3):171–4. Available from: https://doi.org/10.2337/ds17-0015.

7. Tribole E, Resch E. Intuitive eating: a revolutionary program that works. 3rd ed. New York: St. Martin's Griffin; 2012.

8. U.S. Department of Health and Human Services. Office of Disease Prevention and Health Promotion. Cut down on added sugars. [Internet]. 2016 [cited 2018 Aug 12]. Available from: https://health.gov/dietaryguidelines/2015/resources/DGA_Cut-Down-On-Added-Sugars.pdf.

9. U.S. Department of Health and Human Services. Office of Disease Prevention and Health Promotion. Cut down on saturated fats. [Internet]. 2016 [cited 2018 Aug 12]. Available from: https://health.gov/dietaryguidelines/2015/resources/DGA_Cut-Down-On-Saturated-Fats.pdf.

10. U.S. Department of Health and Human Services. Office of Disease Prevention and Health Promotion. Cut down on sodium. [Internet]. 2016 [cited 2018 Aug 12]. Available from: https://health.gov/dietaryguidelines/2015/resources/DGA_Cut-Down-On-Sodium.pdf.

11. U.S. Department of Health and Human Services. Office of Disease Prevention and Health Promotion. How to build a healthy eating pattern. [Internet]. 2017 [cited 2018 Aug 12]. Available from: https://health.gov/dietaryguide-lines/2015/resources/DGA_Healthy-Eating-Pattern.pdf.

12. U.S. Department of Health and Human Services. Office of Disease Prevention and Health Promotion. Shift to healthier food and beverage choices. [Internet]. 2016 [cited 2018 Aug 12]. Available from: https://health.gov/dietaryguidelines/2015/resources/DGA_Shift-to-Healthier-Choices.pdf.

13. U.S. Department of Agriculture. Choose MyPlate.gov. [Internet]. 2018 [cited 2018 Aug 12]. Available from: https://www.choosemyplate.gov/.

14. U.S. Department of Agriculture. Choose MyPlate: all about the fruit group. [Internet]. 2018 [cited 2018 Aug 12]. January 3, 2018. Available from: https://www.choosemyplate.gov/fruit.

15. U.S. Department of Agriculture. Choose MyPlate: all about the vegetable group. [Internet]. 2018 [cited 2018 Aug 12]. Available from: https://www.choosemyplate.gov/vegetables.

16. U.S. Department of Agriculture. Choose MyPlate: all about the grains group. [Internet]. 2017 [cited 2018 Aug 12]. Available from: https://www.choosemyplate.gov/grains.

17. U.S. Department of Agriculture. Choose MyPlate: all about the protein foods group. [Internet]. 2018 [cited 2018 Aug 12]. Available from: https://www.choosemyplate.gov/protein-foods.

18. U.S. Department of Agriculture. Choose MyPlate: all about the dairy group. [Internet]. 2018 [cited 2018 Aug 12]. Available from: https://www.choosemyplate.gov/dairy.

19. U.S. Department of Agriculture. MyPlate plan [Internet]. 2018 [cited 2018 Aug 12]. Available from: https://www.choosemyplate.gov/MyPlatePlan.

20. U.S. Department of Agriculture. MyPlate tip sheets. [Internet]. 2016 [cited 2018 Aug 12]. Available from: https://www.choosemyplate.gov/myplate-tip-sheets.

21. U.S. Department of Agriculture. Tips for vegetarians. [Internet]. 2018 [cited 2018 Aug 12]. Available from: https://www.choosemyplate.gov/tips-vegetarians.

22. U.S. Department of Agriculture. Center for nutrition policy and promotion. USDA food patterns. [internet]. [cited 2018 Aug 12]. Available from: https://www.cnpp.usda.gov/USDAFoodPatterns.

23. U.S. Department of Health & Human Services, President's Council on Sports, Fitness & Nutrition. Eight healthy eating goals. [Internet]. 2017 [cited 2018 Aug 12]. Available from: https://www.hhs.gov/fitness/eat-healthy/how-to-eat-healthy/index.html.

24. U.S. Department of Agriculture. What's on the nutrition facts label. [Internet]. [cited 2018 Aug 12]. Available from: https://www.accessdata.fda.gov/scripts/InteractiveNutritionFactsLabel/factsheets/Whats_On_The_Nutrition_Facts_Label.pdf.

25. U.S. Department of Agriculture. Understanding and using the nutrition facts label. [Internet]. [cited 2018 Aug 12]. Available from: https://www.accessdata.fda.gov/scripts/InteractiveNutritionFactsLabel/factsheets/Understanding_and_Using_the_Nutrition_Facts_Label.pdf.

26. U.S. Department of Agriculture. Food and nutrition information council. [Internet]. [cited 2018 Aug 17]. Available from: https://www.nal.usda.gov/fnic.

27. Institute of Medicine. Dietary reference intakes for water, potassium, sodium, chloride, and sulfate. Washington, DC: National Academy Press; 2004. [Internet]. [cited 2018 Aug 18]. Available from: http://www.nap.edu/read/10925/chapter/1.

28. Khan N, Mukhtar H. Tea and health: studies in humans. Curr Pharm Des. 2013;19(34):6141–7.

29. Higdon JV, Frei B. Coffee and health: a review of recent human research. Crit Rev Food Sci Nutr. 2006;46(2):101–23.

30. Starbucks. Cinnamon Roll Frappuccino Blended Coffee with dolce syrup, white chocolate mocha sauce and vanilla bean, topped with whipped cream and a cinnamon dolce sprinkle. [Internet]. 2018 [cited 2018 Aug 13]. Available from:

https://www.starbucks.com/menu/drinks/frappuccino-blended-beverages/cinnamon-roll-frappuccino-blended-beverage#size=11050792&milk=67&whip=125.

31. Johnson RK, Appel LJ, Brands M, Howard BV, Lefevre M, Lustig RH, Sacks F, Steffen LM, Wylie-Rosett J, on behalf of the American Heart Association Nutrition Committee of the Council on Nutrition, Physical Activity, and Metabolism and the Council on Epidemiology and Prevention. Dietary sugars intake and cardiovascular health: a scientific statement from the American Heart Association. Circulation. 2009;120:1011–20. https://doi.org/10.1161/circulationaha.109.192627.

32. Popkin BM, Armstrong LE, Bray GM, Caballero B, Frei B, Willett WC. A new proposed guidance system for beverage consumption in the United States. Am J Clin Nutr. 2006;83(3):529–42. https://doi.org/10.1093/ajcn.83.3.529.

33. Best Food Facts. Plant waters offer cool alternative. [Internet]. 2017 [cited 2018 Aug 27]. Available from: https://www.bestfoodfacts.org/plant-based-water-vs-plain-water-whats-the-deal/.

34. Food Insight. International Food Information Council (IFIC) Foundation. A closer look at popular "alternative" waters. [Internet]. 2015 [cited 2018 Aug 27]. Available from: https://www.foodinsight.org/closer-look-water-alternatives.

35. Al-Shaar L, Vercammen K, Lu C, Richardson S, Tamez M, Mattei J. Health effects and public health concerns of energy drink consumption in the United States: a mini-review. Front Public Health. 2017;5:225. https://doi.org/10.3389/fpubh.2017.00225.

36. Hoffman J. Caffeine & energy drinks. Strength Cond J. 2010;32(1):15–20.

37. Seifert SM, Schaechter JL, Hershorin ER, Lipshultz SE. Health effects of energy drinks on children, adolescents, and young adults. Pediatrics. 2011;127(3):511–28. https://doi.org/10.1542/peds.2009-3592.

38. U.S. Department of Health and Human Services. mHealth. [Internet]. [cited 2018 July 26]. Available from: http://www.hrsa.aquilentprojects.com/healthit/mhealth.html.

39. Pew Research Center. Demographics of Internet and home broadband usage in the United States. [Internet]. [cited 2018 July 24]. Available from: http://www.pewinternet.org/fact-sheet/internet-broadband/.

40. Pew Research Center. Demographics of mobile device ownership and adoption in the United States. [Internet]. [cited 2018 July 24]. Available from: http://www.pewinternet.org/fact-sheet/mobile/.

41. National Cancer Institute. Health information national trends survey: all HINTS questions. [Internet]. [cited 2018 July 26]. Available from: https://hints.cancer.gov/view-questions-topics/all-hints-questions.aspx.

42. Statista. Global mHealth app downloads 2013–2017. Statistic. [Internet]. [cited 2018 July 26]. Available from: https://www.statista.com/statistics/625034/mobile-health-app-downloads/.

43. Hutchesson MJ, Rollo ME, Callister R, Collins CE. Self-monitoring of dietary intake by young women: online food records completed on computer or smartphone are as accurate as paper-based food records but more acceptable. J Acad Nutr Diet. 2015;115(1):87–94. https://doi.org/10.1016/j.jand.2014.07.036.

44. Sarcona A, Kovacs L, Wright J, Williams C. Differences in eating behavior, physical activity, and health-related lifestyle choices between users and nonusers of mobile health apps. J Health Ed. 2017;45(5):298–305. https://doi.org/10.1080/19325037.2017.1335630.

45. Statista. Fitness & activity tracker. Statistics & Facts. [Internet]. [cited 2018 Aug 10]. Available from: https://www.statista.com/topics/4393/fitness-and-activity-tracker/.

46. Statista. Global fitness tracker shipment share 2013–2016. [Internet]. [cited 2018 Aug 10]. Available from: https://www.statista.com/statistics/795509/fitness-trackers-shipment-share-worldwide/.

47. Intuitive Eating. 10 principles of intuitive eating. [Internet]. [cited 2018 Aug 12]. Available from:http://www.intuitiveeating.org/10-principles-of-intuitive-eating/.

48. Office of Disease Prevention & Health Promotion. Dietary guidelines 2015–2020. Executive summary. [Internet]. [cited 2018 Aug 12]. Available from: https://health.gov/dietaryguidelines/2015/guidelines/executive-summary/.

49. U.S. Department of Agriculture. 10 tips: choose MyPlate. [Internet]. July 18, 2018 [cited 2018 Aug 12]. Available from: https://www.choosemyplate.gov/ten-tips-choose-myplate.

50. Centers for Disease Control and Prevention. Rethink your drink. [Internet]. Sept 3, 2015 [cited 2018 Aug 13]. Available from: https://www.cdc.gov/healthyweight/healthy_eating/drinks.html.

Additional resources

Intuitive Eating. http://www.intuitiveeating.org/.

La Rue K. The simple tool that can help prevent overeating. [Internet]. Nov 22, 2017 [cited 2018 Aug 12]. Available from: https://blog.myfitnesspal.com/the-simple-tool-that-can-help-prevent-overeating/.

The Center for Mindful Eating. https://www.thecenterformindfuleating.org/.

What's Cooking? USDA Mixing Bowl. [Internet]. [cited 2018 Aug 12]. Available from: https://www.choosemyplate.gov/ten-tips-whats-cooking-usda-mixing-bowl. (The USDA has developed an online tool that includes a collection of healthy and budget-friendly recipes and resources that is inspired by the Dietary Guidelines for Americans and MyPlate. Individuals can visit this site to help plan meals and menus.)

Part II
Fitness

Chapter 8
Aerobic Physical Activities

Ilkka M. Vuori

Keywords Walking · Cycling · Health · Aerobic physical activity · Exercise

Key Points
- The list of the health and fitness benefits of aerobic physical activity has continuously expanded, and the evidence supporting those benefits has strengthened. Practicing regular moderate-intensity aerobic physical activities decreases the risk of many of the most common chronic diseases and symptoms, and systematic aerobic exercise training is often a beneficial part of the treatment and rehabilitation of those conditions.
- Walking is the most basic of aerobic activities, and brisk walking brings most of the health and fitness benefits ascribed to aerobic physical activity. Furthermore, walking is acceptable, practical, affordable, cost-effective, and safe activity that can be practiced in many variations. Thus, walking is probably the most suitable physical activity for the largest number of adults.
- Increasing evidence indicates that regular cycling, particularly as a mode of transport, offers health and fitness benefits corresponding to those of walking. However, safe and convenient cycling requires skills, adequate function of many senses, knowledge of traffic rules, and suitable infrastructure.
- Currently there is only fragmentary scientific information of the health benefits of most other aerobic physical activities such as swimming, cross-country and roller skiing, orienteering, ordinary and roller skating, rowing, canoeing, many forms of dancing, and recreationally practiced ballgames such as tennis, badminton, squash, golf, and football.
- Walking and cycling offer substantial possibilities to decrease the wide gap of physical activity among the adults in the USA and most other countries.

Aerobic Physical Activity Definition

Aerobic literally means "with oxygen," referring to the use of oxygen in muscles' energy-generating processes. Oxygen is needed to metabolize carbohydrates and fatty acids to produce adenosine triphosphate (ATP), the basic fuel for all cells. These pathways are the main source of energy for aerobic physical activities that are defined as those in which the body's large muscles move in a rhythmic

I. M. Vuori (✉)
The UKK Institute for Health Promotion Research, Tampere, Finland

© Springer Nature Switzerland AG 2020
J. Uribarri, J. A. Vassalotti (eds.), *Nutrition, Fitness, and Mindfulness*, Nutrition and Health,
https://doi.org/10.1007/978-3-030-30892-6_8

manner for a sustained duration. These modes of physical activity are also called endurance activities. Examples include walking, jogging, running, bicycling, dancing, swimming and other aquatic activities, and rowing. This chapter focuses on the two most scalable and widely practiced modes of aerobic physical activity, walking and cycling.

Principles of Practice and Training of Aerobic Activities

Aerobic activities are the main part of physical activity in domestic chores, going to errands, transport, and leisure. Aerobic activities can also be practiced as planned, structured, repetitive, and purposive "exercise" or "exercise training," generally performed during leisure time to achieve fitness or health benefits.

Aerobic physical activities and exercise can cause gradual changes in body structure and metabolism that enhance health and fitness. These effects can be produced effectively and predictably when the following principles of exercise training are considered:

- Overload: physical activity that exceeds the individual's habitual level is needed to bring health-enhancing adaptive changes. Overload can be regulated by manipulating frequency (how often), intensity (how hard), duration (how long at a time), and type of activity. This is also called the FITT principle (Frequency, Intensity, Time, Type) of training. Because different people have been previously exposed to different physical loading, the overload varies between individuals. Thus, for sedentary individuals and seniors, a smaller absolute loading is required for overload that is necessary for physically active and young people. Therefore, especially the intensity of physical activity or exercise is often expressed as a relative measure, e.g., as percentage of a person's maximal functional capacity or maximal heart rate.
- Progression: when exercise training causes adaptive changes, the same dose of activity will cause gradually less overloading. In order to maintain the sufficient amount of overloading, the exercise dose has to be increased gradually. This is known as the principle of progression of exercise training.
- Diminishing returns: when the exercise dose is continuously increased, the gained benefits in terms of fitness, functional capacity, or health gradually decrease for each increment of the exercise dose. Therefore, the gained benefits are greater in the beginning of an exercise program and decrease with time. The exercise dose of athletes has to be very large in order to achieve small – but often significant – improvements in performance capacity.
- Specificity: adaptive changes develop only or nearly only in the organs and functions that are overloaded by the specific activity. Therefore, aerobic and resistance training produce largely different effects. Many aerobic activities such as walking and cycling load mainly the same muscles and energy-producing functions. Therefore, they can be considered as nonspecific modes of activities regarding their effects on health. However, activities such as walking and rowing distribute the load to partly different muscles and produce partly different specific effects, especially in terms of the musculoskeletal structural change and in the performance capacity.
- Reversibility: all training effects diminish or disappear gradually when the overload decreases or ceases. These changes take place rapidly, in days for metabolic functions, and more gradually, even in months to years, for organ structures, particularly for bones.
- Individual variability: the effects of physical activity and exercise training show large variation between individuals due to genetic factors, age, gender, nutrition, and previous level and modes of physical activities. Given the same physical activity, some individuals may show no effects on aerobic fitness, blood pressure, or blood cholesterol, whereas others may have significant changes in these parameters. Therefore, the recommendations for exercise – intended for populations – should not be implemented broadly but instead should account for variability by tailoring the exercise program to the individual.

Guidelines for Aerobic Physical Activity

In 2008 the US Department of Health and Human Services issued guidelines of aerobic physical activity for adults (https://health.gov/paguidelines/2008/pdf/paguide.pdf). The complete guidelines included also statement on resistance exercise. In 2018 the second edition of the guidelines was issued based on the report and recommendations by the Physical Activity Guidelines Advisory Committee [73]. A summary of the new guidelines was published by Piercy et al. [74]. These guidelines update the previous ones issued in 2008 and expand them by including additional medical conditions for which strong or moderately strong scientific evidence supports physical activity. A summary of the key guidelines for adults, older adults, for women during pregnancy and the postpartum period, and for adults with a chronic health condition or a disability is shown below.

Key guidelines for adults:

- Adults should move more and sit less throughout the day. Some physical activity is better than none. Adults who sit less and do any amount of moderate-to-vigorous physical activity gain some health benefits.
- For substantial health benefits, adults should do at least 150 minutes (2 hours and 30 minutes) to 300 minutes (5 hours) a week of moderate-intensity (such as brisk walking), 75 minutes (1 hour and 15 minutes) to 150 minutes (2 hours and 30 minutes) a week of vigorous-intensity aerobic physical activity, or an equivalent combination of moderate- and vigorous-intensity aerobic activity. Preferably, the aerobic activity should be spread throughout the week.
- Additional health benefits are gained by doing physical activity beyond the equivalent of 300 minutes (5 hours) of moderate-intensity physical activity a week.
- Adults should also do muscle-strengthening activities of moderate or greater intensity that involve all major muscle groups on 2 or more days a week, as these activities provide additional health benefits.

Key guidelines for older adults:
The key guidelines for adults also apply to older adults. In addition, the following key guidelines are just for older adults:

- As part of their weekly physical activity, older adults should do multicomponent physical activity that includes balance training as well as aerobic and muscle-strengthening activities.
- Older adults should determine their level of effort for physical activity relative to their level of fitness.
- Older adults with chronic conditions should understand whether and how their conditions affect their ability to do regular physical activity safely.
- When older adults cannot do 150 minutes of moderate-intensity aerobic activity a week because of chronic conditions, they should be as physically active as their abilities and conditions allow.

Key guidelines for women during pregnancy and the postpartum period:

- Women should do at least 150 minutes (2 hours and 30 minutes) of moderate-intensity aerobic activity a week during pregnancy and the postpartum period. Preferably, aerobic activity should be spread throughout the week.
- Women who habitually engaged in vigorous-intensity aerobic activity or who were physically active before pregnancy can continue these activities during pregnancy and the postpartum period.
- Women who are pregnant should be under the care of a health-care practitioner who can monitor the progress of the pregnancy. Women who are pregnant can consult their health-care practitioner about whether or how to adjust their physical activity during pregnancy and after the child is born.

Key guidelines for adults with chronic health conditions and adults with disabilities:

- Adults with chronic conditions or disabilities, who are able, should do at least 150 minutes (2 hours and 30 minutes) to 300 minutes (5 hours) a week of moderate-intensity (such as walking on brisk pace for them), 75 minutes (1 hour and 15 minutes) to 150 minutes (2 hours and 30 minutes) a week of vigorous-intensity aerobic physical activity, or an equivalent combination of moderate- and vigorous-intensity aerobic activity. Preferably, aerobic activity should be spread throughout the week.

- Adults with chronic conditions or disabilities, who are able, should also do muscle-strengthening activities of moderate or greater intensity that involve all major muscle groups on 2 or more days a week, as these activities provide additional health benefits.
- When adults with chronic conditions or disabilities are not able to meet the above key guidelines, they should engage in regular physical activity according to their abilities and should avoid inactivity.
- Adults with chronic conditions or symptoms should be under the care of a health-care practitioner. People with chronic conditions can consult a health-care professional or physical activity specialist about the types and amounts of activity appropriate for their abilities and chronic conditions.

The key component of the recommended dose is the intensity of physical activity, light, moderate, and vigorous. The intensity can be assessed using objective and subjective measures and in relative and absolute terms. *Relative intensity* refers to the level of effort in relation to the person's maximal capacity required to do the activity. When using relative intensity, people pay attention to how physical activity affects their breathing and heart rate. The talk test is a simple way to measure relative intensity. In general, moderate-intensity activity allows one to talk, but not sing, during the activity. During vigorous-intensity activity, one is not able to say more than a few words without pausing for a breath.

Absolute intensity refers to the amount of energy the person uses per minute of activity, which is commonly expressed as oxygen consumption (VO2). At rest, while sitting quietly, the energy expenditure of a person is typically 3.5 ml/kg per minute or one metabolic unit (MET). Intensity of exercise can be expressed as multiples of the resting energy expenditure in METs. Physical activity requiring 1.6–3 METs is classified as light, 3 to less than 6 METs as moderate, and 6–10 METs as vigorous. Examples of moderate-intensity aerobic activity are walking briskly (3 miles per hour or faster, but not race-walking), bicycling slower than 10 miles per hour, water aerobics, general gardening, tennis (doubles), and ballroom dancing. Examples of vigorous aerobic activities include race-walking, jogging, or running, hiking uphill or with a heavy backpack, bicycling 10 miles per hour or faster, cross-country skiing, high-impact aerobics, heavy gardening (continuous digging or hoeing), snow clearing, swimming laps, tennis (singles), aerobic dancing, and jumping rope. More examples can be found in a comprehensive list of activities [1]. Other methods of measuring intensity of physical activity include various ways to measure and interpret heart rate during the activity and assessment of perceived exertion using some of the standardized rating scales such as the Borg scale [6]. Based on the scientific evidence published since 2008 and summarized below, the report of the Physical Activity Guidelines Advisory Committee emphasizes the value of reducing inactivity even if the 150- to 300-minute weekly target range is not achieved.

- For individuals who perform no or little moderate-to-vigorous physical activity, replacing sedentary behavior with light-intensity physical activity reduces the risk of all-cause mortality, cardiovascular disease incidence and mortality, and the incidence of type 2 diabetes. Before this report, evidence that light-intensity physical activity could provide health benefits had not been clearly stated.
- Individuals who perform no or little moderate-to-vigorous physical activity, no matter how much time they spend in sedentary behavior, can reduce their health risks by gradually adding some or more moderate-intensity physical activity.
- For individuals whose amount of moderate-to-vigorous physical activity is below the current public health target range of 150–300 minutes of moderate-intensity physical activity a week, even small increases in moderate-intensity physical activity provide health benefits. There is no threshold that must be exceeded before benefits begin to occur.

- For individuals whose physical activity is below the current public health target range, greater benefits can be achieved by reducing sedentary behavior, increasing moderate-intensity physical activity, or combinations of both.
- For any given increase in moderate-to-vigorous physical activity, the relative gain in benefits is greater for individuals who are below the current public health target range than for individuals already within the physical activity target range. For individuals below the target range, substantial reductions in risk are available with relatively small increases in moderate-intensity physical activity.
- Individuals already within the physical activity target range can gain more benefits by doing more moderate-to-vigorous physical activity. Individuals within the target range already have substantial benefits from their current volume of physical activity.
- Bouts, or episodes, of moderate-to-vigorous physical activity of any duration may be included in the daily accumulated total volume of physical activity. The 2008 guidelines recommended accumulating moderate-to-vigorous physical activity for 10 minutes or more, because insufficient evidence was available to support the value of activity duration less than 10 minutes. The 2018 Committee concludes that any length of moderate-to-vigorous physical activity contributes to the health benefits associated with the accumulated volume of physical activity. The recent systematic reviews and meta-analyses of Chastin et al. [8] and Amagasa et al. [2] came largely to the same conclusion.

In summary, the revised physical activity guidelines emphasize that some physical activity is better than none.

Health-Enhancing Effects of Aerobic Activities

During the past few decades, the list of the health and fitness benefits of aerobic physical activity has continuously lengthened, and the evidence supporting those benefits has strengthened. Strong or at least moderate scientific evidence indicates that practicing regular moderate-intensity aerobic physical activities such as walking and cycling is associated with a number of preventive benefits by decreasing the risk of many common diseases. A major part of these benefits is shown in Table 8.1. As a therapy, systematic and preferably supervised aerobic exercise training is often beneficial as part of the treatment or rehabilitation of conditions such as coronary artery disease, heart failure, stroke, peripheral arterial disease, obesity, type 2 diabetes, chronic obstructive pulmonary disease, breast, colon and other cancers, chronic kidney disease, fibromyalgia, low back pain, osteoarthritis of the knee and hip, cognitive impairment, dementia, depressive symptoms and depression, and anxiety. Importantly, in the large number of people that already have one or more chronic conditions, regular physical activity can reduce the risk of developing an additional condition, decrease the risk of progression of the existing condition(s), and improve functional capacity and quality of life [29, 36, 68, 71, 73, 82, 88].

Because a wide array of significant benefits for large numbers of adult and elderly people can be achieved with low cost, and relatively safe physical activity, some researchers have named exercise as "the Best Buy of Public Health" [58] or "the Real Polypill" [22]. In addition to the objectively measurable effects discussed above, physical activity and exercise cause several short- and long-term subjective, perceived effects such as improved well-being, relaxation, and stress tolerance. For large numbers of people, these perceived effects are the primary reasons to engage in physical activity or systematic exercise training. However, the scientific evidence to predict these effects especially at the individual level is weak because of the large number of poorly known and poorly understood temporary and long-term individual and environmental factors. Therefore, in physical activity counseling delivered in health-care systems, the biological effects are frequently emphasized rather than the quality of life benefits that may be most valued by the patients.

Table 8.1 Physical activity-related health benefits for the general population and selected populations [73]

Adults, all ages	
All-cause mortality	Lower risk
Cardiometabolic conditions	Lower cardiovascular incidence and mortality (including heart disease and stroke) Lower incidence of hypertension Lower incidence of type 2 diabetes
Cancer	Lower incidence of bladder, breast, colon, endometrium, esophagus, kidney, stomach, and lung cancers
Brain health	Reduced risk of dementia Improved cognitive function Improved cognitive function following bouts of aerobic activity Improved quality of life Improved sleep Reduced feelings of anxiety and depression in healthy people and in people with existing clinical syndromes Reduced incidence of depression
Weight status	Reduced risk of excessive weight gain Weight loss and the prevention of weight regain following initial weight loss when a sufficient dose of moderate-to-vigorous physical activity is attained An additive effect on weight loss when combined with moderate dietary restriction
Older adults	
Falls	Reduced incidence of falls Reduced incidence of fall-related injuries
Physical function	Improved physical function in older adults with and without frailty
Women who are pregnant or postpartum	
During pregnancy	Reduced risk of excessive weight gain Reduced risk of gestational diabetes No risk to fetus from moderate-intensity physical activity
During postpartum	Reduced risk of postpartum depression
Individuals with pre-existing medical conditions	
Breast cancer	Reduced risk of all-cause and breast cancer mortality
Colorectal cancer	Reduced risk of all-cause and colorectal cancer mortality
Prostate cancer	Reduced risk of prostate cancer mortality
Osteoarthritis	Decreased pain Improved function and quality of life
Hypertension	Reduced risk of progression of cardiovascular disease Reduced risk of increased blood pressure over time
Type 2 diabetes	Reduced risk of cardiovascular mortality Reduced progression of disease indicators: hemoglobin A1c, blood pressure, blood lipids, and body mass index
Multiple sclerosis	Improved walking Improved physical fitness
Dementia	Improved cognition
Some conditions with impaired executive function (attention deficit, hyperactivity disorder, schizophrenia, multiple sclerosis, Parkinson's disease, and stroke)	Improved cognition

Walking and Cycling Introduction

Walking is the basic mode of human movement and most prevalent physical activity. In some countries and in some population groups, cycling is also a common mode of movement. Both walking and cycling load mainly the lower extremities; beginning at low and moderate speed, they are nearly exclusively aerobic. As a result, on comparable dose of activity, the health- and performance-related effects of walking and cycling are in large extent similar. However, walking increases performance especially for various walking-type activities and cycling performance especially for activities including some modes of cycling. Both are used for utilities, transport, and leisure.

Walking and Cycling Evidence for Health Benefits

Scientific evidence supporting the benefits of walking comes largely from observational studies and is related especially to cardiovascular health [5, 32, 33, 41, 53, 59, 69] but also metabolic diseases and obesity [26, 40, 52], chronic low back pain [82, 88], chronic musculoskeletal pain [61], low bone mineral density at the femoral neck [51], and hip fracture [18]. Studies analyzing specifically the effects of walking interventions show significant positive effects on many cardiovascular risk factors and physical fitness. These changes are caused by widely varying walking programs and even by modest amounts and light intensity of walking [65]. Thus, the evidence from both observational and intervention studies supports the use of habitual walking as an effective and feasible health-enhancing physical activity.

Evidence of the health benefits of regular cycling has increased and strengthened gradually over time. These benefits are related mainly to cardiovascular, metabolic health, and performance capacity. They are caused especially by cycling done as a mode of transport [7, 12, 13, 23, 28, 30, 41, 42, 45, 62, 67, 76, 77, 81, 89]. At present the accumulated evidence indicates that regular cycling, included in part as a convenient form of transport, offers possibilities to significantly enhance health and fitness.

In the context of many similarities, there are also important differences between walking and cycling. Walking is a natural, inherited way of moving on any solid ground without need of any technology or equipment for most ambulatory patients. For healthy adults, safe walking requires very little attention. The complexity of the synchronized movement pattern is perceptible only to those individuals with deficient muscular coordination, joint disorders, or neurological deficits. Thus, walking can be practiced by most people and in a large variety of environmental conditions, suggesting the potential to increase walking as a large-scale population health intervention. However, in order to attract great numbers of people to choose walking for transport or leisure, the environment must meet several perceived and objective requirements for "walkability" [43, 44, 83, 87].

Bicycling, on the other hand, is a specifically learned skill to move, and it requires use of technology and usually smooth and solid ground. Especially in an urban environment, safe bicycling requires at least intermittent practice, adequate vision, hearing and balance, ability to react promptly, and knowledge of traffic rules and flow. In addition, in order to be a safe and feasible mode of travel, cycling requires special infrastructure [21, 72]. If these conditions are met, the proportion of cyclists in the population may be as large as seen in the Netherlands, for example [19]. Moreover, the accessible distances covered by cycling are much longer than by walking. Cycling is a secondary mode of moving in industrialized societies, but the potential to increase cycling is impressive.

Safety of Cycling

In cycling, the risk of injury is a major concern. However, the health risks of cycling are counterbalanced by health benefits [60, 79]. Furthermore, the risk of accidents in cycling increases less than proportionally to traffic volume for motor vehicles, pedestrians, and cyclists. Thus, when the amount of walking increases by 100%, injuries related to walking increase by 51%, but when cycling increases by 100%, the injuries increase by 43% [15]. Safety of bicycling can be most effectively increased by simultaneously targeting the traffic environment, bicycles, and cyclists, although simple and separate measures alone can substantially decrease the risk of accidents. Thus, evidence from randomized controlled trials show that continuous use of running light decreased accidents leading to injury by 47% overall, wearing a yellow bicycle jacket or other fluorescent cycling garment decreased injuries by 77%, and also reduced the incidence rate for multiparty accidents with personal injury by 38% [46].

The value of using a bicycle helmet is supported by two recent meta-analyses that concluded use decreases overall head injury by 43%, serious head injury by 60%, and cyclist mortality or seriously injury by 34% without serious adverse effects [37, 66]. These studies conclude that use of helmet is highly recommended, especially in situations with an increased risk of single bicycle crashes, such as on slippery or icy roads.

Scalability of Walking and Cycling

In most countries and communities, promoting large increases of both walking and cycling requires substantial and at least in part similar changes in the environmental conditions. Increasing both walking and cycling enhances benefits to individuals in terms of improved health and fitness, decreased risks, and travel costs and time as well as benefits to societies in terms of improved environment, less pollution, and more efficient transport systems [34, 60]. Therefore, the policies and interventions aimed at increasing either regular walking or cycling as modes of transportation act synergistically to enhance conditions for both "walkability" and "bikeability."

Walking and cycling can be done in several modes and for various reasons that widen the possibilities and increase the interest to practice them by different people for different purposes in different environments. Particularly important modes are walking and cycling for transport, because in general they meet the requirements of health-enhancing physical activity in terms of frequency and intensity, and they can make a substantial component or even total amount of the recommended physical activity for most of the year [89]. Substantial scientific evidence supports the potential of walking and especially of cycling for transport as health-enhancing physical activity [7, 13, 23, 30, 41, 45, 60, 67, 76, 77].

Walking and Cycling Variations

Some forms of walking are treadmill-, stair-, mall-, and dog-walking, and the American Medical Association has recommended even "doc-walking" or walking with your doctor [11], pole or Nordic walking, and walking in water. Some of these modes of walking can be incorporated into the daily life of large numbers of people. Treadmill-walking in gym or at home offers possibilities for convenient, safe, and accurately controllable exercise. Stair-walking has been shown to be feasible and effective in improving aerobic fitness and cardiovascular disease risk factors [16, 38, 54], and evidence supports effectiveness of interventions to increase use of stairs [39]. Malls provide safe, accessible, and affordable exercise environments for middle-aged and older adults [17], and detailed guidance on planning, organizing, and using malls for walking is available [9]. A systematic review concluded that 2 in 3 dog owners who walk their dogs are more than 2.5 times more likely to achieve at least 150 mins/week of moderate physical activity compared to non-dog walkers [84]. Pole or Nordic walking adds the muscles of the upper body to the activity, "walking on four legs," may increase the energy expenditure by about one fifth compared to ordinary walking if the poles are used effectively, helps to walk uphill and downhill, supports balance, may decrease loading of the hips, and increases self-confidence in walking [24, 85]. In water-walking the buoyancy takes off about 90% of the body weight, but on the other hand, water increases resistance to movement by about 40% [4]. In addition, water-walking supports joints and balance, and walking in warm water relaxes muscles and mind. Thus, walking, cycling, and other aquatic aerobic activities offer possibilities for effective, safe, and enjoyable physical activity that also may be appropriate for people who have joint disease or mobility limitations.

In addition to cycling outdoors, it can be practiced indoors at home or in gyms as well as in water in the same way as walking. An emerging mode of cycling is the use of electrically assisted bikes. Particularly for elderly people, they offer a feasible mode to cycle for leisure and especially for transport. However, the probability of accidents is increased, and the injuries in accidents are more severe than in accidents on ordinary bike [20].

Other Aerobic Activities

In addition to walking and cycling, other aerobic activities include jogging and running, swimming, cross-country and roller skiing, orienteering, ordinary and roller skating, rowing, canoeing, many forms of dancing, and aerobics in gyms. Many recreationally practiced ballgames such as tennis, badminton, squash, golf, and football are in part aerobic. Currently there is considerable evidence, although fragmentary and of low quality, on the potential health benefits of most aerobic physical activities. A recent review involving 26 different sports disciplines and all major aerobic disciplines found conditional evidence that recreational football and running are associated with health and performance-related benefits, but the evidence for the health benefits of other disciplines was either inconclusive or tenuous [63]. The performance- and health-enhancing effects of running are substantially supported by the findings of recent reviews [35, 48]. The rather surprising results of Oja et al. [63] were mainly due to lack of sufficient high-quality studies. However, absence of evidence is not evidence of absence. More scientifically rigorous studies would probably change the findings.

Indeed, an observational study on a large British adult population cohort found that participation in swimming, basketball, and aerobics (aerobics, keep fit, gymnastics, and dance for fitness) was associated with reduced all-cause and cardiovascular mortality and participation in cycling with all-cause mortality [64]. Further analyses suggested that compared with meeting the generic physical activity guidelines, participation in any sport appeared to be equally protective for all-cause and cardiovascular mortality. In practical terms, this means that at least regarding these outcomes it is not important which aerobic sports one participates, but rather the frequency, intensity, duration, regularity, and continuity of the recreation should meet the criteria of effective aerobic physical activity. On physiological grounds it is highly probable that individuals practicing the aerobic activities mentioned above, e.g., swimming, racket sports, dancing, cross-country skiing, orienteering, skating, and rowing would gain largely the same general health benefits compared to walking and cycling (for transport) on the condition that the training regimens are comparable. Indeed, the 2008 physical activity guidelines recommend tennis, swimming laps, and gardening as health-enhancing aerobic activities. Furthermore, the 2018 Physical Activity Guidelines Advisory Committee Scientific Report as well as the systematic reviews and meta-analyses of Amagasa et al. [2], Chastin et al. [8] emphasize the role of light and short bouts of physical activity. In conclusion, in advising individuals on health-enhancing physical activity, it is justifiable to suggest any aerobic physical activity as either the sole or main activity or in many cases as supplementary activity on the condition that all aspects of the FITT principle of physical activity are met.

Counseling for Aerobic Physical Activity

Insufficient physical activity (PA) is highly prevalent worldwide. In the USA, 40% of adults do not meet the minimum recommended amount of physical activity, when the cumulative activity done at work, at home, for transport, and during leisure is included. Furthermore, the prevalence of insufficient physical activity is increasing [31]. In order to increase PA among the more than 70 million insufficiently active adult Americans [91], interventions are needed immediately and in longer term. One measure that can be immediately used is individual counseling in the health-care system.

Evidence from recent systematic reviews by the US Preventive Services Task Force support lifestyle counseling by health-care professionals to promote PA especially for individuals with CVD risk factors [49] but also for those without CVD or its risk factors [70].

The American Heart Association recommends assessment and promotion of physical activity in health-care settings using brief counseling [50]. This approach has been shown to have a small to moderate positive effect on increasing physical activity levels, at least in the short term. The results have been better when interventions include multiple behavior change resources and target insufficiently active patients with cardiovascular disease risk factors and motivational readiness to change. The number needed to treat for one sedentary adult to meet physical activity recommendations at 1 year was 12. This is comparable to other preventive counseling interventions in primary care such as alcohol (number needed to treat, 9.1) and smoking cessation (number needed to treat, 14). The results can be somewhat improved by integrating the counseling to referral of patients to community-based physical activity resources and programs [50]. Brief advice has been found to be also cost-effective [27, 50]. However, the long-term effectiveness of brief counseling is not well studied [47].

Achieving more durable results would require use of evidence-based approaches that require more resources and lengthy processes such as the transtheoretical model of behavior change [75] or the more recent Behavior Change Wheel [55]. Successful application of these techniques calls for systems approach at least in the health-care units using them [90].

The following discussion is limited to general aspects relevant to brief counseling on aerobic physical activity in the health-care setting. Detailed information for prescribing physical activity and exercise for single diagnoses can be obtained in other sources [25, 36, 71].

A feasible and evidence-based behavioral strategy used widely in counseling for smoking cessation, obesity management, and physical activity promotion is the five A's model: ask, assess, advise, agree, and assist [80, 86]. These A's relate to behavior change theories such as self-management support, readiness assessment, behavior modification, and self-efficacy enhancement.

The first A, Ask, opens the counseling by asking in nonjudgmental way, preferably using the motivational interview technique, about the patient's physical activity behavior and exploring his/her readiness to change it.

The second A, Assess, includes assessment of the patient's PA level habits and health status. Physical activity is recommended to be assessed routinely in medical care as one of the "vital signs" [80], by asking standardized questions such as "On average, how many days per week do you engage in moderate or greater intensity physical activity (like a brisk walk)?" and "On average, how many minutes do you engage in this physical activity on those days?" or objectively using the wearable devices or smartphones [50]. In addition, the major drivers, barriers, and social and other sources of support helping to begin and maintain physical activity are important aspects to explore.

The patient's health status and eventual risks related to physical activity can be assessed by following the ACSM's recommendations for exercise preparticipation health screening [78] or by using the Canadian approach [10].

The third A, Advise, may include discussion of the benefits of physical activity, appropriate regimens to gain them, and relevant aspects that help to increase physical activity.

The A for Agree includes joint explicit acceptance by the patient and physician of the goals and means to increase physical activity. The SMART framework is useful in setting the goals so that they are specific, measurable, achievable, rewarding, and timely for the patient [14].

The A for Assist may include identifying the facilitators and barriers that influence the possibilities the patient has to realize the plan, education, recommendation, and support by the physician on the means and resources that the patient may use [9, 56, 91].

Counseling on Walking and Cycling

In order to lead to adoption or increase of regular physical activity and to its intended benefits, it should meet the APEASE criteria: acceptability, practicability, effectiveness/cost-effectiveness, affordability, safety/side-effects, and equity [3]. Walking is an activity that meets these criteria in large, probably in the largest number of insufficiently active adults. In general, most adults who have not engaged regularly in moderate-to-vigorous physical activity will benefit from walking that is brisk for them. The simplest and potentially most efficient physical activity advice for fitness and health for a great number of adults, and especially for elderly and sick people, might be "keep walking."

Walking is especially indicated as the core habitual physical activity. Walking is an irreplaceable mode for moving around for many hours a day while doing the daily chores, at work and in transport. For most people without serious illnesses, there are no good reasons to minimize the number of steps at home or at work. Especially for elderly and for the chronically ill, rising from the seated position, breaking continuous sitting, and walking at home are important and may be the only accessible PA that helps maintain mobility, independence, and self-confidence. The newly acquired knowledge of the benefits of even light activity in short bouts for otherwise inactive individuals strengthens this concept [2, 73].

Some alternatives to walk in daily life and their effects on health and performance capacity were described above and include domestic chores, walking up or down stairs and escalator, Nordic or pole walking, walking the dog, "doc-walking," running to errands, and walking as part of commuting. Naturally, walks in parks, forests, along marked routes and trails, alone or in company, as such or as part of other activities such as photography or picking fruits or vegetables are excellent examples of alternatives. Information on community-based programs as well as tools and resources related to walking and other health-enhancing physical activities are available at https://millionhearts.hhs.gov/tools-protocols/tools/physical-activity.html [57].

Regular cycling is an effective health-enhancing physical activity as described above. However, in physical activity counseling, cycling can be suggested as well-fitting physical activity much less often than walking because all APEASE criteria are not met due to personal or environmental reasons. However, when these criteria are fulfilled, cycling is highly recommended especially as a mode of regular commuting.

Conclusions

There is great need to increase walking and cycling, because the evidence on their health-enhancing effects is strong and they have the largest potential to decrease the physical activity gap. Much progress could be made by effective communication of the individual and societal value of these simple modes of physical activity and their many feasible variations. In messaging, the health-care professional has great potential that should be fully leveraged. At the same time, there is great need to develop an environment and services to meet the criteria for adequate "walkability" and "bikeability," especially in underserved areas. Promotion of walking and cycling by large-scale, comprehensive, and collaborative measures offers feasible and cost-effective means to improve individual, population, and environmental health.

References

1. Ainsworth BE, Haskell WL, Herrmann SD, et al. Compendium of physical activities: a second update of codes and MET values. Med Sci Sports Exerc. 2011;43:1575–81.
2. Amagasa S, Machida M, Fukushima N, et al. Is objectively measured light-intensity physical activity associated with health outcomes after adjustment for moderate-to-vigorous physical activity in adults? A systematic review. Int J Behav Nutr Phys Act. 2018;15:65.
3. Atkins L. Using the behaviour change wheel in infection prevention and control practice. J Infect Prev. 2016;17:74–8.
4. Becker BE. Aquatic therapy: scientific foundations and clinical rehabilitation applications. PMR. 2009;1:859–72.
5. Boone-Heinonen J, Evenson KR, Taber DR, Gordon-Larsen P. Walking for prevention of cardiovascular disease in men and women: a systematic review of observational studies. Obes Rev. 2009;10:204–17.
6. Borg G. Perceived exertion as an indicator of somatic stress. Scand J Rehabil Med. 1970;2:92–8.
7. Celis-Morales CA, Lyall DM, Welsh P, et al. Association between active commuting and incident cardiovascular disease, cancer, and mortality: prospective cohort study. BMJ. 2017;357:j1456.
8. Chastin SFM, De Craemer M, De Cocker K, et al. How does light-intensity physical activity associate with adult cardiometabolic health and mortality? Systematic review with meta-analysis of experimental and observational studies. Br J Sports Med. 2018;53(6):370–6.
9. https://www.cdc.gov/physicalactivity/downloads/mallwalking-guide.pdf. Accessed 12 Nov 2018.
10. http://www.csep.ca/en/publications/get-active-questionnaire. Accessed Nov 2018.
11. Dan BB. Walk with your doc. JAMA. 1988;13(259):2743–4.
12. Dinu M, Pagliai G, Macchi C, Sofi F. Active commuting and multiple health outcomes: a systematic review and meta-analysis. Sports Med. 2018;49:437. https://doi.org/10.1007/s40279-018-1023-0.
13. Dons E, Rojas-Rueda D, Anaya-Boig E, et al. Transport mode choice and body mass index: cross-sectional and longitudinal evidence from a European-wide study. Environ Int. 2018;119:109–16.
14. Doran GT. There's a S.M.A.R.T. Way to write management's goals and objectives. Manag Rev. 1981;70:35–6.
15. Elvik R, Björnskau T. Safety-in-numbers: a systematic review and meta-analysis of evidence. Saf Sci. 2017;92:274–82.
16. Fardy PS, Ilmarinen J. Evaluating the effects and feasibility of an at work stairclimbing intervention program for men. Med Sci Sports. 1975;7:91–3.
17. Farren L, Belza B, Allen P, et al. Mall walking program environments, features, and participants: a scoping review. Prev Chronic Dis. 2015;12:E129.
18. Feskanich D, Willett W, Colditz G. Walking and leisure-time activity and risk of hip fracture in postmenopausal women. JAMA. 2002;288:2300–6.
19. Fishman E, Schepers P, Kamphuis CB. Dutch cycling: quantifying the health and related economic benefits. Am J Public Health. 2015;105:e13–5.
20. Fishman E, Cherry C. E-bikes in the mainstream: reviewing a decade of research. Transp Rev. 2016;36(1):72–91.
21. Fraser SD, Lock K. Cycling for transport and public health: a systematic review of the effect of the environment on cycling. Eur J Pub Health. 2011;21:738–43.
22. Fiuza-Luces C, Garatachea N, Berger NA, Lucia S. Exercise is the real polypill. Physiology. 2013;28:330–58.
23. Flint E, Webb E, Cummins S. Change in commute mode and body-mass index: prospective, longitudinal evidence from UK biobank. Lancet Public Health. 2016;1:e46–55.
24. Fritschi JO, Brown WJ, Laukkanen R, van Uffelen JG. The effects of pole walking on health in adults: a systematic review. Scand J Med Sci Sports. 2012;22:e70–8.
25. http://www.fyss.se/in-english/chapters-in-fyss/. Accessed 12 Nov 2018.
26. Gao HL, Gao HX, Sun FM, Zhang L. Effects of walking on body composition in perimenopausal and postmenopausal women: a systematic review and meta-analysis. Menopause. 2016;23:928–34.
27. GC V, Wilson EC, Suhrcke M, et al. Are brief interventions to increase physical activity cost-effective? A systematic review. Br J Sports Med. 2016;50:408–17.

28. de Geus B, Joncheere J, Meeusen R. Commuter cycling: effect on physical performance in untrained men and women in Flanders: minimum dose to improve indexes of fitness. Scand J Med Sci Sports. 2009;19:179–87.
29. Gheysen F, Poppe L, DeSmet A, et al. Physical activity to improve cognition in older adults: can physical activity programs enriched with cognitive challenges enhance the effects? A systematic review and meta-analysis. Int J Behav Nutr Phys Act. 2018;15:63.
30. Grøntved A, Koivula RW, Johansson I, et al. Bicycling to work and primordial prevention of cardiovascular risk: cohort study among Swedish men and women. J Am Heart Assoc. 2016;5(11):pii: e004413.
31. Guthold R, Stevens GA, Riley LM, Bull FC. Worldwide trends in insufficient physical activity from 2001 to 2016: a pooled analysis of 358 population-based surveys with 1·9 million participants. Lancet Glob Health. 2018;6:e1077–86.
32. Hamer M, Chida Y. Walking and primary prevention: a meta-analysis of prospective cohort studies. Br J Sports Med. 2008;42:238–43.
33. Hanson S, Jones A. Is there evidence that walking groups have health benefits? A systematic review and meta-analysis. Br J Sports Med. 2015;49:710–5.
34. http://www.heatwalkingcycling.org/#homepage. Accessed 12 Nov 2018.
35. Hespanhol Junior LC, Pillay JD, van Mechelen W, Verhagen E. Meta-analyses of the effects of habitual running on indices of health in physically inactive adults. Sports Med. 2015;45:1455–68.
36. Hoffmann TC, Maher CG, Briffa T, et al. Prescribing exercise interventions for patients with chronic conditions. CMAJ. 2016;188:510–8.
37. Høye A. Bicycle helmets – to wear or not to wear? A meta-analyses of the effects of bicycle helmets on injuries. Accid Anal Prev. 2018;117:85–97.
38. Ilmarinen J, Ilmarinen R, Koskela A, et al. Training effects of stair-climbing during office hours on female employees. Ergonomics. 1979;22:507–16.
39. Jennings CA, Yun L, Loitz CC, Lee EY, Mummery WK. A systematic review of interventions to increase stair use. Am J Prev Med. 2017;52:106–14.
40. Jeon CY, Lokken RP, Hu FB, van Dam RM. Physical activity of moderate intensity and risk of type 2 diabetes: a systematic review. Diabetes Care. 2007;30:744–52.
41. Kelly P, Kahlmeier S, Götschi T, et al. Systematic review and meta-analysis of reduction in all-cause mortality from walking and cycling and shape of dose response relationship. Int J Behav Nutr Phys Act. 2014;11:132.
42. Kelly P, Williamson C, Niven AG, Hunter R, Mutrie N, Richards J. Walking on sunshine: scoping review of the evidence for walking and mental health. Br J Sports Med. 2018;52:800–6.
43. Kerr J, Emond JA, Badland H, et al. Perceived neighborhood environmental attributes associated with walking and cycling for transport among adult residents of 17 cities in 12 countries: the IPEN study. Environ Health Perspect. 2016;124:290–8.
44. Kärmeniemi M, Lankila T, Ikäheimo T, Koivumaa-Honkanen H, Korpelainen R. The built environment as a determinant of physical activity: a systematic review of longitudinal studies and natural experiments. Ann Behav Med. 2018;52:239–51.
45. Knott CS, Panter J, Foley L, Ogilvie D. Changes in the mode of travel to work and the severity of depressive symptoms: a longitudinal analysis of UK Biobank. Prev Med. 2018;112:61–9.
46. Lahrmann H, Madsen TKO, Olesen AV. Randomized trials and self-reported accidents as a method to study safety-enhancing measures for cyclists-two case studies. Accid Anal Prev. 2018;114:17–24.
47. Lamming L, Pears S, Mason D, et al. What do we know about brief interventions for physical activity that could be delivered in primary care consultations? A systematic review of reviews. Prev Med. 2017;99:152–63.
48. Lee DC, Brellenthin AG, Thompson PD, Sui X, Lee IM, Lavie CJ. Running as a key lifestyle medicine for longevity. Prog Cardiovasc Dis. 2017;60:45–55.
49. Lin JS, O'Connor E, Evans CV, Senger CA, Rowland MG, Groom HC. Behavioral counseling to promote a healthy lifestyle in persons with cardiovascular risk factors: a systematic review for the U.S. Preventive Services Task Force. Ann Intern Med. 2014;161:568–78.
50. Lobelo F, Rohm Young D, Sallis R, et al. Routine assessment and promotion of physical activity in healthcare settings: a scientific statement from the American Heart Association. Circulation. 2018;137:e495–522.
51. Ma D, Wu L, He Z. Effects of walking on the preservation of bone mineral density in perimenopausal and postmenopausal women: a systematic review and meta-analysis. Menopause. 2013;20:1216–26.
52. Mabire L, Mani R, Liu L, Mulligan H, Baxter D. The influence of age, sex and body mass index on the effectiveness of brisk walking for obesity management in adults: a systematic review and meta-analysis. J Phys Act Health. 2017;14:389–407.
53. McDermott MM. Exercise training for intermittent claudication. J Vasc Surg. 2017;66:1612–20.
54. Meyer P, Kayser B, Mach F. Stair use for cardiovascular disease prevention. Eur J Cardiovasc Prev Rehabil. 2009;16(Suppl 2):S17–8.

55. Michie S, van Stralen MM, West R. The behaviour change wheel: a new method for characterising and designing behaviour change interventions. Implement Sci. 2011;6:42.
56. https://millionhearts.hhs.gov/tools-protocols/index.html. Accessed 12 Nov 2018.
57. https://millionhearts.hhs.gov/tools-protocols/tools/physical-activity.html. Accessed 12 Nov 2018.
58. Morris JN. Exercise in the prevention of coronary heart disease: today's best buy in public health. Med Sci Sports Exerc. 1994;26:807–14.
59. Morris JN, Hardman AE. Walking for health. Sports Med. 1997;23:306–32.
60. Mueller N, Rojas-Rueda D, Cole-Hunter T, et al. Health impact assessment of active transportation: a systematic review. Prev Med. 2015;76:103–14.
61. O'Connor SR, Tully MA, Ryan B, et al. Walking exercise for chronic musculoskeletal pain: systematic review and meta-analysis. Arch Phys Med Rehabil. 2015;96:724–734.e3.
62. Oja P, Titze S, Bauman A, et al. Health benefits of cycling: a systematic review. Scand J Med Sci Sports. 2011;21:496–509.
63. Oja P, Titze S, Kokko S, et al. Health benefits of different sport disciplines for adults: systematic review of observational and intervention studies with meta-analysis. Br J Sports Med. 2015;49:434–40.
64. Oja P, Kelly P, Pedisic Z, et al. Associations of specific types of sports and exercise with all-cause and cardiovascular-disease mortality: a cohort study of 80 306 British adults. Br J Sports Med. 2017;51:812–7.
65. Oja P, Kelly P, Murtagh EM, Murphy MH, Foster C, Titze S. Effects of frequency, intensity, duration and volume of walking interventions on CVD risk factors: a systematic review and meta-regression analysis of randomised controlled trials among inactive healthy adults. Br J Sports Med. 2018;52:769–75.
66. Olivier J, Creighton P. Bicycle injuries and helmet use: a systematic review and meta-analysis. Int J Epidemiol. 2017;46:278–92.
67. Panter J, Mytton O, Sharp S, et al. Using alternatives to the car and risk of all-cause, cardiovascular and cancer mortality. Heart. 2018;104:1749–55.
68. Pasanen T, Tolvanen S, Heinonen A, Kujala UM. Exercise therapy for functional capacity in chronic diseases: an overview of meta-analyses of randomised controlled trials. Br J Sports Med. 2017;51:1459–65.
69. Patel AV, Hildebrand JS, Leach CR, et al. Walking in relation to mortality in a large prospective cohort of older U.S. adults. Am J Prev Med. 2018;54:10–9.
70. Patnode CD, Evans CV, Senger CA, Redmond N, Lin JS. Behavioral counseling to promote a healthful diet and physical activity for cardiovascular disease prevention in adults without known cardiovascular disease risk factors: updated evidence report and systematic review for the US Preventive Services Task Force. JAMA. 2017;318:175–93.
71. Pedersen BK, Saltin B. Exercise as medicine – evidence for prescribing exercise as therapy in 26 different chronic diseases. Scand J Med Sci Sports. 2015;25(Suppl 3):1–72.
72. Pedroso FE, Angriman F, Bellows AL, Taylor K. Bicycle use and cyclist safety following Boston's bicycle infrastructure expansion, 2009–2012. Am J Public Health. 2016;106:2171–7.
73. 2018 Physical Activity Guidelines Advisory Committee. 2018 physical activity guidelines advisory committee scientific report. Washington, DC: US Department of Health and Human Services; 2018.
74. Piercy KL, Troiano RP, Ballard RM, et al. The physical activity guidelines for Americans. JAMA. 2018;320:2020–8.
75. Prochaska JO, Velicer WF. The transtheoretical model of health behavior change. Am J Health Promot. 1997;12:38–48.
76. Rasmussen MG, Grøntved A, Blond K, et al. Associations between recreational and commuter cycling, changes in cycling, and type 2 diabetes risk: a cohort study of Danish men and women. PLoS Med. 2016;13:e1002076.
77. Rasmussen MG, Overvad K, Tjønneland A, Jensen MK, Østergaard L, Grøntved A. Changes in cycling and incidence of overweight and obesity among Danish men and women. Med Sci Sports Exerc. 2018;50:1413–21.
78. Riebe D, Franklin BA, Thompson PD, et al. Updating ACSM's recommendations for exercise preparticipation health screening. Med Sci Sports Exerc. 2015;47:2473–9.
79. Rojas-Rueda D, de Nazelle A, Tainio M, Nieuwenhuijsen MJ. The health risks and benefits of cycling in urban environments compared with car use: health impact assessment study. BMJ. 2011;343:d4521.
80. Sallis RE, Matuszak JM, Baggish AL, et al. Call to action on making physical activity assessment and prescription a medical standard of care. Curr Sports Med Rep. 2016;15:207–14.
81. Saunders LE, Green JM, Petticrew MP, Steinbach R, Roberts H. What are the health benefits of active travel? A systematic review of trials and cohort studies. PLoS One. 2013;8(8):e69912.
82. Sitthipornvorakul E, Klinsophon T, Sihawong R, Janwantanakul P. The effects of walking intervention in patients with chronic low back pain: a meta-analysis of randomized controlled trials. Musculoskelet Sci Pract. 2018;34:38–46.
83. Smith M, Hosking J, Woodward A, et al. Systematic literature review of built environment effects on physical activity and active transport – an update and new findings on health equity. Int J Behav Nutr Phys Act. 2017;14:158.
84. Soares J, Epping JN, Owens CJ, et al. Odds of getting adequate physical activity by dog walking. J Phys Act Health. 2015;12(Suppl 1):S102–9.

85. Tschentscher M, Niederseer D, Niebauer J. Health benefits of Nordic walking: a systematic review. Am J Prev Med. 2013;44:76–84.
86. Vallis M, Piccinini-Vallis H, Sharma AM, Freedhoff Y. Clinical review: modified 5 as: minimal intervention for obesity counseling in primary care. Can Fam Physician. 2013;59:27–31.
87. Van Cauwenberg J, Nathan A, Barnett A, Barnett DW, Cerin E, Council on Environment and Physical Activity (CEPA)-Older Adults Working Group. Relationships between neighbourhood physical environmental attributes and older adults' leisure-time physical activity: a systematic review and meta-analysis. Sports Med. 2018;48:1635–60.
88. Vanti C, Andreatta S, Borghi S, Guccione AA, Pillastrini P, Bertozzi L. The effectiveness of walking versus exercise on pain and function in chronic low back pain: a systematic review and meta-analysis of randomized trials. Disabil Rehabil. 2017;5:1–11.
89. Vuori IM, Oja P, Paronen O. Physically active commuting to work – testing its potential for exercise promotion. Med Sci Sports Exerc. 1994;26:844–50.
90. Vuori IM, Lavie CJ, Blair SN. Physical activity promotion in the health care system. Mayo Clin Proc. 2013;88:1446–61.
91. Wright JS, Wall HK, Ritchey MD. Million hearts 2022: small steps are needed for cardiovascular disease prevention. JAMA. 2018;320:1857–8.

Chapter 9
Resistance Activities

Jared M. Gollie and Michael O. Harris-Love

Keywords Resistance training · Muscle strength · Aging · Exercise · Sarcopenia · Frailty

Key Points
- The maintenance of neuromuscular health is essential for healthy aging, quality of life, and independence.
- The prescription of resistance activities is an effective treatment for enhancing neuromuscular capacity and physical function with aging.
- Principles of specificity, overload, variation, reversibility, and individuality can be used to inform the design of resistance exercise interventions.
- In addition to healthy older adults, engaging in resistance activities offers numerous health benefits for individuals living with various chronic conditions such as diabetes, cardiovascular disease, and chronic kidney disease.
- Monitoring strategies enhance both adherence and efficacy of resistance activities and provide valuable information to be used by the health-care team to make timely and informed decisions regarding modifications to the prescribe resistance exercise program.

J. M. Gollie (✉)
Muscle Morphology, Mechanics and Performance Laboratory, Human Performance Research Unit, Clinical Research Center, Veterans Affairs Medical Center, Washington, DC, USA

Department of Health, Human Function, and Rehabilitation Sciences, School of Medicine & Health Sciences, The George Washington University, Washington, DC, USA
e-mail: jgollie@gwu.edu

M. O. Harris-Love
Director, Physical Therapy Program, University of Colorado Anschutz Medical Campus, Aurora, CO, USA

Eastern Colorado Geriatric Research Education and Clinical Center, Rocky Mountain Regional VA Medical Center, Aurora, CO, USA
e-mail: Michael.Harris-Love@va.gov

© Springer Nature Switzerland AG 2020
J. Uribarri, J. A. Vassalotti (eds.), *Nutrition, Fitness, and Mindfulness*, Nutrition and Health, https://doi.org/10.1007/978-3-030-30892-6_9

Introduction

As the aging population continues to grow, the ability to maintain or slow the decline in neuromuscular health is essential for the prevention of disability, disease, and premature death. The primary role of the neuromuscular system is the production of force required to perform functional activities. In addition, recent evidence has posited skeletal muscle as an endocrine organ implicated in the promotion of systemic health enhancing effects in response to physical activity. However, adverse changes in skeletal muscle due to physical inactivity may result in endocrine-like responses that contribute to many chronic diseases [44]. Reductions in neuromuscular function and skeletal muscle mass are experienced during the aging process with exponential declines reported to occur around the sixth and seventh decades [2, 28, 38, 66]. The declines in neuromuscular capacity impede upon functional capabilities contributing to limitations in activities of daily living and loss of independence (Fig. 9.1) [73]. Therapeutic interventions to maintain or improve neuromuscular health and function are likely to have a profound effect on reducing the incidence of disability during the later years of life.

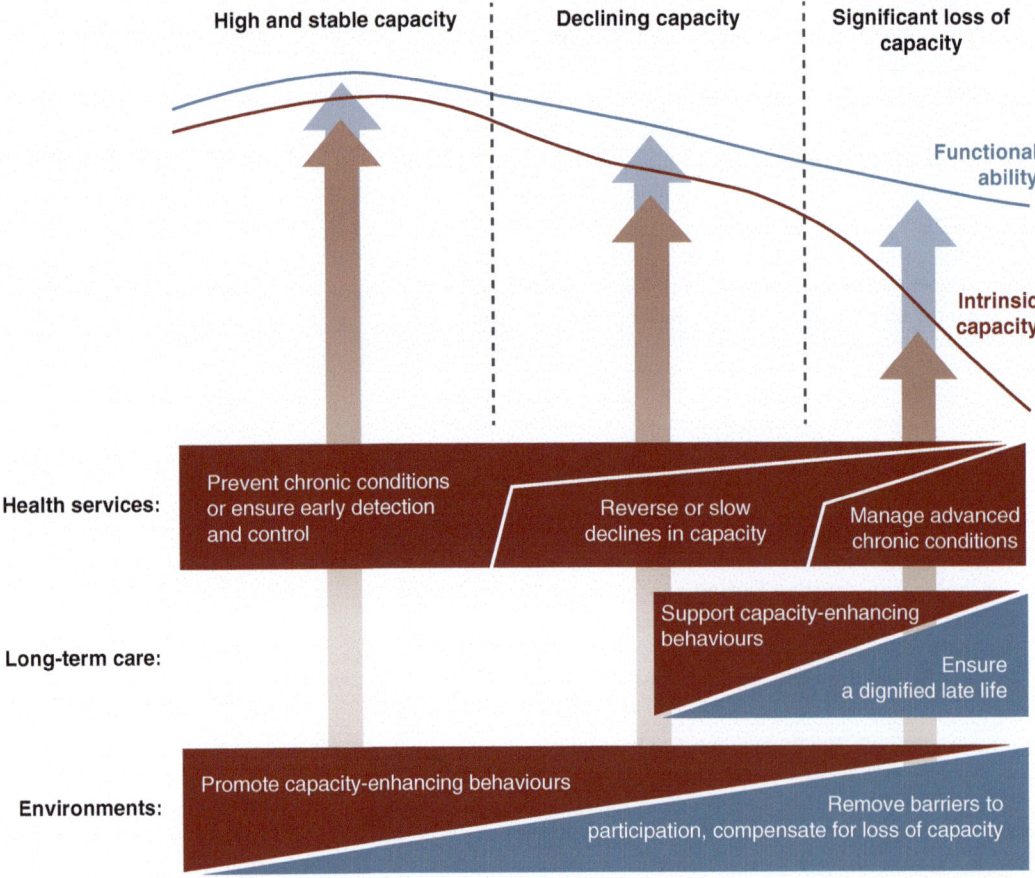

Fig. 9.1 A public health framework for *healthy aging*: opportunities for public health action across the life course proposed by the World Health Organization's *World Report on Health and Aging* [73]

Definition and Characteristics of Resistance Activities

Resistance activities are an effective treatment for maintaining and improving neuromuscular health and physical function. Resistance activities refer to any activity capable of overloading the neuromuscular system to promote specific neuromuscular adaptations [3, 21, 47]. The type, magnitude, and rate of neuromuscular adaptations are dependent on both non-modifiable (e.g., age and gender) and modifiable (e.g., resistance activity workload and modality) factors. Common modalities under the category of resistance activities include weight machines, free weights (dumbbells or barbell), resistance tubing/bands, pneumatic machines, aquatic activities, yoga, and body-weight exercises. Additionally, devices such as neuromuscular electrical stimulation can be used in clinical settings to apply an overload stimulus to maintain or improve muscular health when volitional activity is not possible. For the purposes of this chapter, weight machines, free weights, resistance tubing/bands, pneumatic machines, and body-weight exercises for the prevention of neuromuscular deterioration with aging and disease will be discussed. However, the information provided in section "Prescription of Resistance Activities" is applicable to all activities outlined above as well as to the younger adult.

Neuromuscular Adaptations to Resistance Activities in Older Adults and Chronic Diseases

Aging and the Neuromuscular System

Older adults are more susceptible to clinical syndromes of frailty and sarcopenia due to age-related alterations in the neuromuscular system. Frailty is a state of increased vulnerability to poor resolution of homeostasis after a stress-induced event, which increases the risk of adverse outcomes, including falls, delirium, and disability [14]. Sarcopenia has been characterized as the progressive and generalized loss of skeletal muscle mass and strength with a risk of adverse outcomes such as physical disability, poor quality of life, and death [16] and is considered to be a key component of frailty [14]. Using the World Health Organization's (WHO) definition, healthy aging is the process of developing and maintaining the functional ability that enables well-being in older age [73]. However, in the presence of injury or disease, and without appropriate access to medical resources, declines in physical capacity are accelerated (Fig. 9.2). Thus, it is proposed that the prevention, maintenance, and/or improvement of physical capacity in aging and disease be considered as a primary component for the promotion of healthy aging. In this section we focus our discussion specifically on the mechanisms contributing to neuromuscular decline associated with biological aging in the absence of pathology or disease.

Neuromuscular alterations begin to occur early in life and become accelerated by the sixth and seventh decades [2, 28, 38, 66]. The nervous system undergoes reductions in motor unit number due to apoptosis and an increase in motor unit size as a result of reinnervation of denervated muscle fibers [2, 28]. These changes lead to decreases in voluntary activation, conduction velocity, motor unit discharge rate, and motor unit recruitment range [28]. Together, these age-related adaptations contribute to decreases in muscle activation, lower force-generating capacity, and reduction in rate of force development [2, 28].

The skeletal muscle is lost at an average rate of approximately 0.5–1.0% annually in adults over the age of 70 years [38]. Proposed mechanisms contributing to muscle atrophy with age include reduced levels of anabolic hormones, chronic inflammation, degradation of muscle contractile

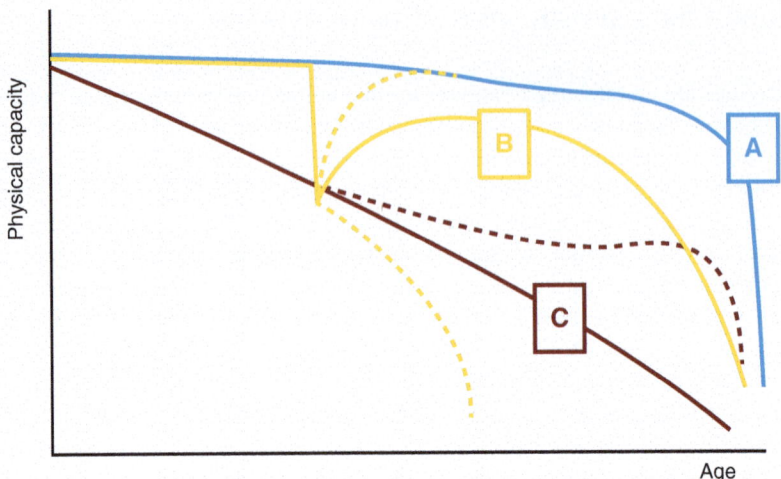

Fig. 9.2 Three hypothetical trajectories of physical capacity as proposed by the World Health Organization (WHO) [73]. (A) Optimal trajectory – intrinsic capacity remains high until the end of life. (B) Interrupted trajectory – an event causes a decrease in capacity with some recovery. Positive trajectory may result for example from access to rehabilitation and a negative trajectory might result from a lack of access to care (yellow dashed lines). (C) Declining trajectory – capacity declines steadily until death. Positive trajectory may result from a change in a health-related behavior or having access to appropriate medical treatment (maroon dashed line)

proteins, loss in regenerative capacity, altered neural activation, and mitochondrial dysfunction [66]. In addition, the aging process is associated with decreases in the number of skeletal muscle fibers and satellite cells, muscle fiber size, and myosin heavy chain IIa, contractile velocity, peak force and power, and calcium sensitivity and concentration [28]. The combination of the loss in skeletal muscle mass, increased intramuscular fat infiltration, alterations in muscle architecture, and compromised metabolic function leads to a reduction in skeletal muscle quality [23, 26]. The processes contributing to neuromuscular dysfunction with aging are exacerbated by skeletal muscle disuse and physical inactivity [66]. Thus, promoting resistance activities to maintain neuromuscular health and function should be viewed as a critical lifestyle component for successful aging.

Neuromuscular Adaptations to Resistance Activities

Both neurological and skeletal muscle adaptations contribute to improved neuromuscular function and health following resistance activities [17, 19, 20, 24, 48]. It is suggested that neurological adaptations occur during the acute stages of a resistance exercise program and precede morphological adaptations seen in skeletal muscle [19, 20]. This is based on findings of disproportionate increases in neuromuscular force in the absence of measurable changes in skeletal muscle size [19, 20]. The mechanisms contributing to neurological enhancement in response to resistance exercise are associated with increases in neural drive (i.e., motor unit recruitment, firing frequency, and synchronization) [17, 19, 20, 29, 65]. Kamen and Knight demonstrated an increase of 49% in maximal motor unit discharge rate as early as 1 week following the initiation of resistance exercise in the vastus lateralis in older adults (67–81 years) [29]. Similarly, Unhjem et al. reported improvements in both force generated during maximal voluntary contraction, rate of force development, and neural drive to the soleus following 8 weeks of heavy resistance activities in aging adults (mean age 74 years) [65]. Thus, resistance activities offer a viable treatment for countering the deleterious effects of aging on neurological function and force-generating capabilities in older adults.

Existing evidence supports skeletal muscle benefits following exposure to resistance activities in older adults [1, 12, 13, 31, 36, 39, 41, 42, 48–51, 57, 64, 67]. Several studies have found increases in lower extremity muscle cross-sectional area (CSA) primarily in type II muscle fibers [1, 13, 31, 36, 39, 57, 62, 67]. For example, Verdijk et al. [67] demonstrated an increase in leg lean mass and quadriceps CSA measured via computed tomography (CT) in healthy older adults (mean age 72 years) who completed 12 weeks of resistance exercise. In addition, greater satellite cell content and capillarization have also been reported concomitantly with increases in skeletal muscle CSA [39, 67]. While improvements in skeletal muscle fiber capillarization following resistance exercise have not been found in all studies [58], capillary density seems to be an important mechanisms for promoting skeletal muscle hypertrophy in older adults [58, 67, 68]. Changes in skeletal muscle architecture have also been demonstrated in addition to increases in muscle CSA [50, 51]. Reeves et al. reported increases in fascicle length and pennation angle both at rest and during maximal isometric contractions after 14 weeks of resistance exercise [51]. Combined, the neurological and morphological adaptations documented after resistance activities in older adults highlight the preserved plasticity of the neuromuscular system with aging.

While this section focused on neuromuscular adaptations in older adults, similar benefits can be expected in younger individuals. It should be noted, however, that the magnitude of the effects of resistance activities on neuromuscular adaptations differs between older and younger individuals. The blunted responses in older individuals may arise due to reductions in exercise intensity, volume, and/or frequency with age, inadequate dietary intake (specifically recommended protein requirements), and altered physiological and metabolic processes. Thus, it becomes important to consider individual responses to resistance activities and not a "one-size-fits-all" approach to exercise prescription.

Health and Functional Benefits of Resistance Activities in Aging and Chronic Diseases

Participation in resistance activities has a positive effect on enhancing neuromuscular strength, power, and physical function in older adults [12, 34, 45, 47, 48, 59, 60]. Peterson et al. performed a meta-analysis of forty-seven studies to examine the effects of resistance exercise in older adults (≥50 years of age) and found that resistance activities improved neuromuscular strength in both the upper and lower extremities [45]. Similarly, in a systematic review and meta-analysis, resistance activities were shown to be efficacious for increasing lower extremity neuromuscular power in adults ≥50 years of age [60]. The strength of evidence is not as robust for enhancing skeletal muscle mass as compared to strength and power; however resistance exercise has been shown to increase lean body mass when performed at sufficient intensities and volumes over longer durations [46]. The effects of resistance activities on physical function demonstrate improvements in functional tasks such as balance, walking speed, and the ability to rise from a chair [12, 34]. In addition to functional benefits, the ability to preserve skeletal muscle mass and quality has major health implications. For example, evidence of skeletal muscle as a secretory organ underscores the importance of maintaining skeletal muscle mass and muscle quality with age [44]. The ability of skeletal muscle to produce, express, and release proteins into circulation during exercise allows for cross-organ communication influencing metabolism and tissue function [44]. Similarly, skeletal muscle mass is shown to be associated with all-cause mortality [33]. Therefore, the maintenance of skeletal muscle mass and quality is essential for healthy aging and disease prevention.

Prescription of Resistance Activities

Goal Setting

Goal setting is the first step of designing an effective resistance exercise treatment [6]. Goal setting should be a collaborative process between the health-care provider, patient, and exercise professionals appropriately trained and certified to work with the respective populations of interest. During the goal setting process the patient should have an opportunity to articulate specific goals they hope to obtain. Based on the goals of the patient as well as any health or functional concerns from a medical standpoint, the interdisciplinary team should educate the patient on what the program will entail, the duration of the program, what the anticipated benefits are and when such benefits may be expected, potential secondary benefits in addition to the primary goals of interest, and potential risks of engaging in such activities. Ideally, a well-constructed goal should be specific, measurable, adjustable, realistic, and time-based [6]. Goal setting can include both short-term (i.e., weeks to months) and long-term (i.e., months to years) expectations and should be re-evaluated periodically to ensure any necessary changes to the resistance program are made to continue to align with the health and functional goals.

Structure and Organization

Resistance exercise programs are structured and organized in accordance with the health and functional goals and the time course in which the specified goals are expected to be achieved. Each individual resistance exercise session should include the following components: (a) warm-up, (b) conditioning (i.e., resistance activities), (c) cooldown, and (d) stretching [3]. The warm-up consists of 5–10 minutes of light-to-moderate intensity activity with the purpose of preparing the body for the demands of the prescribed resistance activity. The warm-up may be completed by cycling on an ergometer or walking on a treadmill, if such equipment is available. If not other light-to-moderate intensity activity can be substituted, such as walking overground or body-weight exercises. The conditioning segment is the main portion of the program. It is during this segment that the types and workloads of resistance activity are performed and may last 20–60 minutes. The duration of the conditioning segment will vary and is determined by the number of activities, exercise volume, and length of rest intervals and should be considered when planning a resistance exercise program (see section "Fundamental Principles of Resistance Activities") [21]. Immediately following the conditioning portion of the program, a brief cooldown period (i.e., 5–10 minutes) including light-to-moderate aerobic or muscular activity should be implemented to allow the body to gradually return to a resting state following exercise [3]. Last, a period of stretching can be prescribed which focuses on improving range of motion and flexibility.

The elements of a resistance exercise plan involve detailing the frequency, intensity, time, type, volume, and progression (i.e., *FITT-VP principle*) [3, 21, 47]. The frequency of exercise refers *how often* resistance activities are to be performed by each major muscle group per week. Intensity or *how hard* someone is exercising can be determined using subjective ratings of effort (i.e., ratings of perceived exertion) or absolute and relative loads lifted (i.e., actual weight lifted or percentage of one repetition maximum). Time (*duration or how long*) can be viewed as the amount of time spent performing muscular activity during an exercise session or over the course of a week. Type (*mode or what kind*) refers to the various resistance activity modalities. Volume is the *amount* of work performed in a given exercise session and is calculated as the number of sets and repetitions completed.

Progression is the *advancement* of the exercise stimulus and can be achieved by increasing volume, frequency, or intensity. Progression will ensure that continued neuromuscular adaptations are experienced; however the rate of progression will be different across individuals and should be prescribed gradually to minimize any potential risks of injury.

Fundamental Principles of Resistance Activities

Specificity, overload, variation, reversibility, and individuality describe the five fundamental principles of resistance activity used to understand neuromuscular adaptation and inform treatment design (Table 9.1) [3, 48]. The principle of specificity states that all exercise adaptations are specific to the stimulus applied [3, 48]. Factors to consider when determining the appropriateness of the stimulus based on specificity include the muscle actions to be performed, speed of the muscle actions, range of motion, muscle groups trained, and energy systems involved. Overload describes the act of exposing the neuromuscular system to increasing demands which are sufficient to elicit disturbances in homeostasis. Variation refers to the process of manipulating one or more variables over time to achieve the desired neuromuscular and/or functional goals. Reversibility describes the loss of neuromuscular adaptations in response to the removal of the exercise stimulus. In one of the most extreme cases, the negative neuromuscular changes associated with bed rest or prolonged periods of inactivity are reflective of the principle of reversibility. This principle describes the loss of neuromuscular function during periods of disuse. Lastly, the principle of individuality describes the unique responses experienced across individuals when exposed to the same exercise stimuli [3, 48].

To increase muscular fitness, resistance activities emphasizing major muscle groups performed at a frequency of ≥2 days per week with at least 48 hours between sessions are recommended [3, 12, 47, 48]. For beginners the intensity should start off light (i.e., 40–50% 1-RM) and progress to higher intensities (i.e., 60–80% 1-RM or rating of perceived exertion of 5–8 on 0–10 scale) in accordance with tolerability of the individual. Those with a previous resistance exercise history may be able to initiate resistance activities at higher intensities or progress at a greater rate. The volume should consist of 8–10 resistance activities involving major muscle groups to be trained for a total of 1–3 sets with 8–12 repetitions per set. Between each completed set of muscular activity, a rest interval of 2–3 minutes will ensure neuromuscular recovery and prevent excessive neuromuscular fatigue. In older adults or deconditioned populations, a resistance exercise regime of ≥1 set of 10–15 repetitions of very light-to-light intensity (i.e., 40–50% 1-RM) activities is sufficient to promote improvements in muscular fitness which can be progressed over time [3, 12, 48].

Table 9.1 Fundamental principles of resistance activities

Principle	Description
Specificity	Neuromuscular adaptations to resistance activities are specific to the stressors imposed by the type of muscle and speed of muscle actions, range of motion, muscle groups, and energy demands required
Overload	Demands are of sufficient level to elicit homeostatic disturbances in order to promote neuromuscular adaptations
Variation	Systematic altering of one or more exercise elements over time in accordance with neuromuscular outcomes of interest
Reversibility	Removal of the exercise stimulus and physical inactivity will result in loss of neuromuscular function
Individuality	Individual responses to a given resistance exercise stimulus

Principles and descriptions adopted from ACSM's Guidelines for Exercise Testing and Prescription Tenth Edition [3]

Recommendations for Improving Neuromuscular Capabilities

While generalized recommendations for engaging in resistance activities are effective for maintaining/improving overall muscular fitness, more specialized exercise prescriptions are necessary to enhance specific neuromuscular characteristics (i.e., hypertrophy, maximal strength, power, endurance) [48]. For increasing skeletal muscle hypertrophy and neuromuscular strength, it is recommended that both single- and multi-joint exercises be prescribed for 1–3 sets per resistance exercise at 60–80% of 1-RM for 8–12 repetitions. These activities should be performed 2–3 days per week with rest periods of 1–3 minutes between sets [48]. In a meta-analysis conducted by Peterson et al., greater increases in lean body mass occurred with higher exercise volumes [46]. Similarly, the effects of progressive resistance exercise on improving maximal strength are dose-dependent with higher intensities (i.e., >75% 1-RM) superior to moderate (i.e., 55–75% 1-RM) and low (i.e., <55% 1-RM) intensities in older adults [45, 59]. Resistance activities emphasizing neuromuscular power development have gained much interest given the relationship between neuromuscular power and physical function [52]. Such activities involve performing high velocity muscle contractions using low-to-moderate intensities (i.e., 30–60% 1-RM) over 1–3 sets of 6–10 repetitions (Table 9.2) [48, 60].

Contraindications and Special Considerations in Chronic Diseases

Despite the overwhelming number of health and functional benefits promoted by physical exercise, there are some risks involved with any exercise program. There is an increased risk of musculoskeletal injuries when participating in resistance activity programs due to the undo stress applied to the neuromuscular system [3]. The intensity and volume of exercise are primary factors contributing to the risk of injury with a greater risk of injury associated with vigorous intensity activity and excessive exercise volumes [3]. Injury risk can be minimized by prescribing gradual progression of intensity and volume as well as tailoring each resistance exercise program to individual responses.

Table 9.2 Recommendations for resistance activities in older adults

Element	Neuromuscular outcome		
	Hypertrophy	Strength	Power
Frequency	2–3 days/week on non-consecutive days	2–3 days/week on non-consecutive days	2–3 days/week on non-consecutive days
Intensity	60–80% 1-RM	60–80% 1-RM	30–60% 1-RM
Time	N/A	N/A	N/A
Type	Free weights; machines	Free weights; machines	Free weights; machines
Volume	1–3 sets/exercise; 8–12 repetitions	1–3 sets/exercise; 8–12 repetitions/set	1–3 sets/exercise; 6–10 repetitions
Progression	Gradual	Gradual	Gradual
Contraction velocity	Slow-to-moderate	Slow-to-moderate	High
Rest intervals	1–3 min between sets	1–3 min between sets	1–3 min between sets
Additional comments	Multiple- and single-joint exercises	Multiple- and single-joint exercises	Should be conducted in combination with training to improve strength; multiple- and single-joint exercises

Resistance exercise recommendations for enhancing muscular hypertrophy, strength, and power for older adults as proposed by the ACSM's Position Stand on Progression Models in Resistance Training for Healthy Adults [48]
Abbreviations: *1-RM* 1 repetition maximum, *min* minute, *N/A* not applicable

To ensure the safety of all individuals engaging in physical exercise, it is critical that all the parties involved have an understanding of the exercise-related events associated with certain populations, especially when working with clinical populations. Individuals with known cardiovascular, metabolic, or renal disease should obtain medical clearance prior to initiating regular exercise under the supervision of a trained professional [3]. Staff should possess the appropriate educational and practical training for managing cardiac emergencies. Exercise personnel should ensure the facilities are equipped with the necessary resources to handle cardiac emergencies in the case one should occur. Furthermore, by ensuring all components of the exercise session are adhered to, specifically the warm-up and cooldown, the potential for adverse events can be dramatically reduced [3].

Prediabetes and Diabetes

Resistance activities performed by individuals with prediabetes and diabetes have been shown to improve insulin action, blood glucose control, and fat oxidation and storage in skeletal muscle and increase muscle mass [15]. Community-dwelling adults with type 2 diabetes mellitus (T2DM) were shown to improve whole-body lean mass following 16 weeks of progressive resistance exercise using three sets of eight repetitions at an intensity of 60–80% 1-RM [7]. In prediabetic obese men, 8 weeks of resistance exercise was reported to increase strength and skeletal muscle fiber hypertrophy while increasing type IIx fiber content with continued improvements up to 16 weeks of exercise [61]. ACSM recommends a minimum of two non-consecutive days per week of resistance activity using 8–10 exercises performed at moderate (i.e., 50–69% of 1-RM)-to-vigorous (i.e., 70–85% of 1-RM) intensities and 1–3 sets of 10–15 repetitions [3].

Cardiovascular Disease

Skeletal muscle mass and strength are inversely associated with mortality and increased risk for cardiovascular disease [4, 27, 69]. For example, in patients with congestive heart failure, knee flexor strength was a strong predictor of long-term survival [27]. In a prospective longitudinal study of hypertensive men, muscular strength was significantly associated with a lower risk of all-cause mortality [4]. Resistance exercise has shown the potential to reduce adjusted absolute HbA1c values, improve lean mass, increase insulin sensitivity and muscle glycogen stores, and reduce dose of prescribed medications [7, 15, 54, 56, 72]. Progressive resistance exercise performed 3 times per week over 16 weeks was shown to increase whole-body lean mass and decrease systolic blood pressure and trunk fat mass in Latino adults with T2DM [7]. Women with type 2 diabetes engaging in resistance activities experienced a 17% risk reduction for cardiovascular disease and 30% rate reduction of type 2 diabetes [54].

Chronic Kidney Disease

Resistance activities, if structured appropriately, may provide a viable treatment to combat muscle wasting, neuromuscular dysfunction, and decreased functional capacity associated with chronic kidney disease (CKD). For example, resistance activities performed in a progressive manner have been shown to positively affect skeletal muscle mass, strength, physical function, and health-related quality of life in both patients with CKD pre-dialysis and end-stage renal disease (ESRD) [9, 11].

In those with CKD stage 3b to 4, 8 weeks of progressive resistance exercise (consisting of 3 sets of 10–12 leg extension repetitions at 70% 1-RM 3 times weekly) increased skeletal muscle anatomical cross-sectional area, muscle volume, knee extensor strength, and exercise capacity [70]. Cheema et al. [10] found that progressive resistance exercise (2 sets of 8 repetitions of 10 exercises at a rate of perceived exertion of 15–17 on a 6–20 point Borg Scale) performed over 24 weeks increased thigh cross-sectional area; however no improvements were observed at 12 weeks in patients with ESRD [10].

Training Throughout the Lifespan

The primary care professional has the important role of facilitating appropriate physical activity and targeted multimodal exercise programs that promote musculoskeletal health and independent functioning [55]. The effort to promote adequate amounts of resistance activity is one element of a comprehensive exercise regimen that demands heightened awareness for older patients [43]. The American Physical Therapy Association's recommendations to the American Board of Internal Medicine's Choosing Wisely® initiative cite the prescription of underdosed resistance exercise regimens to older adults as a problem contributing to lack of strength improvements following resistance exercise [71]. The challenge of maintaining activity levels throughout the lifespan goes beyond issues of attaining optimal exercise intensity/volume thresholds as less than 20% of older adults meet the recommended amounts of physical activity for maintaining overall health [8, 47]. The barriers to exercise faced by older adults include comorbid conditions, the need for greater health education, and accessibility within the built environment [32]. Members of the health-care team can promote increased physical activity and progressive resistance activities by playing an active role in monitoring progress, providing guidance in adjusting the exercise prescription, and understanding the barriers and enablers of program adherence.

Monitoring Progress and Adjusting the Exercise Prescription

Monitoring patient progress is an essential step to maximizing the efficacy of any treatment plan. Measuring and documenting patient progress, or regression, allows for timely adjustments to the exercise prescription and presents opportunities to address gaps in program adherence. The Reach, Effectiveness, Adoption, Implementation, and Maintenance (RE-AIM) framework is a well-known method used to guide program management for those with chronic conditions [22]. This framework considers factors concerning individual and organizational exercise settings and prompts the clinician to consider key patient-level components of any given intervention or exercise program:

1. *Reach*: consider how access limitations, caregiver issues, or health disparities, may impact program participation and progress.
2. *Effectiveness*: ensure that the program outcome measures are aligned with patient goals and values.
3. *Adoption*: determine and assess if the selected exercise setting (e.g., home-based or community-based program) is both feasible and well-suited to the patient over time.
4. *Implementation*: revisit if the exercise program can continue to be executed as designed based on the patient's health status, supervision needs or safety concerns, and equipment availability.
5. *Maintenance*: assess factors that may impact program sustainability such as material or social program support [22].

In moving from general program monitoring to assessing exercise efficacy, monitoring can be based on an evaluation of health risk, the documentation of behavioral change, or an assessment of physical fitness and functional status. Primary care providers may be limited in their approach if monitoring is confined to annual visits. Nevertheless, low-cost serial measures such as grip strength, customary walking speed, body weight, blood pressure, waist-hip ratio, lipid panel, and estimates of insulin sensitivity may provide vital longitudinal health risk data that may help guide exercise goals and inform the clinical management of chronic conditions. In addition, visits with the primary care professional are ideal times to revisit behavioral features of exercise program such as the goals. Unmet goals should receive follow-up by the health-care practitioner or exercise specialist to determine the causative factors and potential strategies to increase goal attainment. Clinical visits should also be used to re-evaluate contraindications to exercise, review safety topics (e.g., rising from a chair, precautions for exercising outdoors during summer months, or exercise technique), and provide further encouragement for program participation.

Monitoring behavioral elements associated with regular exercise or physical activity may also include patient questionnaires. Measures of physical activity vary widely based on the modes or scope of activity under consideration, the method used to estimate intensity or workload, the time frame of the activity period, and the questionnaire testing burden [63]. Common questionnaires used to monitor physical activity and/or program adherence for outpatient populations include the Community Healthy Activities Model Program for Seniors (CHAMPS) Activities Questionnaire for Older Adults, Physical Activity Scale for the Elderly (PASE), and Minnesota Leisure Time Physical Activity Questionnaire. In addition, the Exercise Scale for Older People (AESOP) provides a viable option for older adults with chronic conditions or other significant comorbidities [5, 25]. Nevertheless, all physical activity and exercise monitoring questionnaires have limitations concerning their psychometric properties, theoretical constructs, and adequate representation of activities that represent the specific adaptations to resistance activity [5, 63]. Exercise logs and activity diaries are often used in lieu of lengthy questionnaires and provide specific information concerning resistance training program elements such as volume, frequency, and workload. However, unlike intermittent questionnaires, daily or weekly exercise logs may be perceived as having a greater patient burden, be subject to memory bias, or overestimate activity intensity [63].

Importantly, when exercise specialists are involved in the plan of care, direct observations and fitness assessments may comprise a critical aspect of program monitoring. These tests and measures may include ACSM-recommended assessments of the 1-RM or submaximal 1-RM-estimate equations using a 6–10 repetition test which is easily adopted for older adults or those with comorbid conditions [3]. In addition, more detailed muscle performance measures concerning peak muscle torque and power can be measured using isokinetic dynamometry in clinical settings. In many instances, it may prove to be more practical for a primary care provider or community-based exercise specialist to use simple field-based assessments that include grip strength testing, timed sit to stand, and functional mobility assessments [35, 75].

The exercise prescription may be adjusted after a re-evaluation of the patient's health risks and any new potential barriers to the exercise program. Contact with the primary care professional via annual visits or through episodic care is usually inadequate to adjust the exercise prescription in a timely manner. Changes in a patient's health status, or injuries to specific joints or body regions, may necessitate the primary care provider modifying the exercise program to ensure its safe completion. However, more frequently, the exercise prescription will require regularly occurring adjustment to progress the resistance training regimen. Involvement of an exercise specialist facilitates periodic estimates of strength capacity and a review of proper form for each specific exercise in the program. Nonetheless, the successful execution of a resistance program hinges on appropriate health education that provides the patient with the knowledge to self-regulate the progression of exercise program. The strategy to increase resistance training overload will vary based on the patient goals and abilities. The common approach is a gradual increase in workload when the completed repetitions exceed the prescribed range (e.g., >15 repetitions). The patient may increase the weight used (using approximately 5% increments) until no more than 8–12 repetitions are completed in the absence of volitional fatigue during a given set [3]. Equally important, patients should be advised to reduce the weight used if volitional fatigue or pain is incurred before reaching the targeted repetition range.

Elements of Adherence

Program adherence is a multifaceted aspect of the plan of care that involves the initial identification and assessment of needs, the creation and issuance of the program, monitoring and maintaining the program, and a reassessment process to document improvements and/or identify program barriers. Many theoretical models have been proposed to help understand and improve program adherence. Common elements of the models reflect the interacting dimensions that affect adherence, social and economic status, health-care system and provider factors, severity and rate of progression of disease or comorbid conditions, and treatment burden [74]. Despite the varied ways to understand the factors that influence adherence, there are basic approaches that clinicians may use to enact behavioral changes that engender greater exercise participation [53]. Clinicians should interact with patients to (1) *assess* self-efficacy and social support resources; (2) *advise* regarding exercise benefits and risk management; (3) *agree* on the goals, exercise modes, and rate of progression; (4) *assist* with identifying resources and strategies to maintain consistency; and (5) *arrange* for appropriate referrals and regular reassessment visits [37].

The primary care clinician may proactively address barriers to program adherence through a structured approach such as the information-motivation-behavioral skills model (Fig. 9.3) [18]. The initial stages of this method may be facilitated through *motivation interviewing*, an approach to counseling used to identify, examine, and resolve barriers to an effective change in behavior [30]. In the context of promoting adherence to resistance activities, this approach may involve expressing empathy regarding the patient's health status and concerns about engaging in resistance exercise; supporting the self-efficacy of the patient; allowing the patient to both define their barriers to exercise and suggest potential solutions; and helping patients to see the incongruency between their current health status and their desired health and fitness goals.

These collective strategies allow for primary care professionals to engage in health promotion using individualized methods of behavior change. The decisions related to using of exercise support groups, opting for a home-based exercise program, using supervised exercise sessions, employing variety in the exercise routine, and selecting the method of exercise progress documentation are

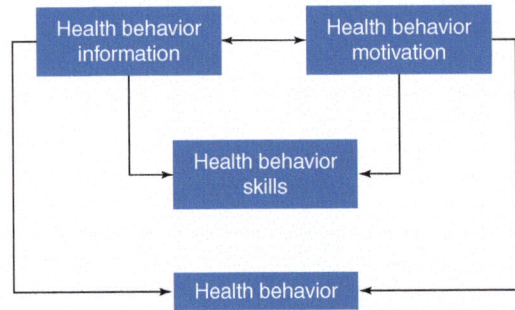

Fig. 9.3 The information-motivation-behavioral skills model. The model depicts the interrelationships among education, motivation, and behavioral factors that are associated with a targeted change in health-related behavior. (Adapted from Fisher et al. [18])

informed by the collaborative interviewing process. Previously sedentary patients who are engaging in a new exercise program may experience general stages of change related to exercise program participation: *contemplation* concerning the need to start an exercise program, *preparation* to attain training goals and improve adherence, *taking action* to enable regular exercise and minimize barriers to program adherence, and reaching a *maintenance phase* when exercise is a regular feature of the weekly routine (e.g., 3–5 times per week over a 6-month period) [40]. The specific health promotion and exercise adherence strategies used by the primary care provider will depend on where the patient resides along this continuum of behavioral change. Finally, it should be noted that an underappreciated aspect of effective exercise adherence is the practical nature of the program – a gradual ramp-up phase and appropriate exercise selection and intensity level minimize the risk of injuries and instill confidence in previously sedentary individuals. Indeed, exercise training programs highlight the importance of both adherence and compliance – consistently participating in the exercise regimen and performing the activities in accordance to the exercise prescription – which are essential to the safe attainment of patient-identified health and fitness goals.

References

1. Aagaard P, Magnusson PS, Larsson B, KjæR M, Krustrup P. Mechanical muscle function, morphology, and fiber type in lifelong trained elderly. Med Sci Sports Exerc. 2007;39:1989–96. https://doi.org/10.1249/mss.0b013e31814fb402.
2. Aagaard P, Suetta C, Caserotti P, Magnusson SP, Kjaer M. Role of the nervous system in sarcopenia and muscle atrophy with aging: strength training as a countermeasure. Scand J Med Sci Sports. 2010;20:49–64. https://doi.org/10.1111/j.1600-0838.2009.01084.x.
3. American College of Sports Medicine. ACSM's guidelines for exercise testing and prescription. 10th ed. Philadelphia: Wolters Kluwer; 2018.
4. Artero EG, Lee D, Ruiz JR, Sui X, Ortega FB, Church TS, Lavie CJ, Castillo MJ, Blair SN. A prospective study of muscular strength and all-cause mortality in men with hypertension. J Am Coll Cardiol. 2011;57:1831–7. https://doi.org/10.1016/j.jacc.2010.12.025.
5. Bollen JC, Dean SG, Siegert RJ, Howe TE, Goodwin VA. A systematic review of measures of self-reported adherence to unsupervised home-based rehabilitation exercise programmes, and their psychometric properties. BMJ Open. 2014;4:e005044. https://doi.org/10.1136/bmjopen-2014-005044.
6. Bovend'Eerdt TJH, Botell RE, Wade DT. Writing SMART rehabilitation goals and achieving goal attainment scaling: a practical guide. Clin Rehabil. 2009;23:352–61. https://doi.org/10.1177/0269215508101741.
7. Castaneda C, Layne JE, Munoz-Orians L, Gordon PL, Walsmith J, Foldvari M, Roubenoff R, Tucker KL, Nelson ME. A randomized controlled trial of resistance exercise training to improve glycemic control in older adults with type 2 diabetes. Diabetes Care. 2002;25:2335–41. https://doi.org/10.2337/diacare.25.12.2335.
8. Centers for Disease Control and Prevention. Nutrition, physical activity and obesity data, trends and maps. Atlanta: Centers for Disease Control and Prevention; 2018.
9. Chan D, Cheema BS. Progressive resistance training in end-stage renal disease: systematic review. Am J Nephrol. 2016;44:32–45. https://doi.org/10.1159/000446847.
10. Cheema B, Abas H, Smith B, O'Sullivan A, Chan M, Patwardhan A, Kelly J, Gillin A, Pang G, Lloyd B, Fiatarone Singh M. Randomized controlled trial of intradialytic resistance training to target muscle wasting in ESRD: the progressive exercise for anabolism in kidney disease (PEAK) study. Am J Kidney Dis. 2007;50:574–84. https://doi.org/10.1053/j.ajkd.2007.07.005.
11. Cheema BS, Chan D, Fahey P, Atlantis E. Effect of progressive resistance training on measures of skeletal muscle hypertrophy, muscular strength and health-related quality of life in patients with chronic kidney disease: a systematic review and meta-analysis. Sports Med. 2014;44:1125–38. https://doi.org/10.1007/s40279-014-0176-8.
12. Chodzko-Zajko WJ, Proctor DN, Fiatarone Singh MA, Minson CT, Nigg CR, Salem GJ, Skinner JS. Exercise and physical activity for older adults. Med Sci Sports Exerc. 2009;41:1510–30. https://doi.org/10.1249/MSS.0b013e3181a0c95c.
13. Claflin DR, Larkin LM, Cederna PS, Horowitz JF, Alexander NB, Cole NM, Galecki AT, Chen S, Nyquist LV, Carlson BM, Faulkner JA, Ashton-Miller JA. Effects of high- and low-velocity resistance training on the contractile properties of skeletal muscle fibers from young and older humans. J Appl Physiol. 2011;111:1021–30. https://doi.org/10.1152/japplphysiol.01119.2010.

14. Clegg A, Young J, Iliffe S, Rikkert MO, Rockwood K. Frailty in elderly people. Lancet. 2013;381:752–62. https://doi.org/10.1016/S0140-6736(12)62167-9.

15. Colberg SR, Sigal RJ, Fernhall B, Regensteiner JG, Blissmer BJ, Rubin RR, Chasan-Taber L, Albright AL, Braun B. Exercise and type 2 diabetes: the American College of Sports Medicine and the American Diabetes Association: joint position statement. Diabetes Care. 2010;33:e147–67. https://doi.org/10.2337/dc10-9990.

16. Cruz-Jentoft AJ, Baeyens JP, Bauer JM, Boirie Y, Cederholm T, Landi F, Martin FC, Michel J-P, Rolland Y, Schneider SM, Topinkova E, Vandewoude M, Zamboni M. Sarcopenia: European consensus on definition and diagnosis: report of the European Working Group on sarcopenia in older people. Age Ageing. 2010;39:412–23. https://doi.org/10.1093/ageing/afq034.

17. Duchateau J, Semmler JG, Enoka RM. Training adaptations in the behavior of human motor units. J Appl Physiol. 2006;101:1766–75. https://doi.org/10.1152/japplphysiol.00543.2006.

18. Fisher JD, Amico KR, Fisher WA, Harman JJ. The information-motivation-behavioral skills model of antiretroviral adherence and its applications. Curr HIV/AIDS Rep. 2008;5:193–203.

19. Folland JP, Williams AG. The adaptations to strength training: morphological and neurological contributions to increased strength. Sports Med. 2007;37:145–68.

20. Gabriel DA, Kamen G, Frost G. Neural adaptations to resistive exercise: mechanisms and recommendations for training practices. Sports Med. 2006;36:133–49.

21. Garber CE, Blissmer B, Deschenes MR, Franklin BA, Lamonte MJ, Lee I-M, Nieman DC, Swain DP. Quantity and quality of exercise for developing and maintaining cardiorespiratory, musculoskeletal, and neuromotor fitness in apparently healthy adults. Med Sci Sports Exerc. 2011;43:1334–59. https://doi.org/10.1249/MSS.0b013e318213fefb.

22. Glasgow RE, Estabrooks PE. Pragmatic applications of RE-AIM for health care initiatives in community and clinical settings. Prev Chronic Dis. 2018;15:170271. https://doi.org/10.5888/pcd15.170271.

23. Goodpaster BH, Park SW, Harris TB, Kritchevsky SB, Nevitt M, Schwartz AV, Simonsick EM, Tylavsky FA, Visser M, Newman AB. The loss of skeletal muscle strength, mass, and quality in older adults: the health, aging and body composition study. J Gerontol A Biol Sci Med Sci. 2006;61:1059–64.

24. Häkkinen K, Kraemer WJ, Newton RU, Alen M. Changes in electromyographic activity, muscle fibre and force production characteristics during heavy resistance/power strength training in middle-aged and older men and women. Acta Physiol Scand. 2001;171:51–62. https://doi.org/10.1046/j.1365-201X.2001.00781.x.

25. Hardage J, Peel C, Morris D, Graham C, Brown C, Foushee HR, Braswell J. Adherence to Exercise Scale for Older Patients (AESOP): a measure for predicting exercise adherence in older adults after discharge from home health physical therapy. J Geriatr Phys Ther. 2007;30:69–78.

26. Heymsfield SB, Gonzalez MC, Lu J, Jia G, Zheng J. Skeletal muscle mass and quality: evolution of modern measurement concepts in the context of sarcopenia. Proc Nutr Soc. 2015;74:355–66. https://doi.org/10.1017/S0029665115000129.

27. Hülsmann M, Quittan M, Berger R, Crevenna R, Springer C, Nuhr M, Mörtl D, Moser P, Pacher R. Muscle strength as a predictor of long-term survival in severe congestive heart failure. Eur J Heart Fail. 2004;6:101–7. https://doi.org/10.1016/j.ejheart.2003.07.008.

28. Hunter SK, Pereira HM, Keenan KG. The aging neuromuscular system and motor performance. J Appl Physiol. 2016;121:982–95. https://doi.org/10.1152/japplphysiol.00475.2016.

29. Kamen G, Knight CA. Training-related adaptations in motor unit discharge rate in young and older adults. J Gerontol A Biol Sci Med Sci. 2004;59:1334–8.

30. Keeley R, Engel M, Reed A, Brody D, Burke BL. Toward an emerging role for motivational interviewing in primary care. Curr Psychiatry Rep. 2018;20:41. https://doi.org/10.1007/s11920-018-0901-3.

31. Kosek DJ, Kim J-S, Petrella JK, Cross JM, Bamman MM. Efficacy of 3 days/wk resistance training on myofiber hypertrophy and myogenic mechanisms in young vs. older adults. J Appl Physiol. 2006;101:531–44. https://doi.org/10.1152/japplphysiol.01474.2005.

32. Lee PG, Jackson EA, Richardson CR. Exercise prescriptions in older adults. Am Fam Physician. 2017;95:425–32.

33. Li R, Xia J, Zhang X, Gathirua-Mwangi WG, Guo J, Li Y, Mckenzie S, Song Y. Associations of muscle mass and strength with all-cause mortality among US older adults. Med Sci Sports Exerc. 2018;50:458–67. https://doi.org/10.1249/MSS.0000000000001448.

34. Liu C, Latham NK. Progressive resistance strength training for improving physical function in older adults. Cochrane Database Syst Rev. 2009. https://doi.org/10.1002/14651858.CD002759.pub2.

35. Lusardi MM, Pellecchia GL, Schulman M. Functional performance in community living older adults. J Geriatr Phys Ther. 2003;26:14–22. https://doi.org/10.1519/00139143-200312000-00003.

36. Martel GF, Roth SM, Ivey FM, Lemmer JT, Tracy BL, Hurlbut DE, Metter EJ, Hurley BF, Rogers MA. Age and sex affect human muscle fibre adaptations to heavy-resistance strength training. Exp Physiol. 2006;91:457–64. https://doi.org/10.1113/expphysiol.2005.032771.

37. Meriwether RA, Lee JA, Lafleur AS, Wiseman P. Physical activity counseling. Am Fam Physician. 2008;77:1129–36.

38. Mitchell WK, Williams J, Atherton P, Larvin M, Lund J, Narici M. Sarcopenia, dynapenia, and the impact of advancing age on human skeletal muscle size and strength; a quantitative review. Front Physiol. 2012;3:260. https://doi.org/10.3389/fphys.2012.00260.

39. Moore DR, Kelly RP, Devries MC, Churchward-Venne TA, Phillips SM, Parise G, Johnston AP. Low-load resistance exercise during inactivity is associated with greater fibre area and satellite cell expression in older skeletal muscle: muscle morphology with exercise and inactivity. J Cachexia Sarcopenia Muscle. 2018;9:747–54. https://doi.org/10.1002/jcsm.12306.

40. Morgan PJ, Young MD, Smith JJ, Lubans DR. Targeted health behavior interventions promoting physical activity: a conceptual model. Exerc Sport Sci Rev. 2016;44:71–80. https://doi.org/10.1249/JES.0000000000000075.

41. Narici MV, Maganaris CN. Adaptability of elderly human muscles and tendons to increased loading. J Anat. 2006;208:433–43. https://doi.org/10.1111/j.1469-7580.2006.00548.x.

42. Narici MV, Reeves ND, Morse CI, Maganaris CN. Muscular adaptations to resistance exercise in the elderly. J Musculoskelet Neuronal Interact. 2004;4:161–4.

43. Oliveira CLP, Dionne IJ, Prado CM. Are Canadian protein and physical activity guidelines optimal for sarcopenia prevention in older adults? Appl Physiol Nutr Metab. 2018;43:1–9. https://doi.org/10.1139/apnm-2018-0141.

44. Pedersen BK. Muscle as a secretory organ. In: Terjung R, editor. Comprehensive physiology. Hoboken: Wiley; 2013. https://doi.org/10.1002/cphy.c120033.

45. Peterson MD, Rhea MR, Sen A, Gordon PM. Resistance exercise for muscular strength in older adults: a meta-analysis. Ageing Res Rev. 2010;9:226–37. https://doi.org/10.1016/j.arr.2010.03.004.

46. Peterson MD, Sen A, Gordon PM. Influence of resistance exercise on lean body mass in aging adults: a meta-analysis. Med Sci Sports Exerc. 2011;43:249–58. https://doi.org/10.1249/MSS.0b013e3181eb6265.

47. Piercy KL, Troiano RP, Ballard RM, Carlson SA, Fulton JE, Galuska DA, George SM, Olson RD. The physical activity guidelines for Americans. JAMA. 2018;320:2020. https://doi.org/10.1001/jama.2018.14854.

48. Ratamess NA, Alvar BA, Evetoch TK, Housh TJ, Kibler WB, Kraemer WJ, Triplett NT. Progression models in resistance training for healthy adults. Med Sci Sports Exerc. 2009;41:687–708. https://doi.org/10.1249/MSS.0b013e3181915670.

49. Raue U, Trappe TA, Estrem ST, Qian H-R, Helvering LM, Smith RC, Trappe S. Transcriptome signature of resistance exercise adaptations: mixed muscle and fiber type specific profiles in young and old adults. J Appl Physiol. 2012;112:1625–36. https://doi.org/10.1152/japplphysiol.00435.2011.

50. Reeves ND, Narici MV, Maganaris CN. Effect of resistance training on skeletal muscle-specific force in elderly humans. J Appl Physiol. 2004;96:885–92. https://doi.org/10.1152/japplphysiol.00688.2003.

51. Reeves ND, Narici MV, Maganaris CN. In vivo human muscle structure and function: adaptations to resistance training in old age. Exp Physiol. 2004;89:675–89. https://doi.org/10.1113/expphysiol.2004.027797.

52. Reid KF, Fielding RA. Skeletal muscle power: a critical determinant of physical functioning in older adults. Exerc Sport Sci Rev. 2012;40:4–12. https://doi.org/10.1097/JES.0b013e31823b5f13.

53. Room J, Hannink E, Dawes H, Barker K. What interventions are used to improve exercise adherence in older people and what behavioural techniques are they based on? A systematic review. BMJ Open. 2017;7:e019221. https://doi.org/10.1136/bmjopen-2017-019221.

54. Shiroma EJ, Cook NR, Manson JE, Moorthy M, Buring JE, Rimm EB, Lee I-M. Strength training and the risk of type 2 diabetes and cardiovascular disease. Med Sci Sports Exerc. 2017;49:40–6. https://doi.org/10.1249/MSS.0000000000001063.

55. Shuval K, DiPietro L, Skinner CS, Barlow CE, Morrow J, Goldsteen R, Kohl HW. "Sedentary behaviour counselling": the next step in lifestyle counselling in primary care; pilot findings from the Rapid Assessment Disuse Index (RADI) study. Br J Sports Med. 2014;48:1451–5. https://doi.org/10.1136/bjsports-2012-091357.

56. Sigal RJ, Kenny GP, Boulé NG, Wells GA, Prud'homme D, Fortier M, Reid RD, Tulloch H, Coyle D, Phillips P, Jennings A, Jaffey J. Effects of aerobic training, resistance training, or both on glycemic control in type 2 diabetes: a randomized trial. Ann Intern Med. 2007;147:357–69.

57. Slivka D, Raue U, Hollon C, Minchev K, Trappe S. Single muscle fiber adaptations to resistance training in old (>80 yr) men: evidence for limited skeletal muscle plasticity. Am J Phys Regul Integr Comp Phys. 2008;295:R273–80. https://doi.org/10.1152/ajpregu.00093.2008.

58. Snijders T, Nederveen JP, Joanisse S, Leenders M, Verdijk LB, van Loon LJC, Parise G. Muscle fibre capillarization is a critical factor in muscle fibre hypertrophy during resistance exercise training in older men. J Cachexia Sarcopenia Muscle. 2017;8:267–76. https://doi.org/10.1002/jcsm.12137.

59. Steib S, Schoene D, Pfeifer K. Dose-response relationship of resistance training in older adults: a meta-analysis. Med Sci Sports Exerc. 2010;42:902–14. https://doi.org/10.1249/MSS.0b013e3181c34465.

60. Straight CR, Lindheimer JB, Brady AO, Dishman RK, Evans EM. Effects of resistance training on lower-extremity muscle power in middle-aged and older adults: a systematic review and meta-analysis of randomized controlled trials. Sports Med. 2016;46:353–64. https://doi.org/10.1007/s40279-015-0418-4.

61. Stuart CA, Lee ML, South MA, Howell MEA, Stone MH. Muscle hypertrophy in prediabetic men after 16 wk of resistance training. J Appl Physiol. 2017;123:894–901. https://doi.org/10.1152/japplphysiol.00023.2017.

62. Suetta C, Aagaard P, Rosted A, Jakobsen AK, Duus B, Kjaer M, Magnusson SP. Training-induced changes in muscle CSA, muscle strength, EMG, and rate of force development in elderly subjects after long-term unilateral disuse. J Appl Physiol. 2004;97:1954–61. https://doi.org/10.1152/japplphysiol.01307.2003.

63. Sylvia LG, Bernstein EE, Hubbard JL, Keating L, Anderson EJ. Practical guide to measuring physical activity. J Acad Nutr Diet. 2014;114:199–208. https://doi.org/10.1016/j.jand.2013.09.018.

64. Trappe S, Williamson D, Godard M. Maintenance of whole muscle strength and size following resistance training in older men. J Gerontol A Biol Sci Med Sci. 2002;57:B138–43.

65. Unhjem R, Lundestad R, Fimland MS, Mosti MP, Wang E. Strength training-induced responses in older adults: attenuation of descending neural drive with age. Age. 2015;37:9784. https://doi.org/10.1007/s11357-015-9784-y.

66. Venturelli M, Reggiani C, Richardson RS, Schena F. Skeletal muscle function in the oldest-old: the role of intrinsic and extrinsic factors. Exerc Sport Sci Rev. 2018;1:188. https://doi.org/10.1249/JES.0000000000000155.

67. Verdijk LB, Gleeson BG, Jonkers RAM, Meijer K, Savelberg HHCM, Dendale P, van Loon LJC. Skeletal muscle hypertrophy following resistance training is accompanied by a fiber type-specific increase in satellite cell content in elderly men. J Gerontol Ser A Biol Med Sci. 2009;64A:332–9. https://doi.org/10.1093/gerona/gln050.

68. Verdijk LB, Snijders T, Holloway TM, VAN Kranenburg J, VAN Loon LJC. Resistance training increases skeletal muscle capillarization in healthy older men. Med Sci Sports Exerc. 2016;48:2157–64. https://doi.org/10.1249/MSS.0000000000001019.

69. Volaklis KA, Halle M, Meisinger C. Muscular strength as a strong predictor of mortality: a narrative review. Eur J Intern Med. 2015;26:303–10. https://doi.org/10.1016/j.ejim.2015.04.013.

70. Watson EL, Greening NJ, Viana JL, Aulakh J, Bodicoat DH, Barratt J, Feehally J, Smith AC. Progressive resistance exercise training in CKD: a feasibility study. Am J Kidney Dis. 2015;66:249–57. https://doi.org/10.1053/j.ajkd.2014.10.019.

71. White NT, Delitto A, Manal TJ, Miller S. The American physical therapy association's top five choosing wisely recommendations. Phys Ther. 2015;95:9–24. https://doi.org/10.2522/ptj.20140287.

72. Willey KA, Singh MAF. Battling insulin resistance in elderly obese people with type 2 diabetes: bring on the heavy weights. Diabetes Care. 2003;26:1580–8. https://doi.org/10.2337/diacare.26.5.1580.

73. World Health Organization. World report on ageing and health. Geneva: World Health Organization; 2015.

74. World Health Organization. Adherence to long-term therapies: evidence for action. Geneva: World Health Organization; 2003.

75. Yorke AM, Curtis AB, Shoemaker M, Vangsnes E. Grip strength values stratified by age, gender, and chronic disease status in adults aged 50 years and older. J Geriatr Phys Ther. 2015;38:115–21. https://doi.org/10.1519/JPT.0000000000000037.

Chapter 10
Yoga as a Mind-Body Practice

Christiane Brems

Keywords Yoga · Mindfulness · Interoception · Neuroception · Embodiment

Key Points
- Yoga includes and integrates a wide range of strategies, categorized into lifestyle and values-related commitments, physical practices, breathing practices, and interior practices.
- Yoga is suitable for individuals of all body shapes, physical abilities, ages, emotional states, cognitive capacities, and demographics. Once a practice has been established with a qualified teacher, yoga can be engaged in by anyone, anywhere, and anytime, at low cost.
- Yoga is a powerful wellness practice and an effective intervention or adjunctive treatment for physical challenges (e.g., musculoskeletal concerns, chronic illness, metabolic disease, cancer, and more) and mental or emotional symptoms (e.g., depression, anxiety, stress, anger, attention deficits, trauma histories).
- Yoga integrates top-down and bottom-up neurobiological processes to help practitioners attain relaxed and calm states in body, breath, and mind, reducing maladaptive emotional, cognitive, behavioral, and relational patterns while increasing capacity for innovative problem-solving and stress tolerance.
- Building a referral network of yoga teachers and therapists will allow clinicians to guide physical and mental health patients to yoga resources that can have a profound effect on their well-being, symptom tolerance, and course of treatment.

A Definition of Yoga: Myths and Realities

The practice of yoga in the United States has seen a tremendous increase in numbers of practitioners [48] and has been identified as among the top ten alternative and integrative practices sought out by patients in physical and mental healthcare settings [4, 5]. Yoga's increase in popularity has been largely due to the strong interest in posture practice as a form of exercise. Posture practice has become a point of focus in gyms, schools, and even work places and is touted as a way of combatting stress, increasing mindfulness, and staying physically healthy. Yoga from that perspective is a physical or

C. Brems (✉)
Department of Psychiatry and Behavioral Sciences, Stanford University School of Medicine, Stanford, CA, USA
e-mail: cbrems@stanford.edu

© Springer Nature Switzerland AG 2020
J. Uribarri, J. A. Vassalotti (eds.), *Nutrition, Fitness, and Mindfulness*, Nutrition and Health,
https://doi.org/10.1007/978-3-030-30892-6_10

exercise-based tradition that helps promote physical health, strength, and balance. Many yoga classes – especially outside of yoga studios and inside conventional venues such as gyms – offer strenuous physical practices that are indeed proven to enhance the physical well-being of practitioner. However, yoga as a holistic practice or life philosophy goes far beyond posture practice alone.

Yoga as traditionally practiced was physical only to prepare practitioners for the more important interior practices (such as concentration and meditation) and interpersonal applications of a thoughtful and deliberate code of life and discipline [12, 37]. Integrated yoga is a holistic practice that combines body, emotion, mind, spirit, and community through a comprehensive lifestyle with implications for individual and collective well-being [35, 49, 114]. It promotes community, self-compassion, and introspection that lead to insights that alter human physiology and anatomy and – perhaps more importantly – emotions, cognitions, behaviors, and relationships. Integrated yoga can be practiced by anyone who can breathe without assistance, almost anywhere, for little to no cost [87]. Yoga motivates practitioners to adhere to the practice more so than a unidimensional posture practice [31] and is freed from Western media stereotypes that tend to limit who seeks access to yoga. Integrated yoga consists of eight sets of ancient practices called *limbs of yoga* [45, 49], grouped into four categories based on modern research [39, 113]. *Values and lifestyle practices* of yoga direct practitioners to ethical and intentional living informed by purposeful values and meaningful life goals. *Physical practices* transform the practitioner's anatomy and physiology, supporting accurate sensory perception of the body from the inside out and of the environment from the outside in. *Breathing practices* stimulate the parasympathetic nervous system, allowing access to a calm, relaxed state from which to become adaptively responsive to inner and outer life demands, achieving systemic homeostasis in body and mind. *Interior practices* draw the practitioner into self-exploration, personal insight, and interpersonal transformation, shedding maladaptive habits, reactivity, and stereotypes while opening space for new choices, adaptive responsiveness, and resilience in body, emotions, mind, and relationships.

Summarized in Table 10.1, all yoga practices are rooted in mindfulness practices, which are the mainstay of yoga philosophy and the foundation on which the entire practice comes to rest. The first aphorism in the *Yoga Sutras of Patanjali*, the millennia-old primary text for yoga teachers and practitioners, states "atha yoga anushasanam" – *now the time for the teachings of yoga*. This aphorism is understood as a reminder that each and every moment – each *now* – is a moment to come into the present; to reflect on body, breath, emotions, and mind; and to be fully in touch with what *is* in a nonjudgmental manner and with deep curiosity. Thus, as each limb is applied, it is important to maintain mindful awareness, an attitude of nonjudgment, and spacious curiosity about effects and sensations that arise from each practice.

Documented Benefits of an Integrated Yoga Practice

Integrated yoga practice [80] and comprehensive, burgeoning research [51, 58, 70] have begun to demonstrate that individuals – if invited into the practice on their terms [54] – can derive substantial benefits. In contrast to Western stereotypes about who practices yoga [85], this includes (but is not limited to) individuals with physical, emotional, and mental challenges; with significant life stress and trauma histories; with aging bodies; in prisons and jails; in hospitals and other healthcare settings; in schools and universities; and more [32, 46, 58]. Positive effects have been documented for a range of physiological, musculoskeletal, and mental health symptoms. Salutary effects have been demonstrated through clinical trials – carefully controlled experiments – as well as case studies, surveys, and other means of establishing the utility of interventions for human health and well-being. Table 10.2 summarizes recent research findings and establishes a compelling evidence base for yoga intervention for a variety of individuals who suffer physically, emotionally, or psychologically.

Table 10.1 An overview of yoga practices

Values and lifestyle practices: limb #1 – life choices for ethical living	
Basic definition	First-person ethics that invite choices based on discernment and mindfulness to result in values-based thought, speech, and action
Central intention	Value clarification to guide moment-to-moment choices in thought, speech, behavior, and relationships
Central principles	Nonharming – nonviolence and peacefulness toward self, other, and everything Truthfulness – honesty with oneself and in all relationships and contexts to create authenticity and integrity in day-to-day life Non-stealing – not taking what is not freely offered Moderation – wise use of personal life energy Non-possessiveness – not being greedy about possessions, relationships, actions, and other aspects of life
Central practices	Nonharming – the practice of living in a manner that seeks not to cause deliberate pain or harm Truthfulness – the practice of living in a manner that is true to a practitioner's real and ideal self Non-stealing – the practice of embracing a sense of abundance, generosity, and reciprocity that eliminates the desires to take or steal from others or to have more than others Moderation – the practice of being neither indulgent nor excessively restrictive when it comes to habits and desires Non-possessiveness – the practice of mindful cultivating gratitude for what life has already provided and thoughtfully relinquishing grasping, desire, and jealousy
Values and lifestyle practices: limb #2 –life choices for purposeful living	
Basic definition	Mindful self-discipline and intentionality to create a meaningful and purposeful life
Central intention	Motivation-to-change goal setting that creates a motivational set for the entire yoga practice that will relate to greater life plans and trajectories, personal development, and contributions to a greater good
Central principles	Purity – simplicity and authenticity in action, speech, and thought Contentment – meeting every moment from a peaceful center that allows for discernment about how to take calm and appropriate action Disciplined use of energy – leading an impassioned life of determined effort and engaged practice Self-reflection – exploring personal reactions, habits, motivations, and intentions to guide toward self-knowledge, insight, and growth Devotion to a greater good – creating meaning for self and others through wise discernment
Central practices	Purity – the practice of finding centered balance in consumption, clutter, toxins, distractions, and overload in all aspects of life, including food, drink, body care, relationships, media use, work, and play Contentment – the practice of taking calm and appropriate action, neither driven by hyper-excitability nor indifference, and of accepting life fully and calmly Disciplined use of energy – the practice of committing to making conscious, not habitual, choices in every moment that are neither hyperactive nor slothful and lead to transformation for self and others Self-reflection – the practice of opening up to new learning from outer sources (like books and teachers) and through quiet introspection Devotion to a greater good – the practice of surrendering ego-driven intentions and committing to positive other-oriented intention and action
Physical practices: limb #3 – physical postures	
Basic definition	Physical discipline of engaging in postures and movements that promote mindfulness of the body and its sensations
Central intention	Mindfulness-based embodied movement to create physical and mental health and fitness, including balance, strength, stamina, flexibility, coordination, and power

(continued)

Table 10.1 (continued)

Central principles	Effort and ease combines in physical practices that integrate form (careful attention to healthful alignment, proprioception, and interoception) and movement (flowing with breath through well-sequenced poses) with breath (see limb# 6) Integration of form and movement invites: Mindful alignment Neuroception of physical safety and containment Interoceptive awareness of how the physical body collaborates with breath and mind Proprioceptive awareness of the body in space Exteroceptive awareness of the body's response to environment stimuli Finding effort and ease allows for restful awareness combined with optimal exertion of effort Integrated posture practice synergistically links to all other limbs of yoga

Central practices	Types of flow practices include, yet are not limited to:
	  Sun and moon salutations
	  Yoga kriyas
	  Vinyasa
	Types of forms include, yet are not limited to:
	  Backbends (e.g., cobra, camel, bridge, wheel)
	  Balancing postures (e.g., tree, eagle)
	  Forward folds (e.g., downward dog, head-to-knee, chair)
	  Inversions (e.g., headstand, handstand, elbow balance)
	  Restorative poses (e.g., relaxation pose, meadow brook, legs-up-the-wall)
	  Seated postures (e.g., staff, hero, lotus, easy seat)
	  Standing postures (e.g., mountain, warrior, triangle, side angle)
	  Twists (e.g., lord of the fishes, supine legs around the belly)

Breathing practices: limb #4 – breath regulation

Basic definition	Breathing exercises and wholesome natural breathing awareness that invites mindfulness, balance, and efficiency in body, breath, mind, and relationships
Central intention	Biofeedback to become mindful of and regulate physiological arousal and emotional reactivity, gain control over the autonomic nervous system, connect to inner sensations, recruit the parasympathetic nervous system, reduce allostatic load, and improve vagal tone
Central principles	Breath timing – attention is given to the number of breaths per minutes and is controlled by either lengthening (slowing down) or shortening (speeding up) the inhalation, exhalation, or both Breath texture – attention is given to smoothness of breath as it travels in and out of the body; includes balance of inhalation, exhalation, and suspension of breath, which is controlled in advanced breathing practices Breath space – attention to where breath is sensed and directed in the body, with mindful awareness of the balance of breath between the right and left side of the body, between front and back, and across the lower, middle, and upper thirds of the torso; also refers to the fullness (or depth) of the breath as it is sensed in the body, filling and emptying the lungs to optimum capacity Breath rest – attention to explorations of the top (between inhalation and exhalation) and bottom (between exhalation and inhalation) of the breath, creating increasing gaps; rest breaks at top and bottom are calibrated to achieve optimal calming of the nervous system and mind

Central practices	Breathing practices range from breath observation (tuning into natural breath) without altering the breath to complex control of the breath.
	Observation of natural breath is a mindful tuning into how breath travels into and out of the body, its timing, texture, space, and natural restfulness
	Samples of breathing practices that consciously alter the breath include, yet are not limited to:
	  Balancing breathing (e.g., same length inhalation/exhalation)
	  Belly breathing (e.g., abdomino-diaphragmatic, thoraco-diaphragmatic)
	  Breath retention (e.g., short break at top of breath)
	  Cleansing breathing (e.g., alternate nostril breathing)
	  Energizing breathing (e.g., breath of fire)
	  Victorious breathing (i.e., ocean-sounding breath)

Interior practices: limb #5 – drawing inward

Basic definition	Disconnecting from the steady flow of sensory input put through the eyes, ears, nose, taste buds, and other sense receptors (e.g., touch, pain, temperature, texture)

Table 10.1 (continued)

Central intention	Directing attention inward to sharpen self-awareness skills of automatic/habitual thoughts, speech, actions, and relational patterns (for top-down regulation) or preparatory sets and to halt the constant flow of stimulation through the senses that leads to overstimulation, poor concentration, and scattered attention
Central principles	Moving inward and tuning out extraneous stimuli allows for mindfully exploring and understanding mental habits and reactivity, becoming attuned to neuroceptive input. It invites stillness and spaciousness in mind and body, without being tossed about on the sea of information that normally streams in through the sense organs When practitioners' attention is focused inward, the mind can become quiet and the body can become calm When the senses become quiet and attention is tuned fully to inner life, awareness emerges of mental habits, preoccupations, fantasies, distortions, and illusions. The lens of perception becomes clean and readies the practitioner for transcending habits, emotional reactivity, and cognitive preoccupations Sense withdrawal is a crucial step toward yet deeper levels of calming the nervous system, reducing emotional reactivity, and resting a ventral vagal space of safety and peace

Central practices	Drawing inward is achieved through practices as uncomplicated as:
	    Sitting still for a moment with the eyes closed to recenter the mind
	    Finding an inner point of focus on the activity of the mind
	    Withdrawing to an inner physical gaze point (e.g., on the third eye)

Interior practices: limb #6 – concentration

Basic definition	Surrendering thought (of which they became aware through sense withdrawal) in exchange for deep inner concentration on a single point of focus to achieve mental one-pointedness
Central intention	Integration of top-down and bottom-up self-regulation invites the mind to become honed and clear, like a still lake, transcending mental states that are disturbing, upsetting, distracting, discouraging, lethargic, heavy, agitated, or restless
Central principles	Single focus of attention emerges through concentration and creates stillness in the nervous system, calming emotions, body, and mind. The practitioner moves into a relaxed ventral vagal space, drawn away from mental chatter, multitasking, and distraction Concentration's a single-pointed focus, the antithesis to multitasking and multiattending. The mind moves into clarity, focus, and even luminosity

Central practices	Concentration practices reduce mental chatter and connect practitioners to their true self beyond thoughts, emotions, and ego-identification
	On the mat, concentration may mean:
	    Focusing on something that is inspiring, such as the image of a revered teacher or a loved one
	    Focusing attention through the chanting of a mantra, the intoning of the syllable "om," or the repetition of a meaningful word (e.g., peace)
	    Finding a physical focus point (such as the breath or the movement of the belly)
	Off the mat, specific practices may include:
	    Practicing an everyday, routine task with full attention and focus
	    An action as uncomplicated and ordinary as being fully focused on washing a dish or peeling a piece of fruit can become a concentration practice
	    Playing a piece of music
	    Being in a state of flow during physical exercise (including yoga posture practice)
	Concentration is also honed through guided imagery exercises, body scans of internal states, loving kindness practices, and other visualizations that keep attention single-pointed, honed, and alert. Although such practices are often called "meditations," in the yogic tradition, they constitute concentration practices

Interior practices: limb #7 – meditation

Basic definition	Achieving an effortless state of awareness and deep concentration that transcends even a single point of focus
Central intention	New neural pathways are forged – neuroplasticity and increased gray matter volume in certain parts of the brain noted in yoga and meditation practitioners are not solely due to meditation; however, meditation is the most effective of the yoga strategies in facilitating new learning and synaptic pathways in the brain

(continued)

Table 10.1 (continued)

Central principles	A decisional gap (between stimulus and response) opens through meditation that helps practitioners to engage in new choices and to exercise conscious authorships over emotions, cognitions, behaviors, and relationships A sense of spaciousness and peacefulness emerges from meditation and ushers in sufficient tranquility so that sensations, emotions, and thoughts that arise while seated no longer become a disturbance. They are observed, noted, and let go. They inform the practitioner more deeply about ingrained emotional and mental habits. Practitioners develop the capacity to observe these stirrings without losing a sense of peace and spaciousness Choice and adaptive, resilient decision-making about new emotional, mental, behavioral, and relational choices emerge when a gap opens in awareness

Central practices	Meditation is a seated (or if physically necessary, reclining) practice in which the skills of all prior limbs come to their full flowering in that they have built the platform upon which the meditator can rest
	
	Meditation is practiced in such a way that:
	    The body is at ease, the breath is calm, and the mind is tuned inward
	    Good posture supports the body
	    Rhythmic breath supports the calming of emotions
	    The mind is still and no longer serves as the constant interpreter and evaluator of experience
	    This combines stillness and prepares the practitioner for moving into a natural state of being and experiencing

Interior practices: limb #8 – absorption	
Basic definition	Once a practitioner has a regular and committed integrated yoga practice, the spontaneous experience of the eighth limb of yoga can arise – absorption. Absorption is not a practice but an experience; it is the spontaneous arising of a felt sense of integration or oneness that is beyond an ordinary state of consciousness
Central intention	Purpose and interconnection arise in absorption. Practitioners gain a clear recognition of the interconnectedness of all sentient beings and a profound connection to a greater whole. Typically, a feeling of being complete, whole, or integrated arises along with the experience of unity with everything. In absorption, practitioners experiences mindful and joyful connection to a greater purpose and a sense of community or belonging

Changes that Emerge from an Integrated Yoga Practice

Research evidence that yoga, in its many manifestations, is helpful for a variety of challenges and with many types of individuals begs the question how this change is facilitated [69, 86]. In fact, the synergy of the multitude of practices within yoga has a profound impact on several human systems that greatly affect day-to-day functioning, wellness, and resilience in times of stress, busyness, challenge, and demand [101]. Yoga optimizes autonomic control, regulates endocrine (e.g., via a decrease in cortisol and an increase in gamma-aminobutyric acid) and immune function, shapes adaptive emotional and behavioral responses, and downregulates reactivity (as evidenced by less widespread arousal, enhanced vagal tone, improved relaxation response, and cardiac variability). It facilitates "optimal physiological conditions" [104], enhances executive functioning and working memory, increases pain tolerance, and facilitates adaptive emotions and behaviors by helping practitioners hold a positive attitude, find new ways of dealing with old inputs, and make accurate discernments in times of stress and challenge [89, 104]. Yoga increases resilience in body, emotion, and mind and brings about self-regulation that supports adaptive responsiveness to meet the needs of the environment, body, emotions, and mind. These salutary benefits arise because yoga affects and integrates bottom-up and top-down pathways in the human brain for coping with internal and external demands, while it recalibrates the nervous system and maintains homeostasis in body and mind (Table 10.3).

Table 10.2 Documented health benefits of yoga

Documented physical health benefits: musculoskeletal disorders and symptoms	
Balance	[82, 91, 107]
Low back pain	[21, 27, 29, 30, 115]
Neck pain	[27, 29, 30, 73]
Musculoskeletal pain	[81]
Posture	[81, 107]
Range of motion	[3, 43, 82]
Documented physical health benefits: pain-related disorders and symptoms	
Arthritis	[6, 27, 29, 30]
Chronic pain	[16, 63, 95]
Restless legs	[47]
Headaches	[52]
Documented physical health benefits: chronic and life-threatening illnesses	
Cardiovascular disease	[3, 8, 24, 25, 84, 96]
Inflammation	[59, 60]
Respiratory illness	[1, 72]
Cancer	[15, 28, 40, 74, 98, 118]
Diabetes	[71, 94]
Digestive/metabolic disorders	[62, 68, 103]
Documented physical health benefits: well-being	
Insomnia	[7, 44]
Fatigue	[10, 43]
Immunity	[2, 41, 43]
Documented mental health benefits: clinical symptoms and disorders	
Anxiety	[57, 66, 88]
Anger	[55, 77, 64]
Depression	[17, 20, 55, 61, 64, 65, 93, 97, 117, 109]
Attention deficit	[22, 50]
Eating disorders	[18, 76]
Trauma spectrum	[19, 33, 75, 99, 106, 111]
Documented mental health benefits: well-being	
Stress perception	[13, 56, 67]
Coping skills	[23, 77, 92]
Emotional well-being	[92, 105]

Table 10.3 Pathways of sensory processing engaged in integrated yoga

Neuroception	The evaluation of current level of safety that results in a felt sense of safety, danger, or life threat, followed by a commensurate nervous system response that activates either the ventral vagal complex (safety), the sympathetic nervous system (danger), or the dorsal vagal complex (life threat)
Interoception	The capacity to attune to, receive, process, and integrate signals about the internal state of the body, including the capacity to sense the physiological state of the body from within via sensations arising from various physiological systems of the body, including but not limited to the respiratory, cardiac, gastrointestinal, thermoregulatory, and nociceptive systems
Exteroception	The ability to attune to stimuli from outside the body, to perceive and take in stimulation from the outside world – conscious and mindful perception of these stimuli can then be integrated with stimuli arising from inside the body (i.e., interoception) and help inform neuroception of safety, danger, or life threat
Proprioception	The ability to grasp the body's movement, directionality, alignment, and positioning in space based on stimuli that arise solely from within the body itself

Top-Down Pathways

Top-down mechanisms or pathways are those that arise from the cerebral cortex of the brain and as such are conscious and intentional. They promote self-regulation through a variety of mechanisms, including cognitive appraisal, reframing, goal setting and follow-through, attention, intentionality, and planning [101, 102, 104]. They decrease the level of engagement of the sympathetic nervous system, decrease habitual emotional and behavioral reactivity, enhance working memory and attentional stability, improve executive functioning, and make stress perception more accurate [36, 38, 39]. Top-down pathways can modulate neuroendocrine output, modulate vagal tone, and affect sympathetic nervous system output. As these changes take effect, even immunity and inflammation are improved [101].

Yoga integrates many practices that strengthen top-down processing and regulation, not the least of which include the exercising of attention, intention, and mindfulness and the ongoing conscious monitoring of the internal states of body, breath, and mind [14]. Further, yoga's first and second limbs as well as other aspects of deeper yoga psychology [35] help practitioners explore motivations, habits, patterns, and predilections [101]; engage in metacognition that allows for decentering and perspective-taking to result in less rigid world views and greater behavioral flexibility [110]; and step out of habits to make conscious choices based on clear intentions and deliberate preparatory plans [79, 80]. Yoga's values clarification practices encourage practitioners to engage in ethical inquiry that supports intentional decision-making and discernment [102]. Yoga's interior practice of drawing awareness inward supports the development of selective attention and response inhibition, facilitating self-regulation and conscious decision-making [39]. Concentration practices, as interior or posture practices (via gaze points or mindful attention of a particular part or state of the body), contribute to strengthening downward self-regulatory control and behavioral flexibility. In fact, all interior practices encourage practitioners to reappraise and reframe their lived experience (e.g., reconceptualizing "discomfort" as "sensation" [90]). Finally, even posture practices in and of themselves can demonstrate positive effects on top-down pathways through demanding planning, problem-solving, set-shifting, and decision-making skills [90].

Bottom-Up Pathways

Bottom-up mechanisms modulate activity in the lower regions of the brain, via ascending pathways that reach from the brain stem, through the limbic system, to the cerebral cortex, including the anterior cingulate and insula [104]. Inputs into the bottom-up circuits arise from somatic, sensory, visceral, cardiovascular, and immune receptors in the body and affect immunity, psychological health, and physical well-being. Bottom-up inputs also arise from the autonomic nervous system (sympathetic and parasympathetic) and the hypothalamic-pituitary-adrenal axis. Bottom-up mechanisms can contribute to self-regulation; however, they do so not via conscious and intentional cognitive processes (as is the case with top-down processing), but via unconscious responsivity to the perceived demand characteristics of a particular input. Symptoms of illness and injury arise from the bottom-up pathways.

Many yoga practices facilitate accurate perception of sensory inputs through careful attention to bodily states, especially as mediated by mindful breath and posture practice. Breathing practices induce calmness in the nervous system with subsequent relaxing responses in the neuroendocrine system via release of oxytocin and prolactin [90]. Successful autonomic nervous system control and decreased endocrine release in turn results in enhanced social bonding and decreased emotional reactivity [83], [101]. Posture practice helps practitioners learn to maintain a balanced nervous system in the face of challenge, as physical and sympathetic arousal from movement is effectively managed by the teacher through careful postural sequencing and processing of exposure, extinction, and adaptive responsiveness [39]. Finally, while not a limb of yoga, chanting or intoning a mantra such as the word "*om*" are additional yogic practices that assert positive autonomic control [102].

Polyvagal System and Top-Down/Bottom-Up Integration

A crucial player in top-down and bottom-up functions is the vagus (tenth cranial) nerve or polyvagal system [83]. The vagus nerve is the primary conduit for communication about the internal state as perceived through various sensory systems to the brain. It relays physical, mental, and environmental sensory input (from the bottom) via the anterior cingulate cortex and the insula to the prefrontal cortex (to the top). It integrates emotion, cognition, and conscious deliberation about sensory input from the top to the bottom, creating a network and integration across brain structures for an integration/collaboration of the top-down and bottom-up pathways. Top-down bottom-up integration facilitates balance in the polyvagal system, allowing for a calm, integrated, and resilient response [39, 90, 101, 102].

The smooth and adaptive integration of bottom-up and top-down pathways is not ingrained, since humans may develop habitual patterns wherein responses are driven reactively by one or the other system [79]. The polyvagal system is the human threat detection system that is unconscious and arises at the sensory receptor level via a process called neuroception; neuroception of the environment or internal state can result in three possible reactions: safety, danger, or life threat (terror). Neuroception of safety activates the ventral vagal complex (VVC) of the polyvagal system. The VVC supports physiological recovery, emotional processing or interoception, mental regulation, and prosocial behavior [104]. The VVC facilitates social engagement and connection through release of oxytocin and prolactin, prosocial behavior, engaging voice and facial expressions, and a relaxed posture. Neuroception of danger activates the sympathetic branch of the autonomic nervous system, readying the organism for fight or flight, mobilizing a response that increases the likelihood of survival. It results in increased muscle tone, redirection of blood flow from the periphery to the core, inhibition of the gastrointestinal system, dilation of the bronchi, and increase in heart rate and respiration (among other physiological responses). Neuroception of life threat activates the dorsal vagal complex (DVC) and results in immobilization of the organism. Human beings in this situation shut down, freeze, or "play dead." An organism in a state of life threat exhibits decreased muscle tone, decreased cardiac output, and reflexive defecation and urination (among other physiological responses) to reduce life functions to the least amount needed for survival.

Humans tend to have habitual or preferred response styles (mediated by the vagus) that develop through experience and learning histories over the developmental span [79, 101, 102]. Some individuals have greater likelihood to perceive safety (living more commonly in their relaxed, engaging, and restorative ventral vagal space); others have a response set for danger (living in a near-constant state of sympathetic arousal, isolation, and physiological overload or breakdown); and some expect life threat and develop a habitual pattern of shrinking back from life, withdrawing – even dissociating – from human experiences. Top-down and bottom-up mechanisms are set in place that perpetuate these preparatory styles and thus can also become the mechanism for change.

As demonstrated above, yoga offers many strategies for top-down and bottom-up processing, most of which work in tandem with each other for a natural integration of these pathways through the synergistic combination of several limbs of yoga. Additionally, yoga facilitates the change of habitual styles by making practitioners more behaviorally flexible, emotionally resilient, and cognitively complex to deal responsively with each input in the moment as it unfolds, rather than reactively based on learning history and experience. Through various integrative practices, yoga facilitates top-down bottom-up integration, ushering in greater response flexibility and decreased reactivity. Yoga creates bidirectional feedback and feedforward loops in the brain that result in greater accuracy of input detection and interpretation and in greater resilience and self-regulation in emotional, mental, and behavioral responses [39, 101, 102]. Yoga stimulates the basal ganglia corticothalamic circuits that help humans unlearn maladaptive behaviors and allow for extinction learning. Simultaneously, yoga (especially through mindfulness practices) creates greater connectivity of the caudate with other (higher and lower) brain regions, facilitating new, goal-directed, flexible learning and behavior [38, 90]. Yoga employs strategies that restore balance to the nervous system through supporting preparatory mind sets that place the organism into the ventral vagal (i.e., calm, relaxed, interpersonally engaged) space. This effect is important as the polyvagal system regulates allostatic load.

Allostasis and Accurate Sensory Processing

Allostasis is the "ability of an organism to maintain stability/homeostasis through change by actively adjusting to both predictable and unpredictable events" [90]. Yoga offers many tools that decrease allostatic load by offering behavioral choices, emotional flexibility, and cognitive reappraisal and restructuring. Resilience in body, emotion, mind, and behavior facilitates a ventral vagal response and promotes successful, integrated (bottom-up and top-down) self-regulation. Allostasis is dependent on the capacity to take self-regulatory action based on accurate internal [26] and external [116] sensory pathways to bring the organism back into balance. Much of what yoga facilitates is exactly that: it prepares the practitioner to take appropriate and adaptive action in response to accurately perceived demands and needs.

Mindfulness (embedded in all yogic practices) encourages accurate perception of sensory input from internal bodily systems and environmental stimuli through conscious awareness of neuroceptive, interoceptive, exteroceptive, and proprioceptive stimuli (see Table 10.3). In other words, yoga encourages conscious and accurate processing of sensory input from inside and outside the body to support self-regulation, bidirectional feedback, and adaptive behavior in support of successful allostasis (ongoing change in the service of stability). Yoga facilitates meta-awareness and in-the-moment lived experience of interoceptive, neuroceptive, exteroceptive, and proprioceptive inputs and thus helps integrate information across top-down and bottom-up systems, a process that is largely coordinated by the insula [38, 39, 108, 104].

These inputs and the capacity to appraise their ebbing and flowing are crucial to psychological well-being, via accurate cognitive appraisal of what is perceived [26], and physical health, via supporting physiological homeostasis [42], as well as to feeling present, effective, and proactive in the world. They become useful – and are applied in the context of yoga – when they are interwoven with mindful and accurate appraisal of the environment or context to result in adaptive behaviors [34] and to break reflexive and reactive cycles of responses. Practitioners of yoga learn to live in a ventral vagal state and to allow for and successfully manage a sympathetic nervous system response during danger. This mindset of *preparedness* allows the individual to maintain or re-achieve ease while being ready to take action when environmental demands arise. In moments of terror or life threat, a mindset of *surrender* may be invoked, wherein the practitioner moves from the ventral vagal to the dorsal vagal space to allow for momentary submission or freezing if the environmental demand is best met by this response. The resultant level of resilient and adaptive self-regulation reduces allostatic load and brings homeostasis or stability to body, emotion, and mind – called equanimity in yoga's language.

The Practical Application of Yoga

Yoga's salutary effects outlined above are mediated by the eight limbs of yoga (Table 10.1). Integrated yoga is a profound journey into body, emotion, mind, and relationship. It is best entered through the guidance of a skilled teacher who can help each practitioner determine an optimal entry point and plot a trajectory for development. Clinicians who wish to help clients augment their physical or mental health journey through yoga practice need to be well-informed about the components and benefits of the practice and how to facilitate a referral to a competent yoga professional who will become a collaborator in the patient's care. Several considerations are crucial.

Referral for Yoga as a Complementary or Integrative Practice

The research evidence is clear: any individual with mental health or physical health challenges can benefit from a tailored yoga practice. Sadly, under-referral is typical as most healthcare professionals do not understand the wide applicability of yoga [100]. However, given the variety of yoga strategies, almost anyone can practice yoga. Lifestyle, breathing, and interior practices are accessible to all bodies; postures come in many forms and can be practiced by nearly everyone. While Western posture practice is often (and counter to traditional yoga) forceful, energetic, and focused on physical beauty and fitness, yoga's physical practices can be modified and adapted. Extant stereotypes about yoga postures limit access to integrated yoga for the very individuals who could benefit [13, 54, 100]. Media depictions imply that yoga is only for those who are already physically adept, slender, White, female, well-to-do, educated, flexible, strong, balanced, and healthy [9, 12, 78, 85]. Nothing could be further from the truth. Integrated posture practice is carefully adapted to individual practitioner's needs by being taught holistically with yoga blocks, straps, bolsters, blankets, pillows, and chairs to allow practitioners of all shapes, ages, sizes, states of health and mobility, and experience to participate fully and reap the benefits of mindful self-expression and self-exploration [11, 53, 112]. Properly modified, nearly all patients, even those with physical challenges and limitations, can experience the benefits of yoga.

Choosing a Yoga Offering and Professional

Making informed choices about selecting a yoga teacher is key to successful referral and practice. To help clinicians make optimal choices about referral to a qualified yoga professional, it is helpful to have facts about yoga as a profession. Three forms of yoga exist: yoga classes, therapeutic yoga, and yoga therapy. Yoga classes take place in gyms, studios, and even online and range widely from being strictly exercise-based to including accessible practices from all yoga limbs. Yoga classes may vary regarding the degree to which they are tailored to individual needs through encouraging props, adaptations, and modification. Therapeutic yoga may happen in the same venues as yoga classes; however, it is practiced in small groups (not to exceed eight to ten practitioners), typically has more than one teacher (and/or assistants), identifies a health or mental health purpose (e.g., yoga for back pain, cancer survivors, stress reduction), and makes demonstrated use of props, adaptations, and modifications. Yoga therapy is offered one-on-one (at most one-on-two if a yoga professional has two patients with very similar clinical presentations) and is completely tailored to the needs and presenting health or mental health concerns of the patient. Yoga therapy is typically collaborative with a referring clinician and presumes a working relationship of the patient with a primary care physician or psychologist (depending on referral). Props, modifications, adaptations, and tailored interventions are a requirement.

Clinicians who draw on the resources of yoga for diagnosable health or mental health challenges are best served by referring to therapeutic yoga or yoga therapy. Some carefully selected yoga classes can also be helpful with the caveats that the patient has manageable symptoms (without significant contraindications for posture practice) and the clinician is familiar with the yoga teachers and their approach to teaching, ascertaining a full eight-limb practice and modifiable posture practice. For clients under preventive care, general yoga classes are an appropriate resource as long as offered classes are sensitive to individual needs by offering props and modifications. Therapeutic yoga can be helpful for preventive care by honing in on particular risk factors of a given individual.

Yoga classes and therapeutic yoga can be offered by a range of qualified yoga teachers. The basic qualification of a yoga teacher is a 200-hour certification, preferably from a yoga school registered with *Yoga Alliance* (www.yogaalliance.org), the national body that registers and reapproves yoga teachers and schools. Yoga teachers with the designation *RYT200* have this certification. Advanced teachers have additional training from at least a 500-hour certification program. If registered by Yoga Alliance, these teachers are designated as *RYT500*. An "*E*" with the *RYT* designation verifies that the teacher has significant experience (with at least 1000 teaching hours). Yoga therapy is offered by qualified yoga therapists, a new profession that requires extensive training and certification by the *International Association of Yoga Therapists* (www.IAYT.org). Yoga therapists have a designation of *C-IAYT* to show their proper training and credentialing from a certified yoga therapy program. Credentials of yoga teachers and therapists can be verified online through the two certification bodies.

Choosing a Yoga Venue

A beneficial yoga venue can serve patients who are presenting either for integrated yoga classes, or therapeutic work may be part of a yoga studio, gym, hospital, mental health center, primary care center, physical therapy practice, and other designated physical space with several key characteristics that include, but may not be limited to, appropriately sized dedicated space, ample offerings of yoga props, proper teacher-to-student ratios, proper lighting, and a harmonious atmosphere conducive to mindful work. Prop offerings include mats, blocks, blankets, and bolsters. Some venues provide straps, chairs, eye pillows, therabands, balls, meditation cushions, meditation beads, hot water bottles, and sandbags. Venues that offer therapeutic yoga likely have most or all of these materials but may be slightly smaller in size, appropriate to the class size that is offered. Yoga therapy venues meet all of the above materials requirements. They may also be located in a private office that is significantly smaller if the provider does not offer yoga classes.

Table 10.4 offers a handout for clinicians and patients that guides successful referral of patients to yoga. It guides the clinician to optimal venues and teachers who apply integrated teaching or therapeutic models. No such guide is perfect; each clinician is encouraged to make personal contact with potential yoga professionals also to assess how well the individual communicates and whether a positive and collaborative working relationship can be established.

How to Talk to Patients About Yoga

As patients likely hold stereotypes about yoga, clinicians are well-served to discuss the principles of an integrated yoga practice before making a referral. Giving patients information about the eight limbs and yoga's accessibility to all types of needs lays a helpful foundation for an informed choice.

Table 10.4 A handout for facilitating a success referral to a yoga professional

Exploring the level of integration of a yoga class
Look for teachers who offer access to all eight limbs of yoga:
The psychology and lifestyle practice of yoga via attending to ethics, dedication to practice, setting intentions, making a commitment to practice, finding a clear purpose in life
Posture practices that are mindful and carefully adapted to your needs (more about this below)
Breathing practices with particular attention to the teaching of mindful breathing in all postures
Concentration practices such as imagery, focusing on an object of attention (e.g., your breath), or being mindful of a particular part of your body
Meditation practices – either guided or silent
Look for teachers who incorporate mindfulness skills by inviting their students to:
Explore how each posture feels in their body, directing them to important sensations that may arise
Explore how the breath moves through the body
Notice all sensations that arise in body, mind, breath, or emotions with curiosity
Notice what is happening inside their body, breath, and mind without judgment
Differentiate for themselves which sensations are "good" or manageable and can be endured versus which sensations are danger signs that suggest that they may want to move out of a posture or away from a particular breath or interior practice
Experience internal sensations – perhaps using the words interoception (feeling their body from the inside out) and proprioception (learning where body parts are in space)
Experience external sensation – perhaps using the word exteroception (sensing stimuli that arise from outside the body, perhaps attending to temperature, air flow, the ground underneath)
Be fully aware of every moment of their practice and be present for every movement and breath
Look for teachers who are most concerned *not* about the outer appearance of a physical posture, but how the posture feels in the practitioners' body by:
Using props to make the pose accessible to your body shape and needs
Inviting postures to be modified, skipped, or adapted in any way that feel optimal to their body, breath, mind, and emotional needs
Adapting the posture to their personal needs, not adapting postures to a particular concept of how a posture *should* look
Offering multiple ways to do each posture that allows them to choose the variation that feels best for them in any given moment
Practicing with mindfulness so that they are fully aware of every movement as they move into a posture, are in a posture, and move out of a posture
Exploring the appropriateness and atmosphere of the physical space
Look for venues that create a conducive atmosphere for integrated yoga:
Adequate room size given the size of the average class
Natural or adjustable lighting
Quiet atmosphere, perhaps using some soft music (but no loud activating exercise music)
Thoughtfulness about chemical sensitivities by being scent-free
Few or no mirrors on the wall – unless teachers can articulate the mirrors' purpose
Privacy during classes (rather than large windows that invite onlookers)
Easy access to restrooms and changing rooms
Look for venues that are inviting to a variety of yoga practitioners as evidenced by:
Sliding fee scales that invite anyone to participate
A varied and diverse student body who comes regularly
Small classes *or* large classes only with multiple teachers and assistants
Therapeutic class offerings that may include adaptive topics such as trauma-sensitive yoga, yoga for aging bodies, yoga for individuals with physical challenges, yoga for particular health conditions

(continued)

Table 10.4 (continued)

Look for venues that can accommodate a range of personal needs as evidenced by:
Yoga props for adapted or modified physical posture practice, such as mats, foam blocks or bricks, bolsters or pillows, blankets, chairs, and straps (if not contraindicated by the clientele), therabands, and other items that can serve to help practitioners' body be more comfortable
Yoga props for breathing practices, such as bolsters and blankets
Yoga props for interior practices, such as bolsters or meditation cushions, blankets, eye pillows, mala beads, or similar items that may be used for meditation, concentration, or introspection
Exploring the personal response to the offered practice
Practitioners are encouraged to assess how they respond to the offered practice by conducting a self-assessment after the first few classes at a new venue or with a new teacher. The following questions are offered as a guide to this self-assessment. There are not definitive answers to the questions below. They are offered to foster an exploration of whether the practitioner felt protected, safe, cared for, and seen as a human being. Yoga classes aim to develop community and support. Yoga classes aim to adapt to individual bodies and needs, not the other way around
1. How do you feel physically? Do you feel as though you worked too hard? Are you sore in a way that is comfortable? Was your body challenged without being hurt?
2. How do you feel emotionally? Did you feel safe? Did you feel vulnerable or unprotected? Do you feel calm and settled at the end of class?
3. Did you connect to other students in the class? Were there positive interactions with others in the class – including students, teacher, or assistants? Do you have a sense of community?
4. Did you feel heard and seen? Were you greeted by the teacher? Was there a farewell? Did the teacher or assistant acknowledge your presence and efforts?
5. Did you receive the support you wanted or needed from the teacher or assistant? Were you offered adaptations or props? Did you receive encouragement? Were you pushed into anything you did not really want to do?
6. Did you feel pushed into anything you did not really want to do? Were you invited to test your own appropriate boundaries? Were you given options about how far to move into your practice? Did you receive invitations not to overdo or over effort?
7. Were you kept physically safe? Did you receive physical adjustments without invitation (against your wishes)? Did the teacher ask for permission to touch before doing so? Did you have the option to decline physical contact?
8. Did you feel encouraged to adapt poses and breathing to your needs? Were you given help to do so? Were you offered props? Were you invited to explore various expressions of the same pose to find the one that fit you best?

Once a referral is made, staying in touch with patients about their experience of yoga is crucial to ascertain that the practice is unfolding as intended, resulting in benefit not harm. Ongoing communication with the yoga professional is indicated, especially if it is a yoga therapist. Clinicians and yoga therapists can be mutually helpful, keeping each other informed of changes, challenges, and improvements in shared clients (with proper releases of information).

Finally, patients and clients can be encouraged to engage in a home practice once they have worked with a yoga teacher or therapist for a while. The teacher or therapist will be the best resource for patients to help them build a successful home practice. Many online resources offer excellent yoga classes at very low cost. Patients can consult with their yoga teacher about how to choose optimal online yoga classes.

Conclusions

Yoga is a lifestyle, a choice, and a commitment. It is a transformative wellness practice that can lead to profound neurophysiological, neurocognitive, and psychological changes; it is a gateway to deep joy, equanimity, compassion, and kindness. Clinicians who want to incorporate yoga as an integrative treatment strategy for their patients can do so by drawing on appropriately trained yoga professionals. Clinicians will also benefit from a personal yoga practice so they too can experience the many benefits the practice has to offer and so they may better understand their patients' yoga experiences.

References

1. Agnihotri S, Kant S, Kumar S, Mishra RK, Mishra SK. Impact of yoga on biochemical profile of asthmatics: a randomized controlled study. Int J Yoga Ther. 2014;7:17–21.
2. Ahmadi A, Nikbakh M, Arastoo A, Habibi AH. The effects of a yoga intervention on balance, speed, and endurance of walking, fatigue, and quality of life in people with multiple sclerosis. J Hum Kinet. 2010;23:71–8.
3. Alexander GK, Innes KE, Selfe TK, Brown CJ. "More than I expected": perceived benefits of yoga among older adults at risk for cardiovascular disease. Complement Ther Med. 2013;21:14–28.
4. Barnes PM, Bloom B, Nahin RL. Complementary and alternative medicine use among adults and children: United States. Natl Health Stat Rep. 2007;12:1–23.
5. Barnett JE, Shale AL, Elkins G, Fisher W. Complementary and alternative medicine for psychologists: an essential resource. Washington, DC: American Psychological Association; 2014.
6. Bedekar N, Prabhu A, Shyam A, Sancheti K, Sancheti P. Comparative study of conventional therapy and additional yogasanas for knee rehabilitation after total knee arthroplasty. Int J Yoga. 2012;5:118–22.
7. Bhaduri T, Kanchan C, Sonali B, Asit PK, Ekta. Evaluation of sirodhara and yoga therapy in management of chronic insomnia. Int Res J Pharm. 2013;4:78–80.
8. Blom K, Baker B, How M, Dai M, Irvine J, Abbey S, et al. Hypertension analysis of stress reduction using mindfulness meditation and yoga: results from the HARMONY randomized controlled trial. Am J Hypertens. 2014;27(1):122–9.
9. Birdee GS, Legedza AT, Saper RB, Bertisch SM, Eisenberg DM, Phillips RS. Characteristics of yoga users: results of a national survey. J Gen Intern Med. 2008;23:1653–8.
10. Bower JE, Garet D, Sternlieb B, Ganz PA, Irwin MR, Olmstead R, Greendale G. Yoga for persistent fatigue in breast cancer survivors: a randomized controlled trial. Cancer. 2012;118:3766–75.
11. Brems C. A yoga stress reduction intervention for university faculty, staff, and graduate students. Int J Yoga Ther. 2015;25:61–77.
12. Brems C, Colgan D, Freeman H, Freitas J, Justice L, Shean M, Sulenes K. Elements of yogic practice: perceptions of students in healthcare programs. Int J Yoga. 2016;9:121–9.
13. Brems C, Justice L, Sulenes K, Girasa L, Ray J, Davis M, Freitas J, Shean M, Colgan D. Improving access to yoga: barriers and motivators for practice among health professions students. Adv Mind Body Med. 2015;29:6–13.
14. Brown KW, Ryan RM, Creswell JD. Mindfulness: theoretical foundations and evidence for its salutary effects. Psychol Inq. 2007;18:211–37.
15. Buffart LM, van Uffelen J, Riphagen II, Bryg J, van Mechelen W, Brown WJ, Chinapaw M. Physical and psychosocial benefits of yoga in cancer patients and survivors, a systematic review and meta-analysis of randomized control trials. BMC Cancer. 2013;12:559.
16. Büssing A, Ostermann T, Ludtke R, Michalsen A. Effects of yoga interventions on pain and pain-associated disability: a meta-analysis. J Pain. 2012;13:1–9.
17. Butler LD, Waelde LC, Hastings TA, Chen X, Symons B, Marshall JJ, et al. Meditation with yoga, group therapy with hypnosis, and psychoeducation for long-term depressed mood: a randomized pilot trial. J Clin Psychol. 2008;64:806–20.
18. Carei TR, Fyfe-Johnson AL, Breuner CC, Brown MA. Randomized controlled trial of yoga in the treatment of eating disorders. J Adolesc Health. 2010;46:346–51.
19. Carter JJ, Gerbarg PL, Brown RP, Ware RS, D'Ambrosio C, Anand L, et al. Multi-component yoga breath program for Vietnam veteran post traumatic stress disorder: randomized controlled trial. Journal of Traum Stress Disord Treat. 2013;2:3. https://doi.org/10.4172/2324-8947.1000108.
20. Chandratrya S. Yoga: an evidence-based therapy. J Mid-Life Health. 2011;2:3.
21. Chang DG, Holt JA, Sklar M, Groessl EJ. Yoga as a treatment for chronic low back pain: a systematic review. J Orthop Rheumatol. 2016;3:1–8.
22. Chaya MS, Nagendra H, Selvam S, Kurpad A, Sirinvasan K. Effect of yoga on cognitive abilities in schoolchildren from a socioeconomically disadvantaged background: a randomized controlled study. J Altern Complement Med. 2012;18:1161–7.
23. Chong CS, Tsunaka M, Tsang HW, Chan EP, Cheung WM. Effects of yoga on stress management in healthy adults: a systematic review. Altern Ther Health Med. 2011;17:32–8.
24. Chu P, Gotink G, Yeh GY, Goldie SJ, Hunink M. The effectiveness of yoga in modifying risk factors for cardiovascular disease and metabolic syndrome: a systematic review and meta-analysis of randomized controlled trials. Eur J Prev Cardiol. 2014;23:291–307.
25. Cohen D, Bower A, Townsend RR. Results of the LIMBS study: yoga, alone or in combination with other lifestyle measures reduces BP in untreated prehypertension and stage 1 hypertension (abstract). Circulation. 2014;130(suppl_2):A11651.

26. Craig AD. How do you feel? An interoceptive moment with your neurobiological self. Princeton: Princeton University Press; 2014.
27. Cramer H, Lauche R, Langhorst J, Dobos G. Yoga for rheumatic diseases: a systematic review. Rheumatology. 2013;52:2025–30.
28. Cramer H, Lange S, Klose P, Paul A, Dobos G. Yoga for breast cancer patient survivors and patients: a systematic review and meta-analysis. BMC Cancer. 2012;12(412):1–13.
29. Cramer H, Lauche R, Haller H, Dobos G. A systematic review and meta-analysis of yoga for low back pain. Clin J Pain. 2013;29:450–60.
30. Cramer H, Lauche R, Haller H, Langhorst J, Dobos G, Berger B. "I'm more in balance": a qualitative study of yoga for patients with chronic neck pain. J Altern Complement Med. 2013;19:536–42.
31. Dittman KA, Freedman MR. Body awareness, eating attitudes, and spiritual beliefs of women practicing yoga. Eat Disord. 2009;17:273–92.
32. Elwy AR, Groessl EJ, Eisen SV, Riley KE, Maiya M, Lee JP, et al. A systematic scoping review of yoga intervention components and study quality. Am J Prev Med. 2014;47:220–32.
33. Emerson D, Hopper E. Overcoming trauma through yoga: reclaiming your body. Berkeley: North Atlantic Books; 2011.
34. Farb N, Duabenmier J, Price CJ, Gard T, Kerr C, Dunn BD, et al. Interoception, contemplative practice, and health. Front Psychol. 2015;6:763. https://doi.org/10.3389/fpsyg.2015.00763.
35. Feuerstein G. The psychology of yoga: integrating eastern and Western approaches for understanding the mind. Boston: Shambala; 2013.
36. Field T. Yoga clinical research review. Complement Ther Clin Pract. 2011;17:1–8.
37. Freeman H, Vladagina N, Razmjou E, Brems C. Yoga in print media: missing the heart of the practice. Int J Yoga. 2017;10:160–6.
38. Gard T, Taquet M, Dixit R, Holzel B, Dickerson B, Lazar S. Greater widespread functional connectivity of the caudate in older adults who practice kripalu yoga and vipassana meditation than in controls. Front Hum Neurosci. 2015;9:137.
39. Gard T, Noggle JJ, Park C, Vago DR, Wilson A. Potential self-regulatory mechanisms of yoga for psychological health. Front Hum Neurosci. 2014;8:770.
40. Geyer R, Lyons A, Amazeen L, Alishio L, Cooks L. Effect of yoga on quality of life of children with cancer. Pediatr Phys Ther. 2011;23:375–9.
41. Gopal A, Mondal S, Gandhi A, Arora S, Bhattacharjee J. Effect of integrated yoga practices on immune responses in examination stress – a preliminary study. Int J Yoga. 2011;4:26–32.
42. Gu J, Strauss C, Bond R, Cavanagh K. How do mindfulness-based cognitive therapy and mindfulness-based stress reduction improve mental health and wellbeing? A systematic review and meta-analysis of meditation studies. Clin Psychol Rev. 2015;37:1–12.
43. Guner S, Inanici F. Yoga therapy and ambulatory multiple sclerosis assessment of gait analysis parameters, fatigue and balance. J Bodyw Mov Ther. 2014;19:72–81.
44. Halpern J, Cohen M, Kennedy G, Reece J, Cahan C, Baharav A. Yoga for improving sleep quality and quality of life for older adults. Altern Ther Health Med. 2014;20:37–46.
45. Hartranft C. The yoga sutra of Patanjali: a new translation with commentary. Boston: Shambala Classics; 2003.
46. Hayes M, Chase S. Prescribing yoga. Prim Care. 2010;37:31–47.
47. Innes KE, Selfe TK, Agarwal P, Williams K, Flack KL. Efficacy of an eight-week yoga intervention on symptoms of restless legs syndrome (RLS): a pilot study. J Altern Complement Med. 2013;19:527–35.
48. IPSOS Public Affairs. 2016 Yoga in America study conducted by Yoga Journal and Yoga Alliance. 2016. Accessed 19 Feb 2019. Retrieved from https://www.yogajournal.com/page/yogainamericastudy.
49. Iyengar BKS. Light on life. New York: Rodale; 2005.
50. Jensen PS, Kenny DT. The effects of yoga on the attention and behavior of boys with attention-deficit/hyperactivity disorder. J Atten Disord. 2004;7:205–16.
51. Jeter PE, Slutsky J, Singh N, Khalsa SB. Yoga as a therapeutic intervention: a bibliometric analysis of published research studies from 1967 to 2013. J Altern Complement Med. 2015;21:586–92.
52. John PJ, Sharma N, Sharma CM, Kankane A. Effectiveness of yoga therapy in the treatment of migraine without aura: a randomized controlled trial. Headache. 2007;47:654–61.
53. Justice L, Brems C, Ehlers K. Bridging body and mind: considerations for trauma-informed yoga. Int J Yoga Ther. 2018;28(1):39–50. Advance online publication. https://doi.org/10.17761/2018-00017R2.
54. Justice L, Brems C, Jacova C. Exploring strategies to enhance self-efficacy about starting a yoga practice. Ann Yoga Phys Ther. 2016;1(2):1–7.
55. Kanojia S, Sharma VK, Gandhi A, Kapoor R, Kukreja A, Subramanian SK. Effect of yoga on autonomic functions and psychological status during both phases of menstrual cycle in young healthy females. J Clin Diagn Res. 2013;7:2133–9.

56. Kauts A, Sharma N. Effect of yoga on academic performance in relation to stress. Int J Yoga. 2009;2:39–43.
57. Khalsa MK, Greiner-Ferris JM, Hoffman SG, Khalsa SBS. Yoga-enhanced cognitive behavioral therapy (Y-CBT) for anxiety management: a pilot study. Clin Psychol Psychother. 2015;22:364–71.
58. Khalsa SBS, Cohen L, McCall T, Telles S. The principles and practice of yoga in healthcare. Edinburgh: Handspring Publishing; 2016.
59. Kiecolt-Glaser JK, Bennett JM, Andridge R, Peng J, Shapiro CL, Malarkey WB, et al. Yoga's impact on inflammation, mood, and fatigue in breast cancer survivors: a randomized controlled trial. J Clin Oncol. 2014;32:1040–9.
60. Kiecolt-Glaser JK, Christian L, Preston H, Houts CR, Malarkey WB, Emery CF, Glaser R. Stress, inflammation, and yoga practice. Psychosom Med. 2010;72:13–21.
61. Kinser PA, Bourguignon C, Whaley D, Hauenstein E, Taylor AG. Feasibility, acceptability, and effects of gentle Hatha yoga for women with major depression: findings from a randomized controlled mixed-methods study. Arch Psychiatr Nurs. 2013;27:137–47.
62. Kuttner L, Chambers CT, Hardial J, Israel DM, Jacobson K, Evans K. A randomized trial of yoga for adolescents with irritable bowel syndrome. Pain Res Manag. 2006;11:217–24.
63. Langhorst J, Klose P, Dobos GJ, Bernardy K, Hauser W. Efficacy and safety of meditative movement therapies in fibromyalgia syndrome: a systematic review and meta-analysis of randomized controlled trials. Rheumatol Int. 2013;33:193–207.
64. Lavey R, Sherman T, Mueser KT, Osborne DD, Currier M, Wolfe R. The effects of yoga on mood in psychiatric inpatients. Psychiatr Rehabil J. 2005;28:399–402.
65. Lavretsy H, Epel ES, Siddarth P, Nazarian N, Cyr NS, Khalsa DS, et al. A pilot study of yogic meditation for family dementia caregivers with depressive symptoms: effects on mental health, cognition, and telomerase activity. Int J Geriatr Psychiatry. 2013;28:57–65.
66. Li AW, Goldsmith CW. The effects of yoga on stress and anxiety. Altern Med Rev. 2013;17:21–35.
67. Luu K, Hall P. Hatha yoga and executive function: a systematic review. J Altern Complement Med. 2015;22:125–33.
68. Manchanda SC, Mehotra UC, Makhija A, Mohanty A, Dhawan S, Sawhney JPS. Reversal of early atherosclerosis in metabolic syndrome by yoga – a randomized controlled trial. J Yoga Phys Ther. 2013;3:1. https://doi.org/10.4172/2157-7595.1000132.
69. McCall MC. How might yoga work? An overview of potential underlying mechanisms. J Yoga Phys Ther. 2013;3(1):1.
70. McCall MC. In search of yoga: research trends in a western medical database. Int J Yoga. 2014;7:4–8.
71. McDermott KA, Rao MR, Nagaranthna R, Murphy EJ, Burke A, Nagendra RH, Hecht FM. A yoga intervention for type 2 diabetes risk reduction: a pilot randomized controlled trial. Complement Altern Med. 2014;14:212. https://doi.org/10.1186/1472-6882-14-212.
72. Mekonnen D, Mossie A. Clinical effects of yoga on asthmatic patients: a preliminary clinical trial. Ethiop J Health Sci. 2010;20:107–12.
73. Michalsen A, Traitteur H, Rainer L, Brunnhuber S, Meier L, Jeiter M, Bussing A, Kessler C. Yoga for chronic neck pain: a pilot randomized controlled clinical trial. J Pain. 2010;13:1122–30.
74. Milbury K, Mallaiah S, Liao ZX, Shannon V, Yang C, Cohen L. Randomized controlled trial (RCT) of a dyadic yoga program for lung cancer patients undergoing radiotherapy and their family caregivers. J Clin Oncol. 2017;35:125. https://doi.org/10.1200/JCO.2017.35.31_suppl.125.
75. Mitchell KS, Dick AM, DiMartino DM, Smith BN, Niles B, Koenen KC, Street A. A pilot study of a randomized controlled trial of yoga as an intervention for PTSD symptoms in women. J Trauma Stress. 2014;27:121–8.
76. Mitchell KS, Mazzeo SE, Rausch SM, Cooke KL. Innovative interventions for disordered eating: evaluating dissonance-based and yoga interventions. Int J Eat Disord. 2006;40:120–8.
77. Noggle JJ, Steiner NJ, Minami T, Khalsa SS. Benefits of yoga for psychosocial well-being in a US high school curriculum: a preliminary randomized controlled trial. J Dev Behav Pediatr. 2012;33:193–201.
78. Park LC, Braun T, Siegel T. Who practices yoga? A systematic review of demographic, health-related, and psychosocial factors associated with yoga practice. J Behav Med. 2015;38:460–71.
79. Payne P, Crane-Gondreau MA. The preparatory set: a novel approach to understanding stress, trauma, and the bodymind therapies. Front Hum Neurosci. 2015;9:178.
80. Payne L, Gold T, Goldman E. Yoga therapy and integrative medicine: where ancient science meets modern medicine. Laguna Beach: Basic Health Publications; 2015.
81. Pimentel do Rosario JL, Orcesi LS, Kobayashi FN, Aun AN, Assumpcao ITD, Blasilio GJ, Hanada ES. The immediate effects of modified yoga positions on musculoskeletal pain relief. J Bodyw Mov Ther. 2013;17:469–74.
82. Polsgrove MJ, Eggleston BM, Lockyer RJ. Impact of 10-weeks of yoga practice on flexibility and balance of college athletes. Int J Yoga. 2016;9:27–34.
83. Porges S. The polyvagal theory: neurophysiological of emotions, attachment, communication, and self-regulation. New York: Norton; 2011.

84. Raghuran N, Rarachuri VR, Swarnagowri MV, Babu S, Chaku R, Kulkarni R, et al. Yoga based cardiac rehabilitation after coronary artery bypass surgery: one-year results on LVEF, lipid profile and psychological states – a randomized controlled study. Indian Heart J. 2014;66:490–502.

85. Razmjou E, Freeman H, Vladagina N, Freitas J, Brems C. Popular media images of yoga: limiting perceived access to a beneficial practice. Media Psychol Rev. 2017;11(2).

86. Riley KE, Park CL. How does yoga reduce stress? A systematic review of mechanisms of change and guide to future inquiry. Health Psychol Rev. 2015;9:379–96.

87. Ross A, Friedmann E, Bevans M, Thomas S. National survey of yoga practitioners: mental and physical health benefits. Complement Ther Med. 2013;21:313–23.

88. Satyapriya M, Nagarathna R, Padmalatha V, Nagendra HR. Effect of integrated yoga on anxiety, depression and well being in normal pregnancy. Complement Ther Clin Pract. 2013;19:230–6.

89. Schmalzl L, Crane-Godreau MA, Payne P. Movement-based embodied contemplative practices: definitions and paradigms. Front Hum Neurosci. 2014;8:205. https://doi.org/10.3389/fnhum.2014.00205.

90. Schmalzl L, Powers C, Blom EH. Neurophysiological and neurocognitive mechanisms underlying the effects of yoga-based practices: towards a comprehensive theoretical framework. Front Hum Neurosci. 2015;9:235.

91. Schmid AA, Puymbroeck M, Koceja DM. Effect of a 12-week yoga intervention on fear of falling and balance in older adults: a pilot study. Arch Phys Med Rehabil. 2010;91:576–83.

92. Sethi JK, Nagendra HR, Ganpat TS. Yoga improves attention and self-esteem in underprivileged girl student. J Educ Health. 2013;2:55.

93. Shahidi M, Motjahed A, Modabbernia A, Motjahed M, Shafiabady A, Delavar A, Honari H. Laughter yoga versus group exercise program in elderly depressed women: a randomized controlled trial. Int J Geriatr Psychiatry. 2011;26:322–7.

94. Shantakumari N, Sequeira S, Eldeeb R. Effects of a yoga intervention on lipid profiles of diabetes patients with dyslipidemia. Indian Heart J. 2013;65:127–31.

95. Sharan D, Manjula M, Urmi D, Ajeesh PS. Effect of yoga on the myofascial pain syndrome of neck. Int J Yoga. 2014;7:54–9.

96. Sharma M, Halder T. Yoga as alternative and complementary treatment for hypertensive patients: a systematic review. J Evid Based Complement Altern Med. 2012;17:199–205.

97. Sharma VK, Das S, Mondal S, Goswami U, Gandhi A. Effects of sahaj yoga on depressive disorders. Indian J Physiol Pharmacol. 2005;49:462–8.

98. Sohl SJ, Danhauer SC, Schnur JB, Daly L, Suslov K, Montgomery GH. Feasibility of a brief yoga intervention during chemotherapy for persistent or recurrent ovarian cancer. J Sci Healing. 2012;8:197–8.

99. Staples JK, Hamilton MF, Uddo M. A yoga program for the symptoms of post-traumatic stress disorder in veterans. Mil Med. 2013;178:854–60.

100. Sulenes K, Freitas J, Justice L, Colgan D, Shean M, Brems C. Underuse of yoga as a referral resource by health professions students. J Altern Complement Med. 2015;21:53–9.

101. Sullivan MB, Erb M, Schmalzl L, Moonaz S, Taylor JN, Porges S. Yoga therapy and polyvagal theory: the convergence of traditional wisdom and contemporary neuroscience for self-regulation and resilience. Front Hum Neurosci. 2018;12:67.

102. Sullivan MB, Moonaz S, Weber K, Taylor JN, Schmalzl L. Toward an explanatory framework for yoga therapy informed by philosophical and ethical perspectives. Altern Ther Health Med. 2018;24:38–47.

103. Taneja I, Deepak KK, Poojary G, Acharya IN, Pandey RM, Sharma MP. Yogic versus conventional treatment in diarrhea-predominant irritable bowel syndrome: a randomized control study. Appl Psychophysiol Biofeedback. 2004;29:19–33.

104. Taylor AG, Goehler LE, Galper DI, Innes KE, Bourguignon C. Top-down and bottom-up mechanisms in mind-body medicine: development of an integrative framework for psychophysiological research. Explore J Sci Healing. 2010;6:29–41.

105. Telles S, Singh N, Bhardwaj AK, Kumar A, Balkrishna A. Effect of yoga or physical exercise on physical, cognitive and emotional measures in children: a randomized controlled trial. Child Adolesc Psychiatry Ment Health. 2013;7:37.

106. Thordardottir K, Gudmundsdottir R, Zoega H, Valdimarsdottir UA, Gudmundsdottir B. Effects of yoga practice on stress-related symptoms in the aftermath of an earthquake: a community-based controlled trial. Complement Ther Med. 2014;22:226–34.

107. Tiedemann A, O'Rourke S, Sesto R, Sherrington C. Community-dwelling people: a pilot randomized controlled trial. J Gerontol. 2013;68:1068–75.

108. Tsakiris M, Tajadura-Jimenez A, Constantini M. Just a heartbeat away from one's body: interoceptive sensitivity predicts malleability of body-representations. Proc R Soc B. 2016. Access Date: February 19, 2019. Available at: https://royalsocietypublishing.org/doi/pdf/10.1098/rspb.2010.2547.

109. Uebelacker LA, Tremont G, Epstien-Lubow G, Gaudiano BA, Gillette T, Kalibatseva Z, Miller IW. Open trial of Vinyasa yoga for persistently depressed individuals: evidence of feasibility. Behav Modif. 2010;34:247–64.
110. Vago DR, Silbersweig DA. Self-awareness, self-regulation, and self-transcendence (S-ART): a framework for understanding the neurobiological mechanisms of mindfulness. Front Hum Neurosci. 2012;6:296. https://doi.org/10.3389/fnhum.2012.00296.
111. van der Kolk BA, Stone L, West J, Rhodes A, Emerson D, Suvak M, Spinazzola J. Yoga as an adjunctive treatment for post-traumatic stress disorder: a randomized controlled trial. J Clin Psychiatry. 2014;75:559–65.
112. Vladagina N, Freeman H, Razmjou E, Freitas J, Sulenes K, Michael P, Brems C. Media images of yoga poses: increasing injury instead of access. Paper presented at the 144th annual American Public Health Association meeting and exposition, Denver. 2016.
113. Ward L, Stebbings S, Sherman K, Cherkin D, Baxter GD. Establishing key components of yoga interventions for musculoskeletal conditions: a Delphi survey. BMC Complement Altern Med. 2014;14(196):1.
114. White G. Yoga beyond belief. Berkeley: North Atlantic Books; 2007.
115. Williams K, Abildso C, Steinberg L, Doyle E, Epstein B, Smith D, Hobbs G, Gross R, Kelley G, Cooper L. Evaluation of the effectiveness and efficacy of Iyengar yoga therapy on chronic low back pain. Spine. 2009;34:2066–76.
116. Witkiewitz R, Roos CR, Colgan DD, Bowen S. Mindfulness: advances in psychotherapy evidence-based practice. Boston: Hogrefe; 2017.
117. Woolery A, Myers H, Sternlieb B, Zeltzer L. A yoga intervention for young adults with elevated symptoms of depression. Altern Ther Health Med. 2004;10:60–3.
118. Wurz A, Chamorro-Vina C, Guilcher GM, Schulte F, Culos-Reed SN. The feasibility and benefits of a 12-week yoga intervention for pediatric cancer out-patients. Pediatr Blood Cancer. 2014;61:1828–34.

**Part III
Mindfulness**

Chapter 11
Health Benefits of Mindful Meditation

Kathleen C. Spadaro and Ingrid M. Provident

Keywords Mindfulness · Stress reduction · Mindfulness-based stress reduction · Evidence-based Practice · Meditation · Mindfulness meditation · Mindfulness-based cognitive therapy

Key Points
- Mindfulness meditation has been studied in numerous populations with physical or mental health conditions with positive findings.
- Consistent practice of mindfulness meditation can improve physical, mental, and cognitive health.
- Mindfulness does not eliminate or cure diseases but rather allows a person to live with these states with less suffering.
- Mindfulness programs offer a variety of meditations for practice that cultivate mindfulness.
- Clinicians can benefit personally from mindfulness as well as use the practices with clients or patients.

Mindfulness

Jon Kabat-Zinn, the creator of the Stress Reduction Clinic at the University of Massachusetts and founding director of the Center for Mindfulness in Medicine, Health Care, and Society, described mindfulness as awareness that arises through paying attention, on purpose, in the present moment, and without judgment [1]. Mindfulness meditation is the application of techniques in practice to change individual "mindless" habits (physical, psychological, psychosocial) to awareness of the experience in the moment, thus allowing the individual to make conscious choices in place of mindless reactions [2].

K. C. Spadaro (✉)
Department of Nursing, Chatham University, Pittsburgh, PA, USA
e-mail: KSpadaro@Chatham.edu

I. M. Provident
Department of Occupational Therapy, Chatham University, Pittsburgh, PA, USA

J. Uribarri, J. A. Vassalotti (eds.), *Nutrition, Fitness, and Mindfulness*, Nutrition and Health,
https://doi.org/10.1007/978-3-030-30892-6_11

Mindfulness Interventions

Grossman et al. [3] described mindfulness-based stress reduction (MBSR) as "a group program that focuses upon the progressive acquisition of mindful awareness, of mindfulness." Jon Kabat-Zinn, a MIT trained molecular scientist, introduced western medicine to mindfulness in 1979 when he developed a program at the University of Massachusetts for chronic pain patients. The 8-week program taught patients mindfulness meditation and other techniques to increase pain management skills when all else had failed. His philosophy blended eastern practices of yoga and Buddhist teachings with science to assist individuals to cope with stress, pain, anxiety, and illness. Skills and techniques taught included mindful eating, awareness of the breath, the body scan, various sitting meditations, walking meditation, guided meditations, yoga, and loving kindness meditation. Currently, there are almost 23,000 certified MBSR instructors that teach mindfulness meditation and techniques with clinics in almost every state and in over 30 countries [4], not including instructors that provide some variation of mindfulness-based approaches in practice or in research settings.

Mindfulness has been used as an intervention in numerous studies. Beside the standard 8-week MBSR intervention (Table 11.1), mindfulness-based cognitive therapy (MBCT), mindful eating, and other modified mindfulness interventions have been studied in various condition-specific populations,

Table 11.1 MBSR 8-week intervention

Week	Content focus	Mindfulness meditations
1	Overview: Mindfulness vs mindlessness, theory, self-regulation	Abdominal breathing Eating meditation Body scan Yoga mountain pose
2	Perceived stress, response vs reaction Practicing being mindful in routine activities	Sitting meditation Standing yoga postures Body scan Awareness of breath sitting meditation
3	Being present, pleasure, and power in being present	Laying down yoga w/ brief body scan Sitting meditation Walking meditation
4	Bringing curiosity and openness to our experiences, cultivate a different relationship with stress	Standing yoga Sitting meditation
5	Awareness of "being stuck," habitual reactions vs mindfulness, perception, and appraisal allows us to respond	Standing yoga Sitting meditation
6	Growing capacity to self-regulate, stressful communication, and relationships	Standing yoga Sitting meditation
All-day class	Silent retreat Cultivating sense of presence in the moment, being open to any experience that arises in the silence	Yoga Sitting meditation Body scan Walking meditation Mountain or lake meditation Eating meditation w/ meal Loving-kindness meditation
7	Integrating mindfulness practice into daily life	Mountain meditation Lake meditation Loving-kindness meditation
8	Keeping the practice going both formal and informal practice	Body scan Yoga Sitting meditation

Note. Adapted from the revised Mindfulness-based stress reduction authorized curriculum guide [5]. All sessions start and end with a brief opening and closing meditation in addition to well populations, and diverse social populations. MBCT is an 8-week group intervention that teaching mindfulness skills and techniques combined with cognitive tools to assist individuals dealing with depression. Mindful eating is a group intervention that targets issues with food, eating, body cues, and sensations to address individuals with poor eating habits or eating disorders. Other mindfulness-based interventions (MBIs) have taken components of these structured programs to address areas of distress, disease, or dysfunction. This chapter will review and summarize research findings on these various health conditions and populations.

Mindfulness Qualities

Mindfulness qualities or attitudes support the practice and are the foundation of mindfulness as a way of life. Kabat-Zinn [1] defined seven qualities, *non-judging*, *patience*, *beginner's mind*, *trust*, *non-striving*, *acceptance*, and *letting go*, that are emphasized and reenforced through mindfulness training. These attitudes are a challenge because typically the opposite of each is how we function on a daily basis, thus creating or increasing our suffering. However, in practicing mindfulness, we can learn to let go of judgments, sit with our "suffering" without reacting, and learn to see each moment with an openness, a new beginning not marred by past experiences. An additional quality that has arisen from the first seven is self-compassion. We can learn to trust ourselves by sitting with thoughts, feelings, and sensations compassionately, without judgment, accepting what is occurring in the moment instead of fighting it, not working so hard for results, and letting go of the need to hold on to what we desire in life. It is learning to accept life as it presents itself in the present moment; as in the words of Kabat-Zinn, "it is what it is." Each of these factors can assist in improving an individual's way of thinking, feeling, sensing, and being regardless of the health issues or symptoms they may be struggling with in the present moment. As a clinician, it is essential to teach patients best practices to improve mood and quality of life, reduce stress, and promote symptom reduction.

Physical Health Benefits

Mindfulness does not eliminate or cure disease states. However, mindfulness has been found to be helpful in symptom reduction of various diseases. Physical health and symptoms of disease are impacted by stress and mood. Numerous mindfulness intervention studies have reported a reduction in stress, improvement in mood, and increased quality of life and symptom-specific improvement related to disease states. The goal of treatment is to improve the individual's functioning. This section will identify the various symptoms and disordered populations that have been studied using mindfulness interventions and discuss their findings.

Stress

Stress can be a physical, mental, or psychological factor that creates tension within an individual. Although stress can be normal and motivating, prolonged stress has a negative impact on individuals. Symptoms of prolonged stress can include but not be limited to chronic headaches, gastrointestinal symptoms, body pain, hypertension, changes in appetite, sleep disturbance, higher risk of infection, irritability, anger, numbness, anxiety, feeling overwhelmed, tearfulness, poor concentration, low motivation, memory issues, and unclear thinking. Prolonged stress impacts an individual's ability to function in everyday life and can lead to ineffective coping such as increased alcohol intake, illegal drug use, overuse of prescription medications, and overeating.

Many reviews of stress and mindfulness on specific populations with a medical or psychiatric diagnosis are cited in this chapter that show significant findings on stress as an outcome. To address healthy adults, a meta-analysis of 17 studies on mindfulness and stress found a positive impact on physiological and psychological measures of stress, including significant findings on the perceived stress scale when used in the studies explored [6]. A meta-analysis of 45 randomized control trials on meditation interventions and stress in a variety of populations found an impact on physiological markers for stress with a reduction in cortisol, C-reactive protein, blood pressure, heart rate, and triglycerides [7]. As clinicians, awareness and management of client stress levels are necessary to promote positive treatment outcomes.

Chronic Pain

The Centers for Disease Control and Prevention (CDC) reported that approximately 20.4% or 50.0 million of US adults surveyed in 2016 met the criteria for chronic pain [8]. The report acknowledged that these individuals are impacted in multiple areas of their life beyond pain: mobility, mood, daily activity functioning, and poor quality of life.

Mindfulness was studied in general chronic pain patients, lower-back pain patients, and patients with fibromyalgia as stress, depression, and anxiety can exacerbate pain symptoms. Several review and meta-analysis articles of randomized control trials (RCT) found in well-designed studies using MBSR were effective in reducing pain intensity and disability significantly with an increased acceptance of the chronic condition, a reduction in depressive symptoms, and in some studies increased quality of life [9, 10]. Teaching mindfulness techniques to patients suffering from chronic pain can improve their functioning and mood while decreasing the amount of pain medication needed. These are important findings given the impact of the opioid crisis facing us today from pain management medical interventions.

Cancer

The second leading cause of death in the USA is cancer, with one in four deaths related to this diagnosis [11]. This statistic alone emphasizes the physical and emotional toll it takes on individuals receiving a cancer diagnosis. In addition, more individuals with cancer are surviving longer due to advances in treatment but still dealing with symptoms of anxiety, depression, sleep disturbances, stress, pain, fatigue, and worry of reoccurrence.

A significant number of studies have explored mindfulness-based interventions to address those symptoms in individuals with various types of cancer. A systematic review and meta-analysis of mindfulness-based interventions in breast cancer patients [12] found significant changes in reducing anxiety, depression, fear of reoccurrence, and fatigue along with significant improvement in physical functioning, physical health, and emotional well-being. Other studies focusing on a variety of cancers noted significance in improvement in mood and stress symptoms, anxiety, pain, and psychological distress [13].

Mindfulness was also explored in biological markers, as stress has been found to be related to cancer outcomes. Studies on cancer patients' sleep, immune system, endocrine, and autonomic functioning demonstrated outcomes of an improved sleep, a reduction in cellular inflammatory response (thought to be more favorable to cancer outcomes), a decrease in cortisol (with higher levels related to poorer clinical outcomes), and a reduction in systolic blood pressure [13]. A systematic review in advanced cancer patients found that MBIs reduced symptoms of depression and anxiety, improved quality of life, and increased acceptance of the disease, while the authors also recommended that the interventions be briefer and more flexible for this population [14]. As a clinician, note that teaching clients mindfulness skills can improve the individual's stress level, mood, quality of life, and sleep and potentially impact their cancer.

Cardiovascular Disease

Cardiovascular disease, including hypertension, coronary artery disease, heart failure, and stroke, is the number one leading cause of preventable death in our country. It is impacted and exacerbated by stress, obesity, diabetes, and smoking as well as other health issues. It can impact an individual's mood and daily functioning, as well as lead to disability and death.

A systematic review of mindfulness interventions on patients with cardiovascular disease reported a significant decrease in systolic and diastolic blood pressure readings and a significant reduction in stress, depression, and anxiety [15]. In another summary of cardiovascular-focused mindfulness studies, findings included significantly improved quality of life in self-report, reduced norepinephrine levels, better cardiopulmonary performance on exercise testing, decreased anxiety, emotion regulation improvement, and healthier coping skills [13]. Obesity, diabetes, smoking, and stress are discussed separately. However, with positive outcomes in those areas combined with these findings, mindfulness interventions can improve cardiovascular health in clients.

Chronic Fatigue Syndrome and Related Disorders

Chronic fatigue syndrome, irritable bowel syndrome, and fibromyalgia are often referred to as functional or somatization disorders, which confound practitioners and patients alike. These disorders are medically challenging and chronic, with treatment-resistant symptoms that combine emotional distress with physical pain or discomfort. Unexplained symptoms may include muscle pain, fatigue, headache, sleep disturbance, depression, and anxiety.

A review and meta-analysis of 13 studies on mindfulness-based interventions (MBSR, MCBT, and MBI) used with this population found significant improvement in reducing pain, symptom severity, depression, and anxiety while improving quality of life [16]. Given the frustration to both the provider and patient, the clinician may find mindfulness a teachable method to cope with the chronicity of the disorder and improve patient mood and symptoms through practicing observing, non-judging, awareness, and acceptance.

HIV/AIDS

Human immunodeficiency virus (HIV) attacks the immune system, damaging its function to fight off illness. Acquired immune deficiency syndrome (AIDS) is the condition or the final stage of HIV progression when the immune system is severely damaged. Individuals with AIDS tend to die of infections or other illnesses because of their compromised immune system. Current antiretroviral drugs have virtually eliminated AIDS in the treated HIV population.

The antiretroviral medication can have distressing side effects including diarrhea, nausea and vomiting, neuropathic pain, and skin rashes that may impact adherence to treatment. A RCT using mindfulness found that the MBSR participants had fewer medication side effects and reduced symptom-related distress [17]. A systematic review showed significance in a reduction in stress and depression using mindfulness-based therapies and a stabilization or improvement in CD4+ T lymphocytes that stimulate the response to fight infection in studies using MBSR or MBCT [18]. Clinicians working with HIV-infected patients may find mindfulness helpful in addressing mood and could potentially impact their immune system to increase ability to fight infection.

Rheumatoid Arthritis

Rheumatoid arthritis (RA) is a chronic, debilitating autoimmune disorder characterized by joint pain, inflammation, and destruction. Other organs can also be affected such as the skin, eyes, lung, and heart as well. Typical symptoms include swelling, tenderness, redness, stiffness, and pain of the joints that may flare and then subside for periods of time. Inflammation in rheumatoid arthritis is partly mediated by cytokines. Increased stress can release more cytokines that increase inflammation and disease activity.

The chronic pain systematic review discussed above included studies of patients with RA. The grouped effects of RA studies found a decrease in pain and depression with an improved quality of life. A RCT using a mindfulness-based intervention with RA patients found significant treatment effects posttreatment and maintained at 12 months in psychological distress, self-efficacy pain and symptoms, emotional processing, fatigue, self-care ability, and overall well-being [12]. Although mindfulness interventions did not impact the disease process, clinicians offer mindfulness interventions for physical and emotional well-being for these individuals.

Diabetes

According to the CDC [19, 20], over 30 million people (9%) in the USA have diabetes. Diabetes is a group of chronic diseases that can be well managed with a prescribed medication regime and lifestyle changes including nutrition and physical activity, but poor adherence increases the risk for devastating complications.

A meta-analysis reported a consistent psychological impact from mindfulness-based interventions of individuals with both type 1 and type 2 diabetes with a decrease in depression, anxiety, and distress [21]. A recent study using the MBSR program with type 2 diabetes (T2DM) patients found significant improvements in overall mental health, depression, anxiety, fasting blood sugars, and hemoglobin A1c compared to the control group both 8 weeks at completion of the MBSR program and 3 months following [22]. These findings support the use of mindfulness-based interventions as an adjunct to medication, nutrition, and physical activity to improve outcomes of patients with diabetes.

Obesity and Disordered Eating

The US population is struggling with an obesity epidemic. Carrying extra weight used to be the sign of wealth and success; now it is classified as a medical disorder and considered the second leading cause of preventable death in the USA after cardiovascular disease [23]. Obesity increases the risk of comorbid conditions such as T2DM, hypertension, high cholesterol, coronary artery disease, stroke, gall bladder disease, some cancers, osteoarthritis, sleep apnea, and physical pain.

Mindfulness-based interventions have been found to significantly improve healthy eating. Benefits include an increase in awareness to make healthier food choices, a decrease in the amount of food intake or restrained eating, a reduction in emotional eating episodes, and a purposeful slow eating process [24, 25]. A systematic review found that out of 19 mindfulness-based studies focused on dietary changes and physical activity, 13 reported significant weight loss [26]. Another review of 15 studies noted an average weight loss of 4.2 kg. with overall effect sizes large for improving eating behaviors; medium for depression, anxiety, and eating attitudes; and small for body mass index (BMI) and meta-cognition [27]. The act of bringing awareness to the present moment without judgment and with compassion can challenge the automatic, mindless eating behaviors by reducing impulsivity, allow for alternative choices besides eating when recognizing emotions, and recognize physiological hunger and satiety cues [28]. Clinician and client resources include the mindful eating meditation from MBSR, the mindful eating program online through the Center of Mindfulness at University of Massachusetts, and the mindfulness-based eating awareness training [MB-EAT] from the Center for Mindful Eating.

Smoking

According to the CDC [19, 20], tobacco use is the leading cause of preventable disease, disability, and death in the USA. Annually, a half million Americans die prematurely of smoking or exposure to secondhand smoke, and another 16 million suffer from a serious illness caused by smoking. Medical care costs are approximately nearly $170 billion to treat smoking-related disease in adults [19, 20].

Several systematic reviews and meta-analyses on smoking and mindfulness-based interventions reported mixed reviews with limited data. One review did report "promising" results with most studies showing the mindfulness had a positive impact on quitting rates, identifying smoking triggers for relapse prevention, reducing cravings, and decreasing the number of cigarettes smoked [29]. The authors found that mindfulness produced positive effects on smokers' mental health that may in turn contribute to smoking cessation and reduction. A meta-analysis of four RCTs using mindfulness with smokers found a moderate effect size, supporting mindfulness for smoking cessation with one study demonstrating a 25% cessation rate for mindfulness group compared to a 13% rate in the comparison group 4 months following [30]. In addition, the authors noted that on the Five Facet Mindfulness Questionnaire (FFMQ) used in several of the studies, there were significant improvements on the components of observing, non-judging, and non-reacting. Those mindfulness skills enhanced by practice can assist smokers in their attempts to quit.

Mental Health Benefits

Mindfulness-interventions have demonstrated positive findings in the domains of stress, physical symptoms, and chronic disorders. Mental health disorders can originate in childhood or adulthood and can be acute or chronic in nature. Just as stress and mental health disorders impact physical health, physical health and stress can also impact the individual's mental health. The goal of treatment for mental health is to maintain or improve the individual's functioning in all areas of life.

Depression

Major depressive disorder affects almost 7% of the nation's population annually and is the leading cause of disability in the age range of 15–44 years [31]. Depression can be acute or recurrent and chronic with psychological and physiological symptoms that can impact daily functioning. Symptoms can include depressed mood, anxiety, guilt, hopelessness, sadness, sleep disturbance, changes in appetite and weight, fatigue, agitation, irritability, tearfulness, social isolation, poor concentration, rumination, and suicidal thoughts.

Mindfulness-based cognitive therapy (MBCT) has been shown to be effective in both acutely depressed individuals and in reducing depression relapse. In a meta-analysis of RCTs using mindfulness-based interventions, including MBCT on individuals in acute depression, findings were significant for depressive symptom reduction [32]. In a meta-analysis and review of MBCT compared to usual treatment for individuals with repeated depressive episodes, MBCT participants had a 34% reduced risk of relapse [33]. A recent meta-analysis of 17 studies that focused on the efficacy of MBCT on individual patients found a reduced risk of relapse within 60 weeks post intervention compared to other active treatments [34]. The qualities that mindfulness practice develops, observing, non-judging, acceptance, and letting go, can assist the individual struggling with depression.

Anxiety

In comparison with depression, 19% of US adults experienced an anxiety disorder in the past year, approximately 40 million adults between the ages of 18 and 54 years with 31% experiencing anxiety at some point in their lifetime [35]. Because many individuals do not seek treatment, the current estimates are closer to 30%. Anxiety is the number one mental health problem with over $42 billion in healthcare expenditures to treat the population that often seeks evaluation for physical disorders instead of or in addition to mental health treatment. Anxiety disorders include generalized anxiety disorder, obsessive-compulsive disorder, social anxiety disorder, panic disorder, specific phobia disorder, separation anxiety disorder, and agoraphobia. Symptoms can include but are not limited to excessive worry about the future, negative thoughts and self-criticism, irritability, restlessness, muscle tension, fatigue, lack of concentration, racing thoughts or unwanted thoughts, fear, feeling of impending doom, insomnia, nausea, palpitations, or trembling.

In a review of 13 RCTs with different anxiety disorders or anxiety symptoms, mindfulness interventions significantly improved anxiety compared to usual treatment [36]. Another review of 16 studies using mindfulness interventions or evaluating mindfulness in the presence of mood and anxiety disorders found that mindfulness was an effective intervention for anxiety and mood disorders [37]. This review included studies using MBSR, MBCT, and other mindfulness-based interventions as well as different delivery modalities (online versus in-person). Practicing observing or detaching from thoughts and emotions, non-judging, acceptance, and staying in the present moment through mindfulness practice can reduce ruminations, acknowledge worrisome thoughts and feelings, decrease critical self-talk, increase self-compassion, and plan to act instead of react in the moment.

ADHD

Attention-deficit hyperactivity disorder has been predominantly a child and adolescence disorder that has been identified more recently in adulthood as well. Symptoms include inattention and/or hyperactivity/impulsivity that impair functioning. ADHD in childhood impacts the child's ability to develop healthy social relationships, function academically, and puts them at higher risk for substance abuse and other mental health issues. In adults, ADHD can impair the individual's ability to focus and function at work, impair relationships, and lead to substance abuse. Both populations can create stress on families and loved ones.

In a systematic review of mindfulness interventions on ADHD, nine studies were evaluated: five with adults, two with adolescents, one with both adults and adolescents, and one with adolescents and children. Mindfulness was studied mostly with adults with ADHD with significant improvement in attention [38]. The authors concluded that they could make no conclusions on the effects on mindfulness on ADHD in children and adolescents due to the limited number of studies and lack of well-designed studies. However, another systematic review and meta-analysis of 11 studies that focused on children with ADHD found statistically significant effects on the outcomes of ADHD symptoms: hyperactivity and inattention (parent and teacher report), as well as parent-child relationship, executive functioning, on-task behavior, parent stress, and parent trait mindfulness ([39], p. 3155). The authors did acknowledge considerable study bias and recommended further studies that are well-designed. These findings do support clinicians offering mindfulness with patients needing attention improvement, given that the practice of mindfulness focuses on paying attention with intention in the present moment.

Addictions

Addiction refers to the physiological and or psychological dependency on substances or actions that drive compulsive behaviors of seeking a pleasurable reward even when there may be severe negative consequences and the reward may no longer be achievable. Addictions for this chapter refer to all substance use disorders, tobacco, and gambling addictions. Although food and other behavioral addictions are not included here, mindfulness could be useful in the treatment of other addictions.

A review of 54 RCTs was conducted that used mindfulness-based interventions on adolescents and adults that struggled with substance use (42), either alcohol, cocaine, opioids, or marijuana, and tobacco (9) or gambling (3) addictions [40]. The review found positive findings that these studies saw a reduction in dependence, craving, and other addiction-related symptoms as well as an improvement in mood: depression, anxiety, and perceived stress. MBIs also appeared to improve emotional dysregulation. Several individual studies within this review also demonstrated specific findings of a reduction in drug use days, reduction in the number of legal issues, and a reduction in relapse, a 54% reduction with drugs and a 59% reduction with alcohol in a 12-month period [9]. Of note, not all positive effects were maintained at follow-up in many of the studies; the authors recommended the use of MBI as an adjunct to usual treatment as the best treatment option. The mindfulness qualities of observing, acceptance, awareness, and non-judging were identified as an important role in reducing cravings. To address addiction cessation and to prevent relapse, clinicians need to provide tools for the client to dealing with their cravings.

Post-traumatic Stress Disorder

Post-traumatic stress disorder (PTSD) can arise from experiencing a traumatic event or repeated events such as combat for soldiers, rape, and other sexual abuse, physical violence, or any other event that is scary, shocking, or dangerous to the individual. PTSD can be acute or chronic with symptoms that can be debilitating: sleep disturbance, nightmares, flashbacks, fear, depression, anxiety, hyperarousal, avoidance, irritability, and anger that can interfere with daily functioning.

In a review of 12 studies using MBSR or trauma-adapted MBSR, MBCT, and other MBIs, the authors recommended that mindfulness interventions had the most evidence and were the best treatment for PTSD [41]. They found significantly reduced symptoms of PTSD and attention difficulties with sustainment over time and a low attrition rate of participants, thus making this intervention highly acceptable. The authors drew correlations between mindfulness and PTSD symptoms reduction findings. Through mindfulness, individuals can view and accept traumatic memories, related thoughts, and stimuli without judgment and have a reduction in shame and improvements in emotion acceptance and regulation. In addition, mindfulness qualities of nonreactivity and acting with awareness appeared to be associated with a reduction in hyperarousal symptoms, seen by staying in the present moment and not reacting to external stimuli.

Other Mental Health Disorders

Patients with either schizophrenia or bipolar disorder were also studied using MBIs. Schizophrenia is a severe and chronic mental health disorder that can be very disabling and affects thinking, emotions, and behaviors, characterized by symptoms of hallucinations, delusions, thought disorders, agitated body movements, reduced expression of emotions, speaking or feelings of pleasure, difficulty beginning and sustaining activities, poor focus, inattention, memory issues, and lack of understanding or processing of information [42]. Individuals with bipolar disorder, (often referred to as manic-depression) experience mood, energy, and behavioral changes, that range from extreme "highs" (manic) to extreme "lows" (depression) or less extreme changes that impair their ability to function [42]. Manic or excessive behaviors such as hypersexuality, religiosity, spending extravagantly, gambling, and other risky behaviors often cause trouble for the individual in work, social, family, and legal situations, while depression can also impact those areas from a lack of activity, social isolation, irritable mood, or suicidal thoughts.

A review of MBIs for psychiatric disorders included 7 studies on patients with schizophrenia that showed strong effects on schizophrenia-specific symptoms [43]. Another review of MBIs and patients with schizophrenia discussed specific research findings: a 50% reduction in rates of hospitalization, significant increases in well-being and global functioning, significant decrease in auditory hallucination distress, reduction in stress, negative self-judging, depression and anxiety, increased self-acceptance, effective coping, and awareness of distressing thoughts [44]. Mindfulness attitudes and qualities are reflected in the findings: awareness, acceptance, non-judging, and stress reduction.

A review of 13 studies on MBCT and patients with bipolar disorder found that the intervention was effective in combination with medication therapy [45]. The analysis of studies found improvements in cognitive functioning and emotional regulation as well as a reduction in anxiety, depression, and mania symptoms that were maintained for a year when mindfulness was practiced regularly. Mindfulness increases awareness of thoughts and feelings, improves concentration and focus, and can reduce reactivity leading to improved choices and behaviors.

Cognitive/Academic Benefits

Learning is a complex process and is a result of what the learner does and thinks [46]. Learners enter into the relationship with a foundation of prior knowledge and some degree of stress and anxiety. Moderate to high levels of anxiety and stress can negatively impact academic performance causing memory impairment that directly affects information recall and attention [47, 48]. Mindfulness meditation has the capacity to assist in reducing test or performance anxiety, improving working memory, and enhancing attention and focus and can lead to overall improved academic performance [49].

Concentration/Selective Attention

The ability to think about only what you are doing without distraction is a common general definition of selective attention or concentration. Concentration is a skill to be mastered and supports learning. Studies have shown that the human mind is estimated to wander roughly half of our waking hours [50]. Learners often find concentration to be difficult due to the myriad of internal or external distractors including one's own thoughts on past or future, multitasking, noises in the environment, and/or the presence of other people.

Foerde et al. [51] studied the effect of multitasking on attention and found that the division of one's concentration between two tasks showed a decreased ability to generalize learned information to new situations. Keeping the learning environment consistent helps to minimize distractions, and consistency of duration that the learner is engaged in the task in regard to time has also been shown to support concentration. Improving sustained attention and concentration takes effort and practice. Mindfulness has been shown to help a person to improve attention and concentration by teaching the learner to be aware of their thoughts and bring themselves back to the task at hand [52–54].

Memory

According to the Merriam-Webster Dictionary, memory is defined as "the power or process of reproducing or recalling what has been learned and retained especially through associative mechanisms." In neuroscience, memory is a complex phenomenon often broken down into subcomponents such as episodic memory, working memory (short term), and long-term memory [55].

A recent study revealed that mindfulness meditation may support memory by increasing the availability of attentional resources and decreasing cognitive distraction as well as presenting a consistent picture of benefit in episodic memory enhancement [56]. A three-arm RCT found using short-term mindfulness training improved the working memory capacity, thus cognitive functioning in adolescents compared to a yoga intervention and a control group [57]. This finding supports the use of brief interventions that are better suited for school-aged students.

Wellness and Optimal Functioning

Perhaps the best documented outcomes of mindfulness meditation are for the purpose of wellness and improving quality of life. Kabat-Zinn's mindfulness-based stress reduction (MBSR) has been reviewed in a systematic review of 101 peer-reviewed publications showing a moderately large effect on outcome measures of mental health, somatic health, and quality of life including social function at post-intervention when compared to an inactive control group [58].

Mindfulness teachings and practice and teaching focus on capturing a quality of consciousness of the current experience. Whereas mindlessness is the state of functioning of being less "awake" or functioning in a state of habitual or automatic behavior which often manifests as reactive functioning. Mindfulness has been shown to shift individuals from automatic thoughts, habits, and unhealthy behavior patterns toward and promoting informed and self-aware behavioral and emotional regulation, which has long been associated with well-being enhancement [59].

Health and Well-Being

As healthcare shifts from disease management to preventative care, mindfulness has become an increasingly sought out intervention for wellness. Reduction of emotional distress, stress management, aiding in sleep improvement, promoting overall health, and quality of life are all outcomes of mindfulness interventions that have been studied and reported in the literature [60]. Mindfulness meditation is taught and practiced to develop within the individual attention to the present surroundings and one's body sensations with a non-judgmental awareness for the benefit of openness and acceptance to the circumstances of one's life. The consistent practice of mindfulness is done for the purpose of acting with more kindness to one's self and others rather than reacting impulsively without thoughtful consideration of the consequences. This basic philosophy of mindful living lends itself to the cultivation of patience, relaxation, and purposeful intentions that at the core embody human wellness.

Stress Management

A certain amount of stress can improve human performance; however intensified stress or prolonged exposure to stress can be damaging to one's health. Continued stress can lead to ruminations that have been shown to consume energy and intensify the stress experience [61]. Mindfulness-based stress reduction has been shown to reduce stress in healthy persons [62] as well as those with diagnosed with chronic conditions [60].

In over 70% of the studies included in a systematic review and meta-analysis, mindfulness interventions were shown to be a superior intervention to controls which included social support, pharmacology, education specific to the patient's condition, and relaxation training [60]. Typical mindfulness interventions used in stress reduction throughout the literature include body scan, which teaches the person to gradually mentally sweep from head to toe to observe sensations, attention on breath awareness, and relaxation as well non-judgmental awareness on the stream of thoughts and distractions that continually flow through the mind [60, 62].

Resilience

Some researchers have described this human quality as the ability to adapt positively to stressful situations or being able to continue your life engagement in a functionally stable manner with a degree of wellness despite ongoing stress [63, 64]. In a general perspective, resilience is seen as a process of "bouncing back" from difficult experiences and having the capacity to adapt to changing circumstances.

A core tenet of mindfulness training is impermanence, that is, the awareness that things do not stay the same and one's emotional reactions to change. Human resilience can be conceptualized on a continuum ranging from low resilience (poor bounce-back ability) to extremely high (strong capacity to recover and or to thrive). Mindfulness interventions in particular have been shown in a recent systematic review to be effective in assisting people with developing or strengthening their resilience [65].

Sports Performance

Athletes have found mindfulness useful to improve their mental fitness and physical performance. Coaches have also integrated mindfulness techniques as a form of psychological training designed to complement physical training [66]. Athletes require common skills such as cognitive ability, concentration, and attention to the sport while playing as well as emotional regulation strategies for peak performance in competitive sports. Traditional psychological techniques used in sports training are geared toward the ability to demonstrate self-control in mind and physical body for developing optimal performance in the athlete's individual sport [67].

While this is useful, mindfulness-based techniques are focused on training a person to accept, feel, and observe the present states of the body and mind without judgment. Once mastered, athletes can employ mindfulness skills to mentally distance themselves from their emotional feelings, thoughts, and perceptions by learning to employ the perspective of observer. The positive effects of mindfulness have recently been studied and shown to be effective suggesting that mindfulness training had, in comparison to a classical sport psychology program, a significant effect [66].

Military Personnel

Military personnel are tasked with protecting our country against harm, often placing themselves at risk both physically and emotionally. Training and performance in the field require attention, focus, and the ability to act, not react. Soldiers are faced with situations that demand multitasking and quick responses, but intrusive thoughts, mind wandering, and off-task thinking may hinder their ability to function effectively and increase the risk of prolonged stress. In addition, PTSD (addressed above) is a common diagnosis for military personnel making this group one of the highest risk occupational groups due to their exposure to traumatic events [68]. Being engaged in combat and deployment away from family and social support increases the likelihood of experiencing mental health problems such as depression or anxiety.

A study using a MBI on marines prior to deployment found an increase in mindfulness and a reduction in stress with correlation between practice time (higher time), mindfulness (greater), and stress (reduced) [69]. In a later study, Jha et al. [70] found that extended periods of high demand experienced during predeployment training may increase attentional lapses; however, soldiers in the mindfulness intervention experienced less lapses in attention, reporting more awareness of their attention in training (improved working memory). Rice et al. [71] utilized both an in-person and virtual MBI with active military personnel and demonstrated clinical reductions in PTSD symptoms and improved attending abilities in ADHD symptoms compared to the control group. Mindfulness research is continuing to focus on the military to enhance resiliency, improve mental health functioning, and increase cognition.

Mindfulness Meditation Practice

Mindfulness is the awareness of the present moment by bringing attention with intention and without judgment. Given that much of the time, individuals function mindlessly, on autopilot, or multitasking, living mindfully does not come naturally to most. To become more mindful in everyday life, one must practice through mindful meditations and techniques.

Mindfulness Meditation Exercises

The MBSR program is a structured process that provides meditation exercises to increase mindfulness in its participants. Over the course of 8 weeks, the MBSR group experiences mindful eating, breathing meditation, the body scan, sitting meditation, mindful yoga, walking meditation, the lake- and mountain-guided imagery exercises, the 3-minute check-in, and the loving kindness meditation. Participants are instructed to practice mindful meditations 45–60 minutes a day. MBCT combines mindfulness meditation with cognitive therapy exercises to focus on thoughts and ruminations. MB-EAT combines mindfulness meditation with specific eating meditations to increase awareness of physical cues of hunger and satiety as well as using all of the senses in the experience of eating. Exercises focus on increasing awareness of emotional triggers to eat, reducing negative thoughts and feelings related to food and weight, and making active choices in food selection, amount, and place of eating. Many of these meditations can be found on CDs, in books, on websites, or in organized trainings.

MBIs typically combine some aspects of the above meditations to cultivate mindfulness while also adding or emphasizing components that specifically address the problem, diagnosis, or population. An example would be in mindfulness relapse prevention programs or substance recovery programs that create exercises and meditations that focus on very specific areas that the individual needs to address, such as identifying triggers of relapse and using mindfulness exercises to acknowledge the thoughts and feelings related to the triggers without acting on them. There are many mindfulness-based programs available in a variety of formats: group, individual, in-person, and online.

One question that always comes up is how much time and practice is necessary to increase mindfulness, given the lack of time everyone complains of in daily life. Although MBSR requires eight weekly sessions with 45–60 minutes of practice a day, other researchers have found that smaller increments of practice, as little as 5–10 minutes a day with three to four weekly mindfulness meditation trainings, can increase mindfulness, reduce impulsive behaviors, and moderate affective reactivity [9]. That said, there are further gains to be had when practice time increases. This is still an area that requires further research.

Potential Risks

As with any intervention, clinicians need to be aware of any potential risks to their clients. While the main focus of the chapter was sharing the evidence of the benefits of mindfulness, it is important to also discuss risks. Some mindfulness practices have the individual experience the positive and or negative states of emotions, thoughts, and physical sensations in the moment. Asking an individual to sit with feelings of joy, excitement, and pleasure can be a positive experience, yet when feelings of intense negative emotions such as anger, guilt, and shame arise, the practice can become quite uncomfortable and even overwhelming. The practice is to assist individuals in accepting all that is being experienced in the present moment, learning to tolerate and accept that experience without judgment. Learning comes from acknowledging the full experience, recognizing the temporary state of the experience, and gaining insight into how one reacts to the experience or can choose to respond differently.

Although mindfulness is a natural human capacity, the clinician still needs to be mindful of the state of the client to do no harm and to recognize when emotional suffering is extended. There has been some concern about the risk of mindfulness interventions on individuals with PTSD triggering flashbacks or a major depressive episode, in individuals with schizophrenia triggering psychosis, or in individuals with epilepsy triggering seizures [9]. However, the literature does not report incidence or prevalence of these events. There is a potential risk in more intensive residential mindfulness retreats that can last 2 weeks to several months. The author pointed out the smaller-spaced dosing of mindfulness as seen in MBSR and MBCT, and most MBIs reported in the literature appear to have minimal risk but also great potential benefit for those under high stress or experiencing physical or emotional trauma.

As a clinician, safety is foremost in treating patients. Two mindfulness researchers addressed safety in an article outlining three key components of a safe practice [72]. These are the intensity of the program, the vulnerability of the individual, and the quality of the instruction (see Table 11.2). Individuals may experience distress over negative feelings, discomfort in sitting meditation or practicing yoga, or challenged by the experience, but it is not lasting or seen as harmful but rather a component of the prac-

Table 11.2 Three key components of safe mindfulness practice

Component	Description/recommendations		
Intensity	Low: self-help books, mindfulness apps, many teacher-led programs	Medium: 8 week MBSR, MBCT, other evidence-based programs with 40+ minutes practice daily	High: mindfulness retreats 1 week or longer, long periods of silence, little instructor interaction
Client vulnerability	Clinician assessment pre-monitoring throughout training and adaptation of mindfulness meditations/techniques as needed		
Quality of instruction	Program-specific instructor training, practice guidelines, certification, and a list of qualified instructors		

tice and growth. There have been rare anecdotal reports of adverse experiences from high level of intensity, with an individual experiencing serious psychological effects that took months or longer to recover. That said, the vulnerability of a client is not always known and is not easily detected based on individual characteristics. Individuals vary in their susceptibility to tolerate intense feelings or experiences. However, the research has shown that even individuals with diagnoses or symptoms that could increase their vulnerability, mindfulness interventions have been delivered safely. The quality and delivery of the instruction rely on the clinician or researcher implementing the mindfulness program. Qualified instructors are trained to know how to address issues and concerns that arise during trainings, adjust and clarify teachings as needed, and act as a support and guide by providing feedback to individuals participating.

Mindfulness Practitioners

To promote and teach mindfulness with patients, it is recommended that the clinician have a personal mindfulness practice. This practice has personal benefits to the clinician and also professional benefits. Bringing a moment-to-moment awareness with a non-judging and accepting attitude promotes trust in the clinician-client relationship and strengthens the client engagement. Letting go of preconceived ideas and being patient as the client explores mindfulness in their time and way can bring about change based on the client's needs, not the clinician's agenda.

There are also trained MBSR and MBCT instructors to refer clients. The Center for Mindfulness in Medicine, Health Care, and Society provides a list of certified instructors at https://www.umassmed.edu/cfm/mindfulness-based-programs/mbsr-courses/find-an-mbsr-program/. There is an option for either a MBSR or MBCT instructor listing. The center also offers an interactive online MBSR program and a self-paced video-recorded MBSR program in partnership with Sounds True for areas that do not have a certified instructor nearby.

However, other healthcare professionals have attended the Center's training and have a mindfulness practice but have not gone through the lengthy certification process. As a clinician, it is important to check on the qualifications of anyone you are referring your patient to. There are important questions to ask. Where did they receive their training? How long they have been practicing? What type of patients they work with and their outcomes with those clients?

Conclusion

This chapter focused on the health benefits of mindfulness meditation with evidence to support the intervention for promoting or maintaining physical and mental health, cognition, and wellness. There are still numerous studies that have a specific focus using mindfulness that could not be covered in this chapter. Evidence cited was mostly based on systematic reviews and meta-analysis of RCTs with a few individual RCTs included. It is important to note that not all studies were robust or well-designed and most reviews still called for further research in these areas. Yet, the amount of evidence presented supports the benefits of mindfulness in health.

References

1. Kabat-Zinn J. Full catastrophe living: how to cope with stress, pain and illness using mindfulness meditation. revised ed. New York: Bantam Books; 2013.
2. Mindful. Jon Kabat-Zinn: defining mindfulness: what is mindfulness? The founder of mindfulness-based stress reduction explains. Mindful. 2017. https://www.mindful.org/jon-kabat-zinn-defining-mindfulness/.
3. Grossman P, Niemann L, Schmidt S, Walach H. Mindfulness-based stress reduction and health benefits: a meta-analysis. J Psychosom Res. 2004;57(1):35–43. https://doi.org/10.1016/S0022-3999(03)00573-7.
4. Sisk D. Mindfulness practices that can be implemented in the regular classroom. J Yoga Physiol. 2017;2(5):555–99. https://doi.org/10.19080/JYP.2017.02.555599.
5. Kabat-Zinn J, Santorelli SF, Meleo-Meyer F, Koerbel L. Mindfulness-based stress reduction (MBSR) authorized curriculum guide. Revised ed. 2017. Retrieved from https://umassmed.edu/globalassets/center-for-mindfulness/documents/mbsr-curriculum-guide-2017.pdf.
6. Sharma M, Rush SE. Mindfulness-based stress reduction as a stress management intervention for healthy individuals: a systematic review. J Evid Based Complementary Altern Med. 2014;9(14):271–86.
7. Pascoe MC, Thompson DR, Jenkins ZM, Ski CF. Mindfulness mediates the physiological markers of stress: systematic review and meta-analysis. J Psychiatr Res. 2017;95:156–78. https://doi.org/10.1016/j.jpsychires.2017.08.004.
8. Dahlhamer J, Lucas J, Zelaya C, Nahin R, Mackey S, DeBar L, Kerns R, et al. Prevalence of chronic pain and high-impact chronic pain among adults — United States, 2016. Morb Mortal Wkly Rep. 2018;67:1001–6. https://doi.org/10.15585/mmwr.mm6736a2.
9. Creswell JD. Mindfulness interventions. Annu Rev Psychol. 2017;68:491–516. https://doi.org/10.1146/annurev-psych-042716-051139.
10. Gotink RA, Chu P, Busschbach JJ, Benson H, Fricchione GL, Hunink MG. Standardised mindfulness-based interventions in healthcare: an overview of systematic reviews and meta-analyses of RCTs. PLoS One. 2015;10(4):e0124344. https://doi.org/10.1371/journal.pone.0124344.
11. Centers of Disease Control and Prevention [CDC]. United States cancer statistics: data visualizations. 2015. https://gis.cdc.gov/Cancer/USCS/DataViz.html.
12. Zhang HA, Mowinckel P, Finset A, Eriksson LR, Høystad TØ, Lunde AK, Hagen KB. A mindfulness-based group intervention to reduce psychological distress and fatigue in patients with inflammatory rheumatic joint diseases: a randomised controlled trial. Ann Rheum Dis. 2012;71(6):911–7. https://doi.org/10.1136/annrheumdis-2011-200351.
13. Shapiro SL, Carlson LE. The art and science of mindfulness: integrating mindfulness into psychology and the helping professions. 2nd ed. Washington, DC: American Psychological Association; 2017.
14. Zimmermann FF, Burrell B, Jordan J. The acceptability and potential benefits of mindfulness-based interventions in improving psychological well-being for adults with advanced cancer: a systematic review. Complement Ther Clin Pract. 2018;30:68–78. https://doi.org/10.1016/j.ctcp.2017.12.014.
15. Abbott RA, Whear R, Rodgers LR, Bethel A, Thompson Coon J, Kuken W, Stein K, et al. Effectiveness of mindfulness-based stress reduction and mindfulness based cognitive therapy in vascular disease: a systematic review and meta-analysis of randomised controlled trials. J Psychosom Res. 2014;76(5):341–51. https://doi.org/10.1016/j.jpsychores.2014.02.012.
16. Lakhan SE, Schofield KL. Mindfulness-based therapies in the treatment of somatization disorders: a systematic review and meta-analysis. PLoS One. 2013;8(8):e71834. https://doi.org/10.1371/journal.pone.0071834.
17. Duncan LG, Moskowitz JT, Neilands TB, Dilworth SE, Hecht FM, Johnson MO. Mindfulnessbased stress reduction for HIV treatment side effects: a randomized, wait-list controlled trial. J Pain Symptom Manage. 2012;43(2):161–71. https://doi.org/10.1016/j.jpainsymman.2011.04.007.
18. Yang Y, Liu YH, Zhang HF, Liu JY. Effectiveness of mindfulness-based stress reduction and mindfulness-based cognitive therapies on people living with HIV: a systematic review and meta-analysis. Int J Nurs Sci. 2015;2:283–94.
19. Centers of Disease Control and Prevention [CDC]. National Diabetes Statistics Report, 2017: estimates of diabetes and its burden in the United States. 2017. https://www.cdc.gov/diabetes/pdfs/data/statistics/national-diabetes-statistics-report.pdf.

20. Centers of Disease Control and Prevention [CDC]. Smoking and tobacco use. 2017. https://www.cdc.gov/tobacco/data_statistics/index.htm?s_cid=osh-stu-home-nav-005.

21. Noordali F, Cumming J, Thompson JL. Effectiveness of Mindfulness-based interventions on physiological and psychological complications in adults with diabetes: a systematic review. J Health Psychol. 2017;22(8):965–83. https://doi.org/10.1177/1359105315620293.

22. Kian AA, Vahdani B, Noorbala AA, Nejatisafa A, Arbabi M, Zenoozian S, Nakhjavani M. The impact of mindfulness-based stress reduction on emotional wellbeing and glycemic control of patients with type 2 diabetes mellitus. J Diabetes Res. 2018;2018:1986820. https://doi.org/10.1155/2018/1986820.

23. National Heart, Lung & Blood Institute. Managing overweight and obesity in adults: systematic evidence review from the obesity expert panel 2013. 2013. http://www.nhlbi.nih.gov/guidelines.

24. Godsey J. The role of mindfulness based interventions in the treatment of obesity and eating disorders: an integrative review. Complement Ther Med. 2013;21:430–9.

25. Katterman SN, Kleinman BM, Hood MM, Nackers LM, Corsica JA. Mindfulness meditation as an intervention for binge eating, emotional eating and weight loss: a systematic review. Eat Behav. 2014;15:197–204. https://doi.org/10.1016/j.eatbeh.2014.01.005.

26. Olson KL, Emory CF. Mindfulness and weight loss: a systematic review. Psychosom Med. 2015;77(1):59–67.

27. Rogers JM, Ferrari M, Mosely K, Lang CP, Brennan L. Mindfulness-based interventions for adults who are overweight or obese: a meta-analysis of physical and psychological health outcomes. Obes Rev. 2017;18(1):51–67. https://doi.org/10.1111/obr.12461.

28. Mantzios M, Wilson JC. Mindfulness, eating behaviors, and obesity: a review and reflection on current findings. Curr Obes Rep. 2015;4:141–6. https://doi.org/10.1007/s13679-014-0131-x.

29. de Souza ICW, de Barros VV, Gomide HP, Miranda TCM, de Paula Menezes V, Kozasa EH, Noto AR. Mindfulness-based interventions for the treatment of smoking: a systematic literature review. J Altern Complement Med. 2015;21(3):129–40.

30. Oikonomou MT, Arvanitis M, Sokolove RL. Mindfulness training for smoking cessation: a meta-analysis of randomized-controlled trials. J Health Psychol. 2017;22(14):1841–50. https://doi.org/10.1177/1359105316637667.

31. National Institute of Health. Mental health information: major depression. 2017. https://www.nimh.nih.gov/health/statistics/major-depression.shtml.

32. Strauss C, Cavanaugh K, Oliver A, Pettman D. Mindfulness-based interventions for people diagnosed with a current episode of an anxiety or depressive disorder: a meta-analysis of randomised controlled trials. PLoS One. 2014;9(4):e96110. https://doi.org/10.1371/journal.pone.0096110.

33. Piet J, Hougaard E. The effect of mindfulness-based cognitive therapy for prevention of relapse in recurrent major depressive disorder: a systematic review and meta-analysis. Clin Psychol Rev. 2011;31:1032–40.

34. Kuyken W, Warren FC, Taylor RS, Whalley B, Crane C, Bondolfi G, Haves R, et al. Efficacy of mindfulness-based cognitive therapy in prevention of depressive relapse: an individual patient data meta-analysis from randomized trials. JAMA Psychiat. 2016;73(6):565–74. https://doi.org/10.1001/jamapsychiatry.2016.0076.

35. National Institute of Health. Mental health statistics: any anxiety disorder. 2017. Retrieved from https://www.nimh.nih.gov/health/statistics/any-anxiety-disorder.shtml.

36. Chen KW, Berger CC, Manheimer E, Forde D, Magidson J, Dachman L, Lejuez CW. Meditative therapies for reducing anxiety: a systematic review and meta-analysis of randomized controlled trials. Depress Anxiety. 2012;29:545–62. https://doi.org/10.1002/da.21964.

37. Rodrigues MF, Nardi AE, Levitan M. Mindfulness in mood and anxiety disorders: a review of the literature. Trends Psychiatry Psychother. 2017;39(3):207–15. https://doi.org/10.1590/2237-6089-2016-0051.

38. Lee CS, Ma MT, Ho HY, Tsang KK, Zheng YY, Wu ZY. The effectiveness of mindfulness-based intervention in attention on individuals with ADHD: a systematic review. Hong Kong J Occup Ther. 2017;30:33–41. https://doi.org/10.1016/j.hkjot.2017.05.001.

39. Chimiklis AL, Dahl V, Spears AP, Goss K, Fogarty K, Chacko A. Yoga, mindfulness, and meditation interventions for youth with ADHD: systematic review and meta-analysis. J Child Fam Stud. 2018;27(10):3155–68.

40. Sancho M, De Gracia M, Rodríguez RC, Mallorquí-Bagué N, Sánchez-González J, Trujols J, Sánchez I, et al. Mindfulness-based interventions for the treatment of substance and behavioral addictions: a systematic review. Front Psych. 2018;9:95. https://doi.org/10.3389/fpsyt.2018.00095.

41. Boyd JE, Lanius RA, McKinno MC. Mindful-ness-based treatments for posttraumatic stress disorder: a review of the treatment literature and neurobiological evidence. J Psychiatry Neurosci. 2018;43(1):7–25. https://doi.org/10.1503/jpn.170021.

42. National Institute of Health. Mental health information: schizophrenia. 2016. https://www.nimh.nih.gov/health/topics/Schizophrenia/index.shtml.

43. Goldberg SB, Tucker RP, Greene PA, Davidson RJ, Wampold BE, Kearney DJ, Simpson TL. Mindfulness-based interventions for psychiatric disorders: a systematic review and meta-analysis. Clinical Psychology Review. 2018;59:52–60. https://doi.org/10.1016/j.cpr.2017.10.011.

44. Davis L, Kurzban S. Mindfulness-based treatment for people with severe mental illness: a literature review. Am J Psychiatr Rehabil. 2012;15:202–32.

45. Bojic S, Becerra R. Mindfulness-based treatment for bi-polar disorder: a systematic review of the literature. Eur J Psychol. 2017;13(3):573–98. https://doi.org/10.5964/ejop.v13i3.1138.
46. Ambrose SA, Bridges MW, DiPietro M, Lovett MC, Norman MK. The Jossey-Bass higher and adult education series. How learning works: seven research-based principles for smart teaching. San Francisco: Jossey-Bass; 2010.
47. Cassady JC. The impact of cognitive test anxiety on test comprehension and recall in the absence of external evaluative pressure. Appl Cogn Psychol. 2004;18(3):311–25. https://doi.org/10.1002/acp.968.
48. Goleman D. Social intelligence. New York: Bantam; 2006.
49. Mrazek MD, Franklin MS, Phillips DT, Baird B, Schooler JW. Mindfulness training improves working memory capacity and GRE performance while reducing mind wandering. Psychol Sci. 2013;24(5):776–81. https://doi.org/10.1177/0956797612459659.
50. Killingsworth MA, Gilbert DA. A wandering mind is an unhappy mind. Science. 2010;330(6006):932. https://doi.org/10.1126/science.1192439.
51. Foerde K, Knowlton BJ, Poldrack R. Modulation of competing memory systems by distraction. PNAS. 2006;103:11778–83.
52. Chambers R, Lo BC, Allen NB. The impact of intensive mindfulness training on attentional control, cognitive style and affect. Cogn Ther Res. 2008;32:303–22.
53. Jha AP, Krompinger J, Baime MJ. Mindfulness training modifies subsystems of attention. Cognit Affective Behav Neurosci. 2007;7:109–19.
54. Valentine ER, Sweet PL. Meditation and attention: a comparison of the effects of concentrative versus mindfulness meditation on sustained attention. Ment Health Relig Cult. 1999;2:59–70.
55. Memory. Merriam-Webster.com.Web. n.d. https://www.merriam-webster.com/dictionary/memory.
56. Brown KW, Goodman RJ, Ryan RM, Anālayo B. Mindfulness enhances episodic memory performance: evidence from a multimethod investigation. PLoS One. 2016;11(4):e0153309. https://doi.org/10.1371/journal.pone.0153309.
57. Quach D, Jastrowski MK, Alexander K. A randomized controlled trial examining the effect of mindfulness meditation on working memory capacity in adolescents. J Adolesc Health. 2016;58(5):489–96. https://doi.org/10.1016/j.jadohealth.2015.09.024.
58. de Vibe M, Bjørndal A, Fattah S, Dyrdal GM, Halland E, Tanner-Smith EE. Mindfulness-based stress reduction (MBSR) for improving health, quality of life and social functioning in adults: a systematic review and meta-analysis. Campbell Syst Rev. 2017;8(1):1–127. https://doi.org/10.4073/csr.2017.11.
59. Ryan RM, Deci EL. Self-determination theory and the facilitation of intrinsic motivation, social development, and well-being. Am Psychol. 2000;55:68–78.
60. Victorson D, Kentor M, Maletich C, Lawton RC, Kaufman VH, Borrero M, Berkowitz C. Mindfulness meditation to promote wellness and manage chronic disease: a systematic review and meta-analysis of mindfulness–based randomized con-trolled trials relevant to lifestyle medicine. Am J Lifestyle Med. 2015;9(3):185–211.
61. Trapnell PD, Campbell J. Private self-consciousness and the five-factor model of personality: distinguishing rumination from reflection. J Pers Soc Psychol. 1999;76:284–304.
62. Chiesa A, Serretti A. Mindfulness-based stress reduction for stress management in healthy people: a review and meta-analysis. J Altern Complement Med. 2009;15:593–600.
63. Bonanno GA. Loss, trauma, and human resilience: have we underestimated the human capacity to thrive after extremely aversive events? Am Psychol. 2004;59:20–8.
64. Luthar SS, Cicchetti D, Becker B. The construct of esilience: a critical evaluation and guidelines for future work. Child Dev. 2000;71:543–62.
65. Joyce S, Shand F, Tighe J, Laurent S, Bryant R, Harvey S. Road to resilience: a systematic review and meta-analysis of resilience training programmes and interventions. BMJ Open. 2018;8:e017858. https://doi.org/10.1136/bmjopen-2017-017858.
66. Jekauc D, Kittler C, Schlagheck M. Effectiveness of a mindfulness-based intervention for athletes. Psychology. 2017;8:1–13. https://doi.org/10.4236/psych.2017.81001
67. Hardy L, Jones JG, Gould D. Understanding psycho-logical preparation for sport: theory and practice of elite performers. New York: Wiley; 1996.
68. Hoge CW, Lesikar SE, Guevara R, Lange J, Brundage JF, Engel CC, et al. Mental disorders among US military personnel in the 1990s: association with high levels of health care utilization and early military attrition. Am J Psychiatr. 2002;159(9):1576–83. https://doi.org/10.3402/ejpt.v3i0.19267.
69. Stanley EA, Schaldach JM, Kiyonaga A, Jha AP. Mindfulness-based mind fitness training: a case study of a high-stress predeployment military cohort. Cogn Behav Pract. 2011;18:556–66.
70. Jha AP, Morrison AB, Dainer-Best J, Parker S, Rostrup N, Stanley EA. Minds "at attention": mindfulness training curbs attentional lapses in military cohorts. PLoS One. 2015;10(2):e0116889. https://doi.org/10.1371/journal.pone.0116889.
71. Rice, V. J., Liu, B. and Schroeder, P. J. (2018). Impact of in-person and virtual world mindfulness training on symptoms of post-traumatic stress disorder and attention deficit and hyperactivity disorder. Mil Med 183, ¾, 413.
72. Baer R, Kuyken W. Is mindfulness safe? Mindful: healthy mind, healthy life. 2016. https://www.mindful.org/is-mindfulness-safe/.

Chapter 12
Health Benefits of Spirituality

Deanna Dragan, Danielle McDuffie, and Martha R. Crowther

Keywords Health · Spirituality · Religiousness

> **Key Points**
> - Addressing the role of spirituality in accordance with physical health symptoms and outcomes
> - Highlighting potential mental health benefits of integrating spirituality into practice
> - Showcasing the current integration of spirituality into communities and potential outcomes on community members
> - Examining potential negative effects of the role in spirituality in the lives of individuals
> - Providing techniques and challenges to the integration of spirituality into practice

Introduction

Health and religion have a long-standing relationship that can be traced back to a time when one's physician was frequently a clergy member as well [25]. Since that early period where health and religion were intertwined, we have seen a push to distance scientific disciplines from addressing religious experiences. Yet, the religiously affiliated are estimated to account for 84% of the global population, and researchers across disciplines have continued to explore the mechanisms between religion and health outcomes [52]. Evidence from decades of research on this relationship suggests a robust and mostly positive association between religion and health. However, before describing the associations, it is important to note that the majority of research that has been conducted has focused primarily on measuring religiousness, not spirituality [10, 12]. Considerable debate regarding the operationalization of these terms continues to persist [12, 17, 42, 59, 60].

Religion is described as having an affiliation with a denomination that has a structured set of beliefs with activities that are organized and reflect long-established traditions [32]. Religion can also encompass a connection to the transcendent in addition to establishing rules and laws for practitioners

D. Dragan · D. McDuffie
Department of Psychology, The University of Alabama, Tuscaloosa, AL, USA

M. R. Crowther (✉)
The University of Alabama, Tuscaloosa, AL, USA
e-mail: mrcrowther@ua.edu

© Springer Nature Switzerland AG 2020
J. Uribarri, J. A. Vassalotti (eds.), *Nutrition, Fitness, and Mindfulness*, Nutrition and Health,
https://doi.org/10.1007/978-3-030-30892-6_12

to follow. Studies frequently assess religiousness by measuring the frequency of engagement in religious activities or rituals (i.e., church attendance, prayer, and reading religious texts). Comparatively, spirituality is described as a broader concept extending beyond religious experiences. It is frequently associated with the search for connection with the sacred or transcendent [32]. Most often, studies measure spirituality by assessing positive psychological and emotional states (meaning, purpose in life, connection, inner peace, etc.), which creates significant overlap between spirituality and mental health indicators [21, 22].

In addition to the difficulties in distinguishing religion from spirituality, there are other common terms used, such as religiosity, faith, the divine, sacred, and more. There is not enough space in this chapter, nor is it the focus, to discuss the differences between the terms. However, the ongoing challenge to reach a consensus on defining and measuring the terms has implications for interpretation of research findings. In clinical settings, it is preferred to appeal to the majority of patients by using a broader term like spirituality [23]. More attention to the importance of word choice in clinical settings will be addressed in the section on integrating religion and spirituality into clinical practice. The field continues to struggle to agree upon delineations of these terms that satisfy both the research and clinical purposes. As this chapter is targeted toward the clinical purpose, we have striven to either match the research evidence's terminology or deferred to using broader terminology as appropriate.

Physical Health

Inherently within the USA, there is a connection between faith and physical health. Faith has proven itself to play an integral role in the medical field overall. Of the healthcare systems in America, there are 654 Catholic hospitals and 1634 Catholic continuing care facilities [4]. Each day, 1 in 6 patients in the USA is cared for in a Catholic hospital [1]. This means in effect that a number of the decisions being made concerning many Americans' day-to-day health are directly influenced by some faith-based structure and guidance. On a more personal level, spirituality and religiosity have been shown to be advantageous in coping with both chronic and terminal illness [31]. During times of health difficulty, many people rely on their faith to help understand their misfortune and to draw strength to weather their condition [36].

Prediabetes and Diabetes

In a sample of 30 African-American men living with type 2 diabetes, it was found that the men frequently engaged in religious behavior to aid with the management of their diabetes [40]. These behaviors included prayer and overall belief in God, turning things over to God, changing unhealthy behaviors, reading the Bible, and gaining support from religious/spiritual individuals. Through prayer, the men often asked God to help them both with managing their diabetes and with aiding them in the change of behaviors that were exacerbating their diabetes. There was also mention made by the men of God giving them diabetes in order to help keep them alive and push them to change their current unhealthy lifestyles [40]. In terms of how healthcare professionals can use this information, it was suggested that clinicians could utilize the role of spirituality in the lives of diabetes patients to help them make sense of their diagnoses. An example of this might be to have a conversation with a spiritual patient suggesting that God had allowed them to contract their condition to help them re-evaluate their lives and their health, rather than it being a punishment.

Cardiovascular Disease

For those experiencing cardiovascular disease, the role of spirituality has been found to have tangible health benefits. Faith in the lives of those with cardiovascular disease has played a role in advanced autonomic cardiac control, reduced blood pressure, and reduced pain [3, 15, 33]. Spirituality, defined as a closeness to and satisfaction with one's relationship with God, was found to be significantly related to parasympathetic and sympathetic cardiac control in middle- and older-aged adults [3]. Further, being more intrinsically religious was also found to be related to experiencing lower blood pressure levels in response to stressors [33]. In a sample of African-American women, prayer was found to be an adaptive strategy for pain management. One example of such highlighted a woman praying to God to remove the pain associated with a heart condition she was facing [15]. Additionally, spirituality can also be used to divert attention from the effects of chronic illness, including heart disease [15]. As an added health benefit for cardiovascular disease patients, engaging in spiritual self-care has been found to mediate the relationship between heart failure and quality of life in African-American adults [57]. Realistically, this means that those who practice more spiritual self-care have a better quality of life despite also having heart failure. These spiritual self-care techniques included practicing yoga or Tai Chi, attending religious services, reading religious texts (e.g., the Bible), praying, meditation, and/or enjoying/cultivating a relationship with nature [57]. Overall, religiousness is associated with lower risk of cardiovascular disease because it is connected to effective coping skills to deal with stressors and rules for engaging in healthy behaviors [25].

Chronic Kidney Disease

Depression has been found to consistently contribute to the reduction of quality of life in those with chronic kidney disease (CKD) and end-stage renal disease (ESRD) [5, 7]. In the context of a high prevalence and severity of depression on those with CKD, it seems necessary that a coping strategy be present to enable successful continuation of life in spite of illness. One of these beneficial coping strategies is spirituality. Darrell [8] found that in a sample of 12 African-American adults living with ESRD, all of the participants endorsed the role of spirituality within their lives. Spirituality was described as having faith that God cares, including utilizing faith to support coping and using prayer to develop strength [8]. Prayer, specifically, was identified as an avenue for participants to come to terms with their ESRD diagnosis, to seek guidance on decisions regarding their treatment (e.g., the use of dialysis), and to generally cope with their illness.

As a special note, some research has called into question the distinction between religion and spirituality in its relation to health outcomes. It has been proposed that religious measures in their relation to health outcomes might be biased, due largely to the fact that most religious outcome measures are predicated on religious service attendance [58]. For those who are more physically impaired, religious service attendance might not be as feasible, thereby those with the physical ability to attend religious services might inherently be healthier than those who cannot, rather than it being a true measure of religion's role in health [58].

Mental Health Benefits

Psychological Distress

Across the most commonly researched diagnoses related to mental health, the evidence suggests inverse relationships between faith and psychological distress. More than 444 studies have reported findings on the relationship between faith and depression; 61% of those studies found significant inverse relationships. Furthermore, 63% of 30 clinical trials found faith interventions produced better outcomes than treatment as usual or control groups [25]. In addition, a review study found that at least 141 studies have assessed the relationship between suicide and religiousness with 75% of the studies reporting inverse relationships. Of the 40 most methodologically rigorous studies, 80% found more religious individuals associated with fewer attempts and more negative attitudes toward suicide [25].

The relationship between religion and symptoms of anxiety is complex. A general trend indicates faith is associated with lower symptoms of anxiety and highlights how people turn to faith to mitigate their anxiety (i.e., fear of death, sense of not being alone, and more). Simultaneously, religious beliefs have the potential to increase anxiety symptoms due to threat of punishment or judgment for sins. It is possible that the increase in anxiety found in some studies may be due to use of the cross-sectional methodology. The evidence from a limited number of longitudinal studies suggests anxiety from religious beliefs may diminish over time, but additional research is needed to confirm this assertion [25].

Religiousness has also been researched as it relates to symptoms of schizophrenia. Many people diagnosed with schizophrenia report delusions and hallucinations that involve religious figures or beliefs. It can be difficult for clinicians to distinguish clinical symptoms of schizophrenia from deeply held religious beliefs. Moreover, the research findings on the relationship between faith and psychotic symptoms suggest no consistent pattern. Religious coping is common among patients with schizophrenia, but the ongoing challenge is to differentiate healthy religious coping behaviors from psychosis [23]. In clinical practice, it is recommended to consider a patient's faith during treatment planning and consult with practitioners of the same faith to clarify the severity of psychotic symptoms.

Psychological Well-Being

In addition to the effect of religion on clinical diagnoses, evidence connecting religion with positive emotional states has also emerged. Most studies have found positive correlations between religious involvement and positive emotions like well-being, happiness, purpose in life, and self-esteem. Based on a systematic review, researchers found that 93% of the 45 studies included reported a positive correlation between faith and sense of purpose in life [23]. Similarly, a review article reported a positive correlation between faith and well-being in 79% of the 326 articles included in the analysis [25]. These results demonstrate the increase in studies devoted to exploring the effects of faith on positive psychology concepts [2]. However, the majority of this evidence comes from cross-sectional studies; thus, it remains unclear as to whether high religiosity precedes psychological well-being or if greater psychological well-being increases religiosity. More complex and longitudinal study designs are being conducted to continue addressing this area of research.

Underlying Theories

Overall, the research on faith and mental health illustrates how religious and spiritual beliefs indirectly contribute to mental health. Evidence suggests that religious involvement influences multiple factors that contribute to mental health, such as chronic inflammation from stress, coping styles, attachment styles, social support, childhood environment, decision-making, and self-control. Further, these factors feed off of one another and amplify the effects of religious involvement. There are 3 primary pathways that religious involvement is associated with positive mental health: (1) religious coping provides a sense of meaning to traumatic experiences; (2) most religious belief systems have rules that protect their believers from risky health behaviors; and (3) most religious belief systems propagate feelings of love toward others, which increases our prosocial behaviors [25, 45]. Given the variety of factors involved, a life span approach offers an encompassing framework to identify the pathways that connects faith and mental health.

Religion and Spirituality in Communities

Health Promotion

Faith communities often act as contexts where spiritual support can give way to the provision of health services through the spread of health information and health promotion [37]. People are often more likely to seek, comprehend, and implement health information when it is framed in accordance with their spiritual beliefs and coming from within their spiritual institutions [37]. It is also the case that healthcare professionals are better able to spread their message when going through faith communities.

Through the socially supportive aspect of religious environments, it has been suggested that having companionships with fellow church members can lead to encouragement of the adoption of positive health behaviors [27]. This is speculated to be due to significant others (including close companions) prompting and/or persuading their loved ones to engage in behavior to enhance their health [54]. Religious involvement has been linked to the tendency to have better health due to engagement in positive health behaviors (e.g., following a healthy diet) and avoidance of negative health behaviors (e.g., excessive alcohol use) [16]. Further, it has been found that those who are more religiously involved (defined by the frequency of church attendance) had significantly better engagement in exercise (including walking), seat belt use, vitamin use, sleep, and usage of preventive healthcare services (e.g., dental and physical checkups) than those who attended church less frequently [16]. It has been suggested that these heightened health behaviors are due largely to religious tenets associating the body with being a temple of God [16].

An applied example of the role of faith-based organizations in health promotion highlights a study conducted on the health information shared over the Internet by four African-American Christian churches in the Atlanta area [14]. In terms of the health resources found on the churches' websites, the themes of (1) online health education, (2) athletic programs, (3) fitness training, (4) fitness facilities, and (5) community outreach and health emerged. Making mention of one specific subheading, under the theme of health education, many of the websites included information for congregants pertaining to certain diseases and illnesses (including obesity and diabetes). Along with provision of general information on these diseases, there were resources on how to manage those diseases and illnesses, tied in conjunction with scripture and teachings from the Bible [14]. In practice, it could be helpful to either assess what types of health information patients living with chronic illnesses could be receiving from their faith communities, and it could be helpful to attempt to establish programs within local faith institutions pertaining to healthy lifestyle factors.

Deleterious Effects of Religion and Spirituality

Negative interactions in the church can come through multiple avenues. A few of the more highlighted examples of negative interactions are unfavorable social interactions with fellow church members, providing excessive help and/or providing ineffective help [53]. Unfavorable social interactions can include disagreements, criticism, rejection, and violations of privacy by other church members [53]. Because it has been found that negative interactions in nonreligious settings can cause adverse health outcomes physically and psychologically [26, 41], it has been suggested that negative social interactions affecting health also extend to religious settings where a wealth of social interaction takes place [27]. As an example of this, having a higher number of negative interactions with other church members is linked to higher endorsement of depressive symptomology and lower endorsement of positive well-being [28]. Further, a larger number of negative interactions within the church have led to members' reporting less overall satisfaction with their health along with greater anxiety [30, 47]. Overall, the resulting effects of negative interactions in the church were found to be greater than the effects of positive interactions [30]. Specifically, excessive demands from other churchgoers are more likely to affect depressive symptoms than other forms of negative interaction such as criticisms [9].

There is also evidence to suggest that going through a religious or spiritual struggle can lead to a greater risk for mortality [46]. This struggle was described as the feeling of being abandoned by God, the questioning of God's love and care, or feeling that malevolent supernatural forces were at work in one's illness. Among those encountering these religious or spiritual struggles, there was a 19–28% increased risk of mortality [46]. Further confirmation of this trend comes from the finding that individuals who have more doubts regarding their faith also report being less satisfied with their health [29]. For clinicians, it is important to be cognizant of the fact that having a patient report on their faith might not always mean it is acting as an advantageous factor in their lives.

Integration into Practice

Given the scope of the research findings presented throughout this chapter, it may seem daunting to integrate clients' religiousness and spirituality into practice. First and foremost, it is recommended to include a spiritual history assessment in your clinic's standard intake procedures across clinical settings. While this should be presented from a neutral perspective (i.e., not implying that one "should be religious"), collecting a spiritual history creates space for patients to share their personal beliefs, preferences, and the value they attribute to faith in their life. The number of items in the assessment may differ based on time constraints and clinical settings. Collecting a spiritual history sets the foundation for the clinician to be able to respect the patient's beliefs simply by taking the time to ask about them. Currently, there is no standardized tool for spiritual histories; but several have been suggested to guide clinicians in choosing a set of questions that fits their clinical needs and the treatment setting [11, 18, 19, 24, 34, 39]. For many people, it may be beneficial to spend smaller amounts of time over several sessions to fully explore the role their faith plays in their life. In particular, this can help patients feel more comfortable if they desire to share a religious struggle or a behavior they feel ashamed of because of their faith.

In addition to conducting a spiritual assessment, treatment professionals can support patients' religious beliefs, and, when appropriate, practitioners can sparingly challenge beliefs that seem to be acting as barriers to reaching treatment goals. Being supportive of a patient's faith can be accomplished by encouraging that individual to continue engaging in religious activities that are effective coping strategies. Also, clinicians can consider using treatment approaches that are adapted to fit a patient's faith, such as cognitive behavioral therapy that has been developed to integrate the Bible into treatment [6, 49, 51]. Professionals can also support patients' faith by praying with them; however, this is a very controversial practice that requires consideration of the power dynamic [23]. Similar to the ethics concerning physical contact with clients, praying with patients can be a powerful tool if appropriately timed and if initiated by the patient. If the clinician suggests praying together, it could put the patient into a position where they feel coerced into praying. For those who are interested in further study of this practice, guidelines have been developed [50].

Integrating a client's faith into practice in a supportive way can simply involve matching the patient's terminology and illustrating your openness to discussing the importance of their faith. In contrast, determining appropriate times to challenge a client's belief system because it is impeding treatment goals or exacerbating symptoms is more difficult. For some, reaching out to family members, religious community members, or religious leaders can help with the identification of such patients and serve to lend credibility to the treatment approach from the patient's perspective. This is especially true when trying to lessen the rigidity of a patient's beliefs by demonstrating other practitioners of the same faith tradition are open to modifying certain beliefs to remove the barrier to treatment. Therefore, it is possible to intervene when a client's faith is serving to exacerbate symptoms or disrupt therapy; however, the practitioner should approach this cautiously and strive to maintain good rapport with the patient.

Lastly, knowing when to refer a patient to another clinician can be challenging, especially for those who are less familiar with integrating faith into their practice. Familiarizing oneself with the different types of clergy that can provide counseling can be a useful first step. For example, knowing the differences between a pastoral counselor and a chaplain can help determine which clergyperson would be better fit for a particular patient. Similarly, clergy may find it difficult to know when to refer a medical or mental health practitioner; it is equally as important for them to familiarize themselves with the differences in training across health professionals to make appropriate referrals. The spiritual history assessment can help the clinician to identify patients who should be referred based on exploring the following factors: severity of the symptoms, conflict between the patient's religious beliefs and treatment goals, depth of rapport built with the patient, pervasiveness of the patient's faith influencing treatment, and the availability of clergy members for referral [23].

Even on a basic level, patients' spiritual concerns can begin to be addressed by asking a question as simple as: "is there anything about your spiritual beliefs you think it is important for me to know in order to help me care for you better?"

Challenges to Integrating

One relevant challenge to the integration of faith with health could be the role of the faith institution, including its clergy, in the lives of spiritual patients. Mentally and emotionally, there is evidence to suggest that about one-fourth of people primarily look to clergy for aid when encountering psychological difficulties [56]. Clergymen have been shown to frequently reference mental health disturbances such as anxiety, depression, and worry within their sermons [35]. Specifically, these illnesses can often be described in sermons as being the result of external supernatural forces (e.g., the devil) or the result of internal spiritual shortcomings (e.g., not being in adherence to one's faith or the biblical teachings) [35]. Presumably, for individuals who turn to religious leaders for help with mental disturbances and received a message that partially placed blame for their disturbance on the individual's own religiosity, this could increase the individual's resistance to seek treatment from mental health professionals.

In similar manner, the receptiveness of the clinician to engage in discussions on the patient's faith could hinder the integration of faith in clinical practice. There seems to be an overall trend indicating a lack of receptiveness by professionals to gather spiritual histories of patients. While most healthcare professionals feel they should be aware of patients' spirituality, an additional majority said they would not directly ask about spiritual topics unless the patient was dying [38]. Thereby, clinicians and practitioners should be aware of how their own receptiveness (or lack thereof) to the conversation of spirituality might be a barrier to addressing and meeting patients' spiritual needs.

Clinicians' personal religious or spiritual beliefs can also serve as a barrier to providing competent treatment that involves faith. People commonly turn to their religious or spiritual beliefs to aid in decision-making processes, which can similarly be extended to apply to treatment providers [25].

For example, personal faith beliefs on topics like abortion may influence physicians' and other healthcare professionals' comfort with performing procedures or prescribing medications. The influence of personal beliefs on providing clinical care can become particularly problematic when there is a significant difference between the provider's faith and that of the patient. Further, psychologists are more likely to identify as religiously unaffiliated (agnostic, atheist, and none) when compared to the general public [13, 20]. Thus, there is an even higher chance the psychologist may have little personal experience with the benefits of religion and be less inclined to recognize the significance of faith in a patient's life. In a study with members from the Association for Behavioral and Cognitive Therapies (ABCT), 64% of respondents indicated that they felt mostly or very comfortable addressing faith in practice [55]. Based on social desirability and respondents self-selecting to participate in studies like these, investigators have likely underestimated the discomfort clinicians feel when addressing religion or spirituality in practice. Therefore, it can be challenging for practitioners to integrate faith into their practice due to conflicts between their personal belief system and that of their patients. Tenets of cultural competency and ethical practice indicate the need for treatment providers to identify potential biases related to religious beliefs. Through increased awareness and client-centered practice, practitioners can find ways to integrate religion and spirituality into their practice and respect patients' beliefs.

An additional challenge to integration addresses the nature of the individual's style of religious coping. It has been proposed that there are three styles by which people utilize their relationship with a higher being to cope with stressors in life (including illness): collaborative religious coping, active religious surrender, and passive religious deferral [43–45]. Collaborative religious coping is the notion by the individual that they are in partnership with God in resolving their problems and that both the individual and God have active problem-solving roles [43–45]. This style has been associated with better physical health in individuals when facing stressors. The active religious surrender coping style involves the individual initiating efforts to aid with their stressors; however instead of working collaboratively with the higher being, they manage some aspects of their situation and then leave the rest for the higher being to control [43–45]. While active religious surrender has also been found to be positively associated with well-being, the associations are weaker than with the collaborative coping style [45]. In the passive religious deferral coping style, the individual leaves the responsibility of full resolution of the situation to the higher being. This style has the weakest associations of all three styles with well-being. Contrary to the benefits that are associated with religious coping, negative religious coping styles and spiritual struggles have been correlated with increasing psychological distress [48]. For integrating faith with practice, it is important to note which of these relational styles the client might be engaging in and to understand how their religious coping style might affect their willingness to engage in prescribed treatments such as taking medicine or compliance with other medical interventions.

In instances where religious affiliations might come in clear contradiction to accepted patterns of treatment (e.g., a Jehovah's Witness patient who might refuse a blood transfusion), it is important to consider the well-being of the patient despite what accepted medical practices might be. It could be the case that imposing treatments on patients who are unwilling to comply due to religious restrictions could lead to the patient feeling defensive and denying all means of care, thereby potentially worsening their condition. It is important for the professional to potentially check his or her own biases and negative feelings related to a religious practice that might contradict the professional's scientific background, as to not adversely harm the patient by inadvertently neglecting other care options.

Conclusion

There is a growing evidence to support clinicians integrating faith into clinical practice to reach treatment goals, enhance adherence to medical treatments, and encourage engagement in healthy behaviors. It is recommended to gather a spiritual history early to guide treatment planning. Practitioners face several challenges to integrating faith into their practice. Yet, research detailing the physical and mental health benefits associated with being religious or spiritual illustrates the powerful role faith can play in a client's life. As research on this topic utilizes more complex methodological study designs, it is expected that evidence will more comprehensively describe the relationship between faith and health.

References

1. American Hospital Association. American Hospital Association annual survey, 2016. 2016. Retrieved September 9, 2018, from https://www.aha.org/system/files/research/reports/tw/chartbook/2016/2016chartbook.pdf.
2. Barton Y, Miller L. Spirituality and positive psychology go hand in hand: an investigation of multiple empirically derived profiles and related protective benefits. J Relig Health. 2015;54(3):829–43. https://doi.org/10.1007/s10943-015-0045-2.
3. Berntson GG, Norman GJ, Hawkley LC, Cacioppo JT. Spirituality and autonomic cardiac control. Ann Behav Med. 2008;35:198–208.
4. Catholic Health Association of the United States. Catholic health care in the United States. 2018. Retrieved from https://www.chausa.org/about/about/facts-statistics.
5. Chilcot J, Wellsted D, Da Silva-Gane M, Farrington K. Depression on dialysis. Nephron Clin Pract. 2008;108:256–64.
6. CSTH. Religiously-integrated cognitive behavioral therapy (RCBT) manuals and workbooks (including training video). Durham: Duke University Center for Spirituality, Theology and Health; 2014. Retrieved from http://www.spiritualityandhealth.duke.edu/index.php/religious-cbt-study/therapy-manuals.
7. Cukor D, Peterson RA, Cohen SD, Kimmel P. Depression in end-stage renal disease hemodialysis patients. Nat Clin Pract Nephrol. 2006;2:678–87.
8. Darrell L. Faith that god cares: the experience of spirituality with African American hemodialysis patients. Soc Work Christ. 2016;43:189–212.
9. Ellison CG, Zhang W, Krause N, Marcum JP. Does negative interaction in the church increase depression? Longitudinal findings from the Presbyterian Panel Survey. Sociol Relig. 2009;70:409–31.
10. Flannelly KJ, Jankowski KB, Flannelly LT. Operational definitions in research on religion and health. J Health Care Chaplain. 2014;20(2):83–91. https://doi.org/10.1080/08854726.2014.909278.
11. Gomi S, Starnino VR, Canda ER. Spiritual assessment in mental health recovery. Community Ment Health J. 2014;50(4):447–53.
12. Hall DE, Meador KG, Koenig HG. Measuring religiousness in and health research. J Relig Health. 2008;47(2):134–83.
13. Harris KA, Spengler PM, Gollery TJ. Clinical judgment faith bias: unexpected findings for psychology research and practice. Prof Psychol Res Pract. 2016;47(6):391–401. https://doi.org/10.1037/pro0000113.
14. Harris TM, Lee CN. Health promotion from within: a platform for advancing a health agenda for and by the church body. In: Miller AN, Rubin DL, editors. Health communication and faith communities. New York: Hampton Press; 2011. p. 143–61.
15. Harvey IS. Self-management of a chronic illness: an exploratory study on the role of spirituality among older African American women. J Women Aging. 2006;18:75–88.
16. Hill TD, Burdette AM, Ellison CG, Musick MA. Religious attendance and health behaviors of Texas adults. Prev Med. 2006;42:309–12.
17. Hill PC, Pargament KI, Hood JW, McCullough ME, Swyers JP, Larson DB, Zinnbauer BJ. Conceptualizing religion and spirituality: points of commonality, points of departure. J Theory Soc Behav. 2000;30(1):51–77.
18. Hodge DR. Implicit spiritual assessment: an alternative approach for assessing client spirituality. Soc Work. 2013;58(3):223–30.
19. Huguelet P, Mohr S, Betrisey C, Borras L, Gillieron C, Marie AM, et al. A randomized trial of spiritual assessment of outpatients with schizophrenia: patients' and clinicians' experience. Psychiatr Serv. 2011;62(1):79–86.
20. Hyman C, Handal PJ. Definitions and evaluation of religion and spirituality items by religious professionals: a pilot study. J Relig Health. 2006;45(2):264–82.
21. Koenig HG. Concerns about measuring "spirituality" in research. J Nerv Ment Dis. 2008;196(5):349–55.
22. Koenig HG, McCullough ME, Larson DB. Handbook of religion and health. New York: Oxford University Press; 2001.
23. Koenig HG. Religion and mental health: research and clinical applications. San Diego: Academic Press; 2018.
24. Koenig HG. Spirituality in patient care: why, how, when, and what. Philadelphia: Templeton Foundation Press; 2013.
25. Koenig HG. Religion, spirituality, and health: the research and clinical implications. ISRN Psychiatry. 2012;2012:1. https://doi.org/10.5402/2012/278730.

26. Krause N. Negative interaction and heart disease in late life: exploring variations by socioeconomic status. J Aging Health. 2005;17:28–55.

27. Krause NM. Aging in the church: how social relationships affect health. West Conshohocken: Templeton Foundation Press; 2008.

28. Krause N, Ellison CG, Wulff KM. Church-based social support, negative interaction, and psychological well-being: findings from a national sample of Presbyterians. J Sci Study Relig. 1998;40:637–56.

29. Krause N, Wulff KM. Religious doubt and health: exploring the potential dark side of religion. Sociol Relig. 2004;65:35–56.

30. Krause N, Wulff KM. Church-based social ties, a sense of belonging in a congregation, and physical health status. Int J Psychol Relig. 2005;15:73–93.

31. Larson DB, Larson SB. Spirituality's potential relevance to physical and emotional health: a brief review of quantitative research. J Psychol Theol. 2003;31:37–52.

32. Lucette A, Ironson G, Pargament KI, Krause N. Spirituality and religiousness are associated with fewer depressive symptoms in individuals with medical conditions. Psychosomatics. 2016;57:505–13.

33. Masters KS, Hill RD, Kircher JC, Benson TLL, Fallon JA. Religious orientation, aging, and blood pressure reactivity to interpersonal and cognitive stressors. Ann Behav Med. 2004;28:171–8.

34. Mathai J, North A. Spiritual history of parents of children attending a child and adolescent mental health service. Australas Psychiatry. 2003;11(2):172–4.

35. Mattox R, McSweeney J, Ivory J, Sullivan G. A qualitative analysis of Christian clergy portrayal of anxiety disturbances in televised sermons. In: Miller AN, Rubin DL, editors. Health communication and faith communities. New York: Hampton Press; 2011. p. 187–202.

36. McCombs HG. The spiritual dimension of caring for people affected by disasters. In: Dass-Brailsford P, editor. Crises and disaster counseling: lessons learned from Hurricane Katrina and other disasters. Newbury Park: Sage; 2009. p. 131–47.

37. Miller AN, Yrisarry N, Rubin DL. Introduction: health communication in, by, and through communities of faith. In: Miller AN, Rubin DL, editors. Health communication and faith communities. New York: Hampton Press; 2011. p. 1–26.

38. Monroe MH, Bynum D, Susi B, Phifer N, Schultz L, Franco M, MacLean CD, Cykert S, Garrett J. Primary care physician preferences regarding spiritual behavior in medical practice. Arch Intern Med. 2003;163:2751–6.

39. Moreira-Almeida A, Koenig HG, Lucchetti G. Clinical implications of spirituality to mental health: review of evidence and practical guidelines. Rev Bras Psiquiatr. 2014;36(2):176–82.

40. Namageyo-Funa A, Muilenburg J, Wilson M. The role of religion and spirituality in coping with type 2 diabetes: a qualitative study among black men. J Relig Health. 2015;54:242–52.

41. Okun MA, Keith VM. Effects of positive and negative social exchanges from various sources on depressive symptoms in younger and older adults. J Gerontol Psychol Sci. 1998;53B:4–20.

42. Oman D. Defining religion and spirituality. In: Paloutzian RF, Park CL, editors. Handbook of the psychology of religion and spirituality. 2nd ed. New York: Guilford Press; 2013. p. 23–47.

43. Pargament KI, Ensing DS, Falgout K, Olsen H, Reilly B, van Haitsma K, Warren R. God help me: (I): religious coping efforts as predictors of the outcomes to significant negative life events. Am J Community Psychol. 1990;18:793–824.

44. Pargament KI, Kennell J, Hathaway W, Grevengoed N, Newman J, Jones W. Religion and the problem-solving process: three styles of coping. J Sci Study Relig. 1988;27:90–104.

45. Pargament KI, Koenig HG, Perez LM. The many methods of religious coping: development and initial validation of the RCOPE. J Clin Psychol. 2000;56:519–43.

46. Pargament KI, Koenig HG, Tarakeshwar N, Hahn J. Religious coping methods as predictors of psychological, physical and spiritual outcomes among medically ill elderly patients: a two-year longitudinal study. J Health Psychol. 2004;9:713–30.

47. Pargament KI, Zinnbauer BJ, Scott AB, Butter EM, Zerowin J, Stanik P. Red flags and religious coping: identifying some religious warning signs among people in crisis. J Clin Psychol. 1998;54:77–89.

48. Park C, Masters K, Salsman J, Wachholtz A, Clements A, Salmoirago-Blotcher E, et al. Advancing our understanding of religion and spirituality in the context of behavioral medicine. J Behav Med. 2017;40(1):39–51. https://doi.org/10.1007/s10865-016-9755-5.

49. Pearce M. Cognitive behavioral therapy for Christians with depression: a practical tool-based primer. Conshohocken: Templeton Foundation Press; 2016.

50. Pearce M, Chiaramonte D. When a patient asks you to pray: what's a provider to do? Int J Palliat Nurs. 2017;23(7):316.

51. Pearce MJ, Koenig HG, Robins CJ, Nelson B, Shaw SF, Cohen HJ, King MB. Religiously integrated cognitive behavioral therapy: a new method of treatment for major depression in patients with chronic medical illness. Psychotherapy. 2015;52(1):56.

52. Pew Research Center. The global religious landscape. 2012. Retrieved from http://www.pewforum.org/global-religiouslandscape.aspx.
53. Rook KS. The negative side of social interaction: impact on psychological well-being. J Pers Soc Psychol. 1984;46:1097–108.
54. Rook KS. Stressful aspects of older adults' social relationships: current theory and research. In: Stevens MAP, Crowther JH, Hobfoll SE, Tennenbaum DL, editors. Stress and coping in later life. Washington, DC: Hemisphere; 1990. p. 172–92.
55. Rosmarin DH, Pirutinsky S, Green D, McKay D. Attitudes toward spirituality/religion among members of the Association for Behavioral and Cognitive Therapies. Prof Psychol Res Pract. 2013;44(6):424–33.
56. Wang PS, Demler O, Kessler RC. Adequacy of treatment for serious mental illness in the United States. Am J Public Health. 2002;92:92–8.
57. White ML. Spirituality self-care effects on quality of life for patients diagnosed with chronic illness. Self-Care Depend Care Nurs. 2013;20:23–32.
58. Zimmer Z, Jagger C, Chiu C-T, Ofstedal MB, Rojo F, Saito Y. Spirituality, religiosity, aging and health in global perspective: a review. SSM- Popul Health. 2016;2:373–81.
59. Zinnbauer BJ, Pargament KI, Cole B, Rye MS, Butter EM, Belavich TG, et al. Religion and spirituality: unfuzzying the fuzzy. J Sci Study Relig. 1997;36(4):549–64. https://doi.org/10.2307/1387689.
60. Zinnbauer BJ, Pargament KI. Religiousness and spirituality. In: Paloutzian RF, Park CF, editors. Handbook of the psychology of religion and spirituality. New York: Guilford Press; 2005. p. 21–42.

Chapter 13
The Health Benefits of Resilience

Lauren A. Peccoralo, Darshan H. Mehta, Gabrielle Schiller, and Lia S. Logio

Keywords Resilience · Wellness · Adaptability

Key Points
- Resilience is defined as one's "ability to adapt or rebound quickly from change, illness, or bad fortune."
- In the GROW framework of resilience, the four key components are (1) good emotions, (2) reason and purpose, (3) others (social connections), and (4) wellness flexibility.
- Evidence supports that having higher levels of resilience may improve health outcomes in chronic disease, decreases incidences of certain illnesses, and increases one's ability to cope with certain medical diagnoses.
- Practicing gratitude, identifying one's core values, depending relationships and goal setting are all simple ways to coach patients to enhance their levels of resilience.

L. A. Peccoralo
Department of Medicine, Department of Medical Education, Icahn School of Medicine at Mount Sinai, New York, NY, USA

D. H. Mehta
Department of Medicine, Benson-Henry Institute for Mind Body Medicine at Massachusetts General Hospital|Osher Center for Integrative Medicine at Brigham & Women's Hospital and Harvard Medical School, Boston, MA, USA

G. Schiller
Department of Geriatric and Palliative Medicine, Icahn School of Medicine at Mount Sinai, New York, NY, USA

L. S. Logio (✉)
Department of Medicine, Drexel University College of Medicine, Philadelphia, PA, USA
e-mail: lsl45@drexel.edu

© Springer Nature Switzerland AG 2020
J. Uribarri, J. A. Vassalotti (eds.), *Nutrition, Fitness, and Mindfulness*, Nutrition and Health,
https://doi.org/10.1007/978-3-030-30892-6_13

Introduction

Definition of Resilience

Resilience is defined as one's "ability to adapt or rebound quickly from change, illness, or bad fortune." Resilient people are those that pick themselves up in the face of adversity and push forward: a woman with breast cancer whose positive mindset gets her through treatment to then volunteer to help other women fighting the disease or the war veteran who loses a lower leg in battle but learns to walk again with a prosthetic limb. What are the characteristics that make these individuals able to move forward from such adversity? Can being resilient really improve health and quality of life? How can one learn how to be more resilient to promote health and well-being?

Elements of Resilience

Steven Southwick and Dennis Charney describe ten elements of resilience in their book *Resilience: The Science of Mastering Life's Greatest Challenges*. Through their interviews with former prisoners of war, special forces, and civilians who survived traumatic events, they found evidence to support the following ten components of resilience: optimism, confronting fears, moral compass, religion/spirituality, social support, role models, physical fitness, brain fitness, cognitive and emotional flexibility, and meaning, purpose, and growth [71].

Table 13.1 describes each of Southwick and Charney's elements of resilience. These elements of resilience help define the relationship between resilience and overall health and well-being, especially following a traumatic event [71].

Seligman's Positive Psychology Theory and Resilience

Another model of resilience is offered by Martin Seligman through his work in the field of positive psychology. In his book, *Authentic Happiness*, Seligman describes happiness analyzed into three specific domains: positive emotion, engagement, and meaning [65]. The first of these he terms the

Table 13.1 Southwick and Charney's ten elements of resilience

Optimism	To see a bright future and believe that things will turn out well, giving an individual a reason to pick up and move on
Confronting fears	To identify what makes an individual afraid, helps to move beyond a traumatic event, and eliminates the need to avoid triggers and reminders
Moral compass	To know right from wrong and to be altruistic
Religion/spirituality	A connection to something larger than oneself
Social support	A network of others to lean on during time of need and to care for when those others are in need
Role models	Individuals who have defined a path out of difficulty through experience provide a guide to those struggling to find their way
Physical fitness	The ability to physically recover
Brain fitness	The ability to mentally recover
Cognitive and emotional flexibility	Active problem solving, finding humor in situations, seeing whatever light exists in the most dark of circumstances
Meaning, purpose, and growth	The recognition of personal responsibility in life, including one's own importance and commitment to personal growth

pleasant life full of as many pleasures as possible and raw positive feelings of cheerfulness, happiness, and joy. Second, the *good life* is one of high engagement or flow, where individuals feel so absorbed in something that time stands still. The good life is not one of feeling pleasure but more of feeling enormously capable. The third domain allows for the *meaningful life* where individuals act in the service of something larger than themselves. This theory of authentic happiness defines life satisfaction (or authentic *happiness*) as the sum of these three domains: positive emotion, engagement, and meaning [65].

More recently, Seligman modified his thinking around happiness as a state of mind and instead shifted toward the concept of flourishing or well-being. Happiness was not an attainable constant nor an end goal but rather a part of a larger concept of *well-being*. His new well-being theory remedies the gap of his authentic happiness theory by defining *well-being* more as a construct made up of several other elements (versus happiness which is a recognizable inconstant emotional state). The five elements of well-being, each a measurable parameter, are interrelated but remain distinct. In his updated book, *Flourish*, he states that well-being theory is a theory of unforced choice, that is, the five elements comprise what individuals will choose freely *for their own sake* [66].

The five elements can be remembered through the mnemonic **PERMA** [66, 77]:

P: Positive emotion
E: Engagement or *flow*
R: Relationships
M: Meaning
A: Accomplishment

The first two of these components are measured only subjectively, i.e., as experienced by the individual and not measurable from an observer. Positive emotion includes in the present a sense of pleasure, ecstasy, comfort, warmth, and joy. Engagement, measured retrospectively, is equally measured only subjectively through questions like "Were you completely absorbed in that task?" or "Did you lose track of time by what you were doing?" In this new model, Seligman is clear that while positive emotion and engagement are still part of life satisfaction or authentic happiness, the new model of well-being includes these important elements, but they no longer become the overarching goal [66].

Supportive relationships make up the third element, focusing on connection with others. Human beings seek to be loved; loneliness can be a major barrier to well-being. Few high points in life are solitary. Acts of celebration and having a sense of pride both require other people to share in the good feeling. The fourth element is the meaningful life and is related to service in the name of something bigger than self. The final component is accomplishment; individuals pursue success and mastery for their own sakes.

In this comprehensive model, Seligman asserts the goal of positive psychology is to increase the amount of "flourishing." Originally defined by Felicia Huppert and Timothy So of the University of Cambridge, flourishing is having the core features of positive emotions, engagement, and meaning as well as three of the six additional features self-esteem, optimism, resilience, vitality, self-determination, and positive relationships. Each is cultivated and developed with deliberate practice and targeted interventions [29].

GROW Framework: Four Components of Resilience

Resilience, as a complex entity, includes several interdependent but distinct domains whether using the model of Southwick and Charney or the theories of Seligman. Deconstructing resilience can serve as an important tool to help both clinicians and their patients understand how to enhance their own

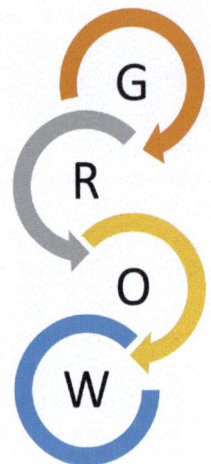

Good emotion:
Optimism, joy, pleasure, positive emotions, happiness

Reason:
Purpose, meaning, having worthwhile goals in life, contributing to something larger than self

Others:
Social connectedness, positive relationships, altruism (abandonment of self), achievement and mastery (of something Other)

Wellness:
Flexibility, emotional learning, self awareness, reflection, ability to grow, gratitude, humor, curiosity

Fig. 13.1 GROW framework: four components of resilience

ability to bounce back from adversity. We offer here a new simplified framework taken from the overlap between the two theories described above which define the four core ingredients of emotional resilience. The four areas are good emotions (**G**), reason and purpose (**R**), others and connection to the world (**O**), and wellness flexibility (**W**). Physical fitness and spirituality are part of resilience, but their benefits are covered in other chapters in this book.

This chapter will focus on these four (**GROW**) components of resilience and provide the evidence for how each of these domains affects health and health outcomes (see Fig. 13.1).

Good Emotions

Good emotions include optimism, joy, pleasure, and positive emotions that individuals identify as part of happiness. Good emotion maps to Seligman's pleasant life, with the focus on considering ways to amplify raw positive feelings. Optimism is included in this domain as *realistic* optimism, not *blind* optimism. Realistic optimism considers the actual probability of a hopeful outcome, whereas blind optimism underestimates risk, overestimates ability, and/or leads to inadequate preparation. Several exercises that will be described later in this chapter can aid in enhancing good emotions.

Reason and Purpose

The second domain, reason and purpose, links resilience to meaning, often one that contributes to a larger view of the world. Victor Frankl, a physician and Holocaust survivor, articulated this most poignantly in his book, *Man's Search for Meaning*, where he wrote, "Deep down, in my opinion, man is dominated neither by the will-to-pleasure nor by the will-to-power, but by what I like to call man's will to meaning; that is to say, his deep-seated striving and struggling for a higher and ultimate meaning to his existence" [21]. Reason and purpose help to frame difficulties in a larger context, creating more perseverance and a stronger willingness to endure challenges for the ultimate goal of overcoming them. Achievement and mastery are embedded in this element as well; if a person's actions reach a level of achievement or mastery, meaning and purpose are reinforced.

Others and Connection to the World

Others and connection to the world combine the concepts of social connectedness and support and a person's capacity for altruism. This component of resilience celebrates an individual's enormous capability and capacity to abandon self and help others. To achieve this third domain requires altruism with an intentional and complete orientation away from self, a commitment to someone or something else. In addition, this element highlights an individual's ability to form deep lasting relationships and to accept help and love from others especially in times of need and despair. If a person's actions are driven by social connection or love, it enhances the connection to others and to the world.

Wellness Flexibility

Wellness flexibility can be best described as learning those skills necessary to develop emotional awareness. In today's fast paced world, there is less time for pause and reflection and less mindfulness. Technologies such as mobile smartphones have squeezed out moments of "down time"; moments that used to be filled with thought and reflection are now filled with checking emails or playing games. A posture of learning, growing, and working hard toward goals is required for wellness flexibility in lieu of choosing a fixed mindset that believes basic abilities, intelligence, talents, and an individual's " lot in life" are fixed traits that cannot be changed. Carol Dweck defined the growth mindset as the belief that effort and persistence will result in improved outcomes [19]. Reflective practice is an intentional effort to understand how to adapt to different situations combined with a willingness to try new things and learn about coping which are strong predictors of wellness flexibility and thus resilience. Other elements of wellness flexibility include accepting one's current state, creative problem solving, and utilizing strategies such as humor and gratitude to cope with adversity. These practices of reflection, curiosity, humor, and learning from mistakes facilitate the adaptation and growth elements of resilience.

Measures of Resilience

Given the multiple dimensions within the definition of resilience, experts agree that there are challenges in operationalizing this dynamic construct, given the interactive and interdependent nature of each contributor [53]. Even defining what it means to "bounce back from adversity" is difficult. Additional variables exist across a life span (i.e., what resilience means as a child versus what it means as an older adult). Finally, there are cultural contexts that must be considered. Presently, there are more than 15 measures that have been described in the literature [84]. We describe three validated published scales here that have been shown to have internal consistency and content validity and are reliably reproducible (test-retest) [14].

Connor-Davidson Resilience Scale (CD-RISC)

This is a 25-item self-report scale that was developed for clinical practice and studied in adult populations. The scale measures 5 dimensions using a 5-point scale on each item: personal competence, trust/tolerance/strengthening effects of stress, acceptance of change and secure relationships, control, and spiritual influences. There is a 10-item, as well as a 2-item, short version of the scale that has been used to measure stress coping ability. It has been used to evaluate changes in response to pharmacologic interventions [13].

Resilience Scale for Adults (RSA)

This was originally a 37-item self-report scale that measured 5 dimensions using a 5-point scale on each item: personal competence, social competence, family coherence, social support, and personal structure. Experts in the field find it most useful for assessing the protective factors that inhibit or provide a buffer against psychological disorders. There is an updated 33-item self-report scale that also measures 5 dimensions: personal strength, social competence, structured style, family cohesion, and social resources. The RSA is unique in its measurement of social and family aspects of resilience [22].

Brief Resilience Scale (BRS)

This is a 6-item self-report scale that is designed to measure the ability to bounce back or recover from stress. It is a unidimensional construct and has been studied in adult populations with clinical conditions [70].

Resilience and Health Outcomes in the GROW Framework

Good Emotions

Consistently experiencing good emotions such as optimism, joy, and happiness benefits physical health for a host of medical conditions and improves overall physical health outcomes [57]. Optimism seems to both protect against the development of cardiovascular disease and improve outcomes for those that develop it. With regard to primary prevention, the Women's Health Initiative study of over 95,000 healthy women found that optimistic women were less likely to develop cardiac disease or die from any cause [79]. The VA Normative Aging Study found similar results in that optimistic individuals had 25% less cardiovascular disease than average [81]. The effect of optimism includes secondary and tertiary prevention benefits, including those who have had acute coronary syndrome (heart attack), open heart surgery, or a heart transplant [24, 59, 62]. In addition, for individuals who underwent coronary bypass, optimists experienced less pain and fewer postoperative symptoms [59, 60]. Finally, for individuals with cardiac disease, higher reported optimism was associated with lower mortality and fewer hospitalizations [7, 18, 65].

Positive emotions may also predict better outcomes in metabolic and kidney diseases. In one study, a positive affect was associated with lower mortality rates in individuals with diabetes [49]. In patients with chronic kidney disease, resilience and optimism were associated with higher rates of adherence to medical therapies [52] and with more healthy behaviors [42, 52]. Furthermore, a greater sense of hope predicts adjustment to hemodialysis in end-stage renal patients [5].

Individuals with high levels of optimism and joy also show improved outcomes in other medical conditions. Optimism is associated with higher levels of physical health and lower levels of distress in breast cancer patients [8]. Optimism can protect against the development of PTSD (following a trauma) and is associated with higher quality of life in patients with Parkinson's disease [25, 64, 87]. A more positive affect can also dampen the experience of pain; interventions aiming to improve affect can reduce the sensation of pain [26]. Finally, in subjects exposed to an upper respiratory viral infection, those with higher levels of optimism were less likely to develop cold symptoms; if they did get sick, the symptoms were attenuated compared to the more pessimistic subjects [12]. At the cellular level, optimism has been shown to be associated with higher levels of immunity and immune markers [36, 63, 73].

Interventions to Improve Good Emotions

Changes that can improve positive emotions improve resilience to adversity, increase happiness, lower levels of cortisol, reduce inflammatory markers, improve depression and anxiety symptoms, reduce physical pain, augment immune responses, and change cardiovascular health. Clinical providers can facilitate these processes through a more intentional process of enhancing optimism and positive emotion. One powerful prescriptive process is to guide patients in the cultivation of gratitude [67]. The following approaches are simple examples of suggestions that can be used in the clinical setting:

- Keep a daily journal about things for which to be grateful.
- Mindful thinking about gratitude.
- Write down on a weekly basis three things for which you are grateful.
- Write one thank you note per week to a person who has impacted your life in a positive way.
- Identify, reflect, and show gratitude for one's own signature strengths.

Reason and Purpose

Individuals that believe there is a reason and purpose in life as well as those who have a sense of control over their lives are likely to have more favorable health outcomes. A higher sense of purpose is associated with greater use of preventive health services, such as cholesterol screening [34]. It has also been associated with improved surgical recovery as well as increased physical activity [46]. For patients with cardiovascular disease, having a sense of purpose in life was associated with a reduced risk of macrovascular events and a decrease in all-cause mortality [85]. Satisfaction with one's life has also been associated with a reduced risk of developing diabetes; a sense of life control is correlated with better glucose control in patients with diabetes [6, 75]. In patients with terminal cancer, a sense of hope and meaning in life and, in turn, higher psycho-spiritual health improved individuals' ability to cope with and find meaning in the experience of terminal illness [40].

Having a reason for living also correlates with improved outcomes for older adults and in individuals with mental health conditions. In older adults, a purpose in life was associated with both positive affect and perceived cognitive function [3]. Moreover, Musich and colleagues demonstrated that older adults with a higher sense of purpose in life had better physical and mental health outcomes as well as lower healthcare costs, higher usage of preventive health services, and better quality of life [50]. Finally, a greater reason/purpose in life is associated with improved mental health outcomes following stressful events. For example, Tsai and colleagues studied a group of US veterans and found that those who reported growth in personal strength from trauma were protected against detriment from future trauma [81].

Interventions to Improve Reason and Purpose

According to Drageset, Haugan, and Tranvåg, there are four main experiences that encourage meaning and purpose in life: (1) physical and mental well-being, (2) belonging and recognition, (3) personally treasured activities, and (4) spiritual closeness and connectedness [17]. In addition, identifying core values and setting goals can help guide one's sense of meaning and purpose [20]. The following approaches can be prescribed to patients to enhance their sense of reason and purpose:

- Do a simple chair-based yoga or qigong movement practice (physical and mental well-being).
- Participate in a community or group activity based upon a mutual interest, such as a book club (belonging and recognition).
- Listen to music (experiencing personally treasured activities).

- Go outside to enjoy the sunrise/sunset (spiritual closeness and connectedness).
- Identify one's core values and choose to do something that enhances one of those values.
- Set goals for doing a purposeful activity once per week.

Others and Connection to the World

Having connections with others and a strong support network can improve one's health and lead to better health outcomes. In patients with recent myocardial infarctions, having close friendships decreased the risk of death following the cardiac events [83]. It has been shown that social connectedness can be protective against cardiovascular disease, while a lack of social support confers an increased risk of coronary heart disease [2, 39]. Social connectedness can also improve outcomes in cancer patients. Patients with small social networks experienced higher risk of recurrence and mortality, while those with increased contact with friends and family post diagnosis had a lower risk of death [4, 10, 37, 38, 55]. In addition, supportive family types are associated with higher quality of life in individuals with cancer [51].

Individuals with metabolic and kidney disease also experience improved outcomes when they have strong social networks. In adolescents with type 1 diabetes, higher levels of peer support were associated with better outcomes [16]. Litchman and colleagues found that diabetic patients who consistently participated in a diabetes online community were more likely to have improved glycemic control as well as higher quality of life and better self-care than those who did not participate consistently [41]. Rashid also found that social support was associated with patients' self-efficacy in diabetes medication management [56]. In a community health worker program, peer support resulted in improvements in diabetes outcomes (lower hemoglobin A1c levels) and lower levels of distress [72]. It also appears that social support may be protective in the development of obesity [48, 68]. In chronic renal disease, social support is associated with improved disease self-management, and the presence of a supportive caregiver improves the quality of life in hemodialysis patients [9, 54]. In addition, varied social support networks protect against developing common colds with individuals exhibiting fewer symptoms when they do develop them [11].

Finally, social support is associated with improved mental health outcomes. Higher levels of social support are associated with decreased depressive symptoms, increased recovery rates, and better outcomes after trauma [35, 80]. Social support may improve response to stressful or traumatic events because individuals feel more confident and in control, practice healthier behaviors, use active coping strategies (talking), and are less likely to see these events as insurmountable [28, 61]. Social connectedness and support is also associated with decreased depression in patients with cancer, heart disease, rheumatoid arthritis, and multiple sclerosis [28, 44, 47, 58].

Interventions to Improve Connections with Others

There are several targets within this domain to help improve social support. First is the notion that having strong social circles provides patients with people to help them and to lean on when health is challenging or faltering. Then, there is the complementary notion of moving beyond the self and toward the service of others, which includes fostering altruism. There are strong correlations between the well-being, happiness, health, and longevity of people who are behaviorally compassionate, so long as helping does not overwhelm them —economically, emotionally, or physically. In addition, building relationships through enhancing communication and working through conflicts can strengthen resilience [23, 31]. A simple prescription could be one of the following to develop altruism or build strong social connections:

- Do a loving-kindness meditation by imagining a loved one and sending that individual love and wishing them health, happiness, and well-being.
- Encourage simple random acts of kindness (e.g., buying a cup of coffee for the person in line behind you).
- Volunteer (e.g., tutoring students at the local school).
- Practice active constructive responding – "that is wonderful, tell me more."
- Participate in a disease-specific peer-support program.
- Reflect on conflicts and develop strategies for improved communication.
- Act to deepen relationships with family and community through communication participation.

Wellness Flexibility

Individuals who are emotionally flexible via acceptance, reflection, and growth are likely to demonstrate better self-efficacy behaviors, improved mental health, and better ability to cope with stress. For patients with cancer, acceptance was correlated with lower rates of depression [43], and for families of children with cancer, acceptance was associated with better ability to cope [32]. Adaptive strategies, like the use of humor, have been associated with lower levels of distress in cancer patients [8]. In patients with diabetes, emotional vitality, the ability to regulate one's behaviors and emotions, and one's engagement in life were all associated with lower rates of diabetes diagnoses [6]. In addition, in patients with diabetes, belief in one's abilities (self-efficacy) predicted adherence to diet, exercise, blood glucose testing and medication adherence, as well as diabetic control [1, 82]. Finally in hemodialysis patients, self-efficacy was associated with lower levels of symptoms [54].

Wellness flexibility and emotional vitality can also improve outcomes in patients with mental illness or trauma. In survivors of 9/11, those who accepted the event had lower rates of developing PTSD [69]. The use of humor also improves outcomes for individuals with depression and high levels of stress [27]. In addition, the use of cognitive reappraisals as a form of reflection demonstrates improved psychological health and outcomes [30, 45]. Acceptance is also an effective strategy for families coping with loved ones with mental illness [86]. In those who stutter, higher levels of emotional vitality and self-efficacy protected against developing psychologic distress from their stutter [15].

Interventions to Enhance Wellness Flexibility

Posttraumatic growth as a form of wellness flexibility was defined by Calhoun and Tedeschi as a positive change experienced as a result of the struggle with a major life crisis or a traumatic event [76]. It reflects the idea that human beings can be changed by their encounters with life challenges, sometimes in radically positive ways. Health coaching in self-efficacy can improve health outcomes in cancer, cardiovascular disease, and diabetes [74, 78]. Wellness flexibility practices such as mindfulness, gratitude, acceptance, and learning from failure can all improve health outcomes [30, 33, 45, 74, 86]. In addition, cognitive behavioral approaches can also improve wellness flexibility [74]. One might encourage enhancing wellness flexibility with patients by inviting them to try the following techniques:

- Encourage patients to work with a health coach, someone who works with patients to improve self-efficacy and self-confidence around certain disease goals.
- Create "bite-size" goals with patients to create opportunities for change.
- See Interventions to Improve Good Emotions above.

- Tackle cognitive distortions – reflect on one's insecurities and negative, self-doubting thoughts; replace with more realistic thoughts.
- Practice acceptance – reflect on a current transition, challenge, or feedback; accept it, and brainstorm on the possibilities for growth and opportunity in the change.

Summary and Recommendations

Resilience, an individual's ability to bounce back following a setback, is often characterized by overcoming adversity and learning from and finding meaning in a challenging situation. In the GROW framework of resilience, the four key components are good emotions, reason and purpose, others (social connectedness), and wellness flexibility. An individual with high levels of these elements of resilience is often less likely to suffer severe consequences of disease. Higher resilience has been associated with improved outcomes in cardiovascular disease, diabetes and kidney disease, a better ability to cope with a cancer diagnosis, and decreased mental health consequences. Physicians can guide patients in practices that can improve resilience in these four areas. Providing brief advice to patients on small behavioral changes can improve resilience and, in turn, health outcomes.

References

1. Al-Khawaldeh OA, Al-Hassan MA, Froelicher ES. Self-efficacy, self-management, and glycemic control in adults with type 2 diabetes mellitus. J Diabetes Complicat. 2012;26:10–6. https://doi.org/10.1016/j.jdiacomp.2011.11.002.
2. Barefoot JC, Grønbaek M, Jensen G, et al. Social network diversity and risks of ischemic heart disease and total mortality: findings from the Copenhagen City Heart Study. Am J Epidemiol. 2005;161:960–7. https://doi.org/10.1093/aje/kwi128.
3. Bartrés-Faz D, Cattaneo G, Solana J, et al. Meaning in life: resilience beyond reserve. Alzheimers Res Ther. 2018;10(1):47. https://doi.org/10.1186/s13195-018-0381-z.
4. Beasley JM, Newcomb PA, Trentham-Dietz A, et al. Social networks and survival after breast cancer diagnosis. J Cancer Surviv. 2010;4:372–80. https://doi.org/10.1007/s11764-010-0139-5.
5. Billington E, Simpson J, Unwin J, et al. Does hope predict adjustment to end-stage renal failure and consequent dialysis? Br J Health Psychol. 2008;13:683–99. https://doi.org/10.1348/135910707X248959.
6. Boehm JK, Trudel-Fitzgerald C, Kivimaki M, Kubzansky LD. The prospective association between positive psychological well-being and diabetes. Health Psychol. 2015;34:1013–21. https://doi.org/10.1037/hea0000200.
7. Buchanan GM, Seligman MEP, Seligman M, et al. Explanatory style. New York: Routledge; 2013.
8. Carver CS, Pozo C, Harris SD, et al. How coping mediates the effect of optimism on distress: a study of women with early stage breast cancer. J Pers Soc Psychol. 1993;65:375–90.
9. Chen Y-C, Chang L-C, Liu C-Y, et al. The roles of social support and health literacy in self-management among patients with chronic kidney disease. J Nurs Scholarsh. 2018;50:265–75. https://doi.org/10.1111/jnu.12377.
10. Chou AF, Stewart SL, Wild RC, Bloom JR. Social support and survival in young women with breast carcinoma. Psychooncology. 2012;21:125–33. https://doi.org/10.1002/pon.1863.
11. Cohen S, Doyle WJ, Skoner DP, et al. Social ties and susceptibility to the common cold. JAMA. 1997;277:1940–4.
12. Cohen S, Doyle WJ, Turner RB, et al. Emotional style and susceptibility to the common cold. Psychosom Med. 2003;65:652–7.
13. Connor KM, Davidson JRT. Development of a new resilience scale: the Connor-Davidson Resilience Scale (CD-RISC). Depress Anxiety. 2003;18:76–82. https://doi.org/10.1002/da.10113.
14. Cosco TD, Kaushal A, Richards M, et al. Resilience measurement in later life: a systematic review and psychometric analysis. Health Qual Life Outcomes. 2016;14:16. https://doi.org/10.1186/s12955-016-0418-6.
15. Craig A, Blumgart E, Tran Y. Resilience and stuttering: factors that protect people from the adversity of chronic stuttering. J Speech Lang Hear Res. 2011;54:1485–1496A. https://doi.org/10.1044/1092-4388(2011/10-0304).
16. Doe E. An analysis of the relationships between peer support and diabetes outcomes in adolescents with type 1 diabetes. J Health Psychol. 2018;23:1356–66. https://doi.org/10.1177/1359105316656228.
17. Drageset J, Haugan G, Tranvåg O. Crucial aspects promoting meaning and purpose in life: perceptions of nursing home residents. BMC Geriatr. 2017;17:254. https://doi.org/10.1186/s12877-017-0650-x.

18. DuBois CM, Lopez OV, Beale EE, et al. Relationships between positive psychological constructs and health outcomes in patients with cardiovascular disease: a systematic review. Int J Cardiol. 2015;195:265–80. https://doi.org/10.1016/j.ijcard.2015.05.121.

19. Dweck CS. Mindset: the new psychology of success. New York: Random House Publishing Group; 2006.

20. Locke E, Latham G. Goal setting theory. In: Organizational behavior. Armonk: M. E. Sharpe; 2005. p. 175–81.

21. Frankl VE, Winslade WJ. Man's search for meaning. Boston: Beacon Press; 2006.

22. Friborg O, Hjemdal O, Rosenvinge JH, Martinussen M. A new rating scale for adult resilience: what are the central protective resources behind healthy adjustment? Int J Methods Psychiatr Res. 2003;12:65–76.

23. Gable SL, Reis HT, Downey G. He said, she said: a quasi-signal detection analysis of daily interactions between close relationship partners. Psychol Sci. 2003;14:100–5. https://doi.org/10.1111/1467-9280.t01-1-01426.

24. Giltay EJ, Kamphuis MH, Kalmijn S, et al. Dispositional optimism and the risk of cardiovascular death: the Zutphen Elderly Study. Arch Intern Med. 2006;166:431–6. https://doi.org/10.1001/archinte.166.4.431.

25. Gison A, Dall'Armi V, Donati V, et al. Dispositional optimism, depression, disability and quality of life in Parkinson's disease. Funct Neurol. 2014;29:113–9.

26. Hanssen MM, Peters ML, Boselie JJ, Meulders A. Can positive affect attenuate (persistent) pain? State of the art and clinical implications. Curr Rheumatol Rep. 2017;19:80. https://doi.org/10.1007/s11926-017-0703-3.

27. Hendin H, Hass AP. Wounds of war: the psychological aftermath of combat in Vietnam. Philadelphia: Basic Books; 1984.

28. Holahan CJ, Valentiner DP, Moos RH. Parental support, coping strategies, and psychological adjustment: an integrative model with late adolescents. J Youth Adolescence. 1995;24:633–48. https://doi.org/10.1007/BF01536948.

29. Huppert FA, So TTC. Flourishing across Europe: application of a new conceptual framework for defining well-being. Soc Indic Res. 2013;110:837–61. https://doi.org/10.1007/s11205-011-9966-7.

30. John OP, Gross JJ. Healthy and unhealthy emotion regulation: personality processes, individual differences, and lifespan development. J Pers. 2004;72(6):1301–34.

31. Johnson DW, Johnson RT. Conflict resolution and peer mediation programs in elementary and secondary schools: a review of the research. Rev Educ Res. 1996;66:459–506. https://doi.org/10.3102/00346543066004459.

32. Kazak AE, Simms S, Barakat L, et al. Surviving cancer competently intervention program (SCCIP): a cognitive-behavioral and family therapy intervention for adolescent survivors of childhood cancer and their families. Fam Process. 1999;38:176–91. https://doi.org/10.1111/j.1545-5300.1999.00176.x.

33. Kenne Sarenmalm E, Mårtensson LB, Andersson BA, et al. Mindfulness and its efficacy for psychological and biological responses in women with breast cancer. Cancer Med. 2017;6:1108–22. https://doi.org/10.1002/cam4.1052.

34. Kim ES, Strecher VJ, Ryff CD. Purpose in life and use of preventive health care services. Proc Natl Acad Sci U S A. 2014;111:16331–6. https://doi.org/10.1073/pnas.1414826111.

35. King AC, Rejeski WJ, Buchner DM. Physical activity interventions targeting older adults. This paper was a background paper for the Cooper Institute Conference Series Physical Activity Interventions, an ACSM Specialty Conference. A critical review and recommendations. Am J Prev Med. 1998;15:316–33. https://doi.org/10.1016/S0749-3797(98)00085-3.

36. Krafft-Ebing R, Chaddock CG. Psychopathia sexualis. Valley Cottage: F.A. Davis Company; 1894.

37. Kroenke CH, Kwan ML, Neugut AI, et al. Social networks, social support mechanisms, and quality of life after breast cancer diagnosis. Breast Cancer Res Treat. 2013;139:515–27. https://doi.org/10.1007/s10549-013-2477-2.

38. Kroenke CH, Michael YL, Poole EM, et al. Postdiagnosis social networks and breast cancer mortality in the After Breast Cancer Pooling Project. Cancer. 2017;123:1228–37. https://doi.org/10.1002/cncr.30440.

39. Lett HS, Blumenthal JA, Babyak MA, et al. Social support and coronary heart disease: epidemiologic evidence and implications for treatment. Psychosom Med. 2005;67:869–78. https://doi.org/10.1097/01.psy.0000188393.73571.0a.

40. Lin H-R, Bauer-Wu SM. Psycho-spiritual well-being in patients with advanced cancer: an integrative review of the literature. J Adv Nurs. 2003;44:69–80.

41. Litchman ML, Edelman LS, Donaldson GW. Effect of diabetes online community engagement on health indicators: cross-sectional study. JMIR Diabetes. 2018;3(2):e8. https://doi.org/10.2196/diabetes.8603.

42. Ma L-C, Chang H-J, Liu Y-M, et al. The relationship between health-promoting behaviors and resilience in patients with chronic kidney disease. ScientificWorldJournal. 2013;2013:124973. https://doi.org/10.1155/2013/124973.

43. Manne SL. Prostate cancer support and advocacy groups: their role for patients and family members. Semin Urol Oncol. 2002;20:45–54.

44. Manne SL. Intrusive thoughts and psychological distress among cancer patients: the role of spouse avoidance and criticism. J Consult Clin Psychol. 1999;67:539–46.

45. Martin RE, Ochsner KN. The neuroscience of emotion regulation development: implications for education. Curr Opin Behav Sci. 2016;10:142–8. https://doi.org/10.1016/j.cobeha.2016.06.006.

46. Mavros MN, Athanasiou S, Gkegkes ID, et al. Do psychological variables affect early surgical recovery? PLoS One. 2011;6:e20306. https://doi.org/10.1371/journal.pone.0020306.

47. Mohr DC, Classen C, Barrera M. The relationship between social support, depression and treatment for depression in people with multiple sclerosis. Psychol Med. 2004;34:533–41.
48. Moore S, Daniel M, Paquet C, et al. Association of individual network social capital with abdominal adiposity, overweight and obesity. J Public Health (Oxf). 2009;31:175–83. https://doi.org/10.1093/pubmed/fdn104.
49. Moskowitz JT, Epel ES, Acree M. Positive affect uniquely predicts lower risk of mortality in people with diabetes. Health Psychol. 2008;27:S73–82. https://doi.org/10.1037/0278-6133.27.1.S73.
50. Musich S, Wang SS, Kraemer S, et al. Purpose in life and positive health outcomes among older adults. Popul Health Manag. 2018;21:139–47. https://doi.org/10.1089/pop.2017.0063.
51. Nissen KG, Trevino K, Lange T, Prigerson HG. Family relationships and psychosocial dysfunction among family caregivers of patients with advanced cancer. J Pain Symptom Manag. 2016;52:841–849.e1. https://doi.org/10.1016/j.jpainsymman.2016.07.006.
52. Noghan N, Akaberi A, Pournamdarian S, et al. Resilience and therapeutic regimen compliance in patients undergoing hemodialysis in hospitals of Hamedan, Iran. Electron Physician. 2018;10:6853–8. https://doi.org/10.19082/6853.
53. Pangallo A, Zibarras L, Lewis R, Flaxman P. Resilience through the lens of interactionism: a systematic review. Psychol Assess. 2015;27:1–20. https://doi.org/10.1037/pas0000024.
54. Perales-Montilla CM, Duschek S, Reyes-Del Paso GA. The influence of emotional factors on the report of somatic symptoms in patients on chronic haemodialysis: the importance of anxiety. Nefrologia. 2013;33:816–25. https://doi.org/10.3265/Nefrologia.pre2013.Aug.12097.
55. Pinquart M, Duberstein PR. Associations of social networks with cancer mortality: a meta-analysis. Crit Rev Oncol Hematol. 2010;75:122–37. https://doi.org/10.1016/j.critrevonc.2009.06.003.
56. Rashid AA, Zuhra H, Tan CE. Social support, self-efficacy and their correlation among patients with Type 2 Diabetes Mellitus: a primary care perspective. Med J Malaysia. 2018;73:197–201.
57. Rasmussen HN, Scheier MF, Greenhouse JB. Optimism and physical health: a meta-analytic review. Ann Behav Med. 2009;37:239–56. https://doi.org/10.1007/s12160-009-9111-x.
58. Revenson TA. The role of social support with rheumatic disease. Baillieres Clin Rheumatol. 1993;7:377–96. https://doi.org/10.1016/S0950-3579(05)80095-0.
59. Ronaldson A, Molloy GJ, Wikman A, et al. Optimism and recovery after acute coronary syndrome: a clinical cohort study. Psychosom Med. 2015;77:311–8. https://doi.org/10.1097/PSY.0000000000000155.
60. Ronaldson A, Poole L, Kidd T, et al. Optimism measured pre-operatively is associated with reduced pain intensity and physical symptom reporting after coronary artery bypass graft surgery. J Psychosom Res. 2014;77:278–82. https://doi.org/10.1016/j.jpsychores.2014.07.018.
61. Rozanski A, Blumenthal JA, Kaplan J. Impact of psychological factors on the pathogenesis of cardiovascular disease and implications for therapy. Circulation. 1999;99:2192–217.
62. Scheier MF, Matthews KA, Owens JF, et al. Dispositional optimism and recovery from coronary artery bypass surgery: the beneficial effects on physical and psychological well-being. J Pers Soc Psychol. 1989;57:1024–40. https://doi.org/10.1037/0022-3514.57.6.1024.
63. Segerstrom SC, Sephton SE. Optimistic expectancies and cell-mediated immunity: the role of positive affect. Psychol Sci. 2010;21:448–55. https://doi.org/10.1177/0956797610362061.
64. Segovia F, Moore JL, Linnville SE, Hoyt RE. Optimism predicts positive health in repatriated prisoners of war. Psychol Trauma. 2015;7:222–8. https://doi.org/10.1037/a0037902.
65. Seligman M. Authentic happiness. Boston: Nicholas Brealey Publishing; 2011.
66. Seligman MEP. Flourish: a visionary new understanding of happiness and well-being. Delran: Simon and Schuster; 2012.
67. Seligman MEP, Steen TA, Park N, Peterson C. Positive psychology progress: empirical validation of interventions. Am Psychol. 2005;60:410–21. https://doi.org/10.1037/0003-066X.60.5.410.
68. Serlachius A, Elovainio M, Juonala M, et al. High perceived social support protects against the intergenerational transmission of obesity: the Cardiovascular Risk in Young Finns Study. Prev Med. 2016;90:79–85. https://doi.org/10.1016/j.ypmed.2016.07.004.
69. Silver RC, Holman EA, McIntosh DN, et al. Nationwide longitudinal study of psychological responses to September 11. JAMA. 2002;288:1235–44. https://doi.org/10.1001/jama.288.10.1235.
70. Smith BW, Dalen J, Wiggins K, et al. The brief resilience scale: assessing the ability to bounce back. Int J Behav Med. 2008;15:194–200. https://doi.org/10.1080/10705500802222972.
71. Southwick S, Charney D. Resilience: the science of mastering life's greatest challenges. New York: Cambridge University Press; 2018.
72. Spencer MS, Kieffer EC, Sinco B, et al. Outcomes at 18 months from a community health worker and peer leader diabetes self-management program for Latino adults. Diabetes Care. 2018;41:1414–22. https://doi.org/10.2337/dc17-0978.
73. Stellar JE, John-Henderson N, Anderson CL, et al. Positive affect and markers of inflammation: discrete positive emotions predict lower levels of inflammatory cytokines. Emotion. 2015;15:129–33. https://doi.org/10.1037/emo0000033.

74. Sudhir PM. Advances in psychological interventions for lifestyle disorders: overview of interventions in cardio-vascular disorder and type 2 diabetes mellitus. Curr Opin Psychiatry. 2017;30:346–51. https://doi.org/10.1097/YCO.0000000000000348.
75. Surgenor LJ, Horn J, Hudson SM, et al. Metabolic control and psychological sense of control in women with diabetes mellitus. Alternative considerations of the relationship. J Psychosom Res. 2000;49:267–73.
76. Tedeschi RG, Calhoun LG. The posttraumatic growth inventory: measuring the positive legacy of trauma. J Trauma Stress. 1996;9:455–71.
77. The Trustees of the University of Pennsylvania. Authentic happinesslauthentic happiness. In: Authentic happiness; 2019. https://www.authentichappiness.sas.upenn.edu/. Accessed 22 Jan 2019.
78. Thomas ML, Elliott JE, Rao SM, et al. A randomized, clinical trial of education or motivational-interviewing-based coaching compared to usual care to improve cancer pain management. Oncol Nurs Forum. 2012;39:39–49. https://doi.org/10.1188/12.ONF.39-49.
79. Tindle HA, Chang Y-F, Kuller LH, et al. Optimism, cynical hostility, and incident coronary heart disease and mortality in the Women's Health Initiative. Circulation. 2009;120:656–62. https://doi.org/10.1161/CIRCULATIONAHA.108.827642.
80. Tsai J, Harpaz-Rotem I, Pietrzak RH, Southwick SM. The role of coping, resilience, and social support in mediating the relation between PTSD and social functioning in veterans returning from Iraq and Afghanistan. Psychiatry. 2012;75:135–49. https://doi.org/10.1521/psyc.2012.75.2.135.
81. Tsai J, Mota NP, Southwick SM, Pietrzak RH. What doesn't kill you makes you stronger: a national study of U.S. military veterans. J Affect Disord. 2016;189:269–71. https://doi.org/10.1016/j.jad.2015.08.076.
82. Venkataraman K, Kannan AT, Kalra OP, et al. Diabetes self-efficacy strongly influences actual control of diabetes in patients attending a tertiary hospital in India. J Community Health. 2012;37:653–62. https://doi.org/10.1007/s10900-011-9496-x.
83. Weiss-Faratci N, Lurie I, Benyamini Y, et al. Optimism during hospitalization for first acute myocardial infarction and long-term mortality risk: a prospective cohort study. Mayo Clin Proc. 2017;92:49–56. https://doi.org/10.1016/j.mayocp.2016.09.014.
84. Windle G, Bennett KM, Noyes J. A methodological review of resilience measurement scales. Health Qual Life Outcomes. 2011;9:8. https://doi.org/10.1186/1477-7525-9-8.
85. Yu L, Boyle PA, Wilson RS, et al. Purpose in life and cerebral infarcts in community dwelling older persons. Stroke. 2015;46:1071–6. https://doi.org/10.1161/STROKEAHA.114.008010.
86. Zauszniewski JA, Bekhet AK, Suresky MJ. Indicators of resilience in family members of adults with serious mental illness. Psychiatr Clin North Am. 2015;38:131–46. https://doi.org/10.1016/j.psc.2014.11.009.
87. Zeidner M, Hammer AL. Coping with missile attack: resources, strategies, and outcomes. J Pers. 1992;60:709–46. https://doi.org/10.1111/j.1467-6494.1992.tb00271.x.

Chapter 14
The Value of Sleep for Optimizing Health

Matthew A. Tucker

Keywords Sleep · Health · Cognition · Memory processing · Sleep deprivation · Sleep disorders

Key Points
- Sleep is necessary for survival, and adequate sleep is necessary for optimal daytime function. Unfortunately, societal demands and increasing rates of sleep disorders prevent individuals from obtaining enough quality sleep.
- Despite attempts to manipulate sleep quality and quantity, either pharmacologically or behaviorally, sleep patterns are surprisingly challenging to modify.
- Each of us has an optimal sleep duration that, if uninterrupted, can optimize daytime function. Living a healthy lifestyle, reducing stress, and adopting a consistent bedtime routine are the best ways to achieve this goal.
- Even though people can become adept at concealing the effects of compromised sleep on daily function, there are simple steps the clinician can take to identify whether an individual is obtaining adequate sleep quality and quantity.
- Understanding the myriad ways in which sleep can be compromised, and learning how to identify the signs of poor or inadequate sleep, will help clinicians formulate a plan to improve patients' sleep and overall health.

The Importance of Sleep

Sleep is an essential biological process, a fact that has been confirmed in the seminal findings of several sleep research laboratories. For example, in extensive research in rodents, Allan Rechtschaffen and colleagues studied the effects of sleep deprivation in rats, using the "disk-over-water" technique, in which the rat sits on a motorized disk situated just above a shallow pool of water [52]. Each time the rat falls asleep, the disk starts to rotate, causing the rat to wake up. A control rat can be placed on a disk that is yoked to the experimental rat's disk. Each time the experimental rat falls asleep, both disks rotate, allowing the control rat to obtain sleep while the disks are motionless (i.e., while the

M. A. Tucker (✉)
Department of Biomedical Sciences, University of South Carolina School of Medicine, Greenville, Greenville, SC, USA
e-mail: MATUCKER@greenvillemed.sc.edu

© Springer Nature Switzerland AG 2020
J. Uribarri, J. A. Vassalotti (eds.), *Nutrition, Fitness, and Mindfulness*, Nutrition and Health,
https://doi.org/10.1007/978-3-030-30892-6_14

experimental rat is awake). The two rats experience the same conditions, except that the experimental rat is sleep deprived, while the control rat obtains adequate sleep. Using this protocol, total sleep deprivation over a 3-week period leads to rapid weight loss even with increased food intake, markedly increased energy expenditure/hyperactivity, skin lesions, body temperature dysregulation, organ failure, and compromised immune response. Between 3 and 5 weeks of total sleep deprivation, death is inevitable. Surprisingly, the same physical deterioration occurs after 4–6 weeks of selective deprivation of rapid eye movement (REM) sleep, the stage of sleep associated with vivid dreaming [39]. These findings conclusively demonstrate the importance of sleep for survival. However, what they do not provide, even after decades of intensive scientific study, are clear answers about why sleep is so biologically important [51].

Sleep Stages: What Kinds of Sleep Do We Need?

Mammals cycle through several stages of sleep multiple times each night (4–5 times per night in humans), including stage 2 sleep (~45%), slow wave sleep (SWS; ~25%), and REM sleep (~25%) (Fig. 14.1). A sleep cycle starts with a brief period of Stage 1 sleep, followed by Stage 2 sleep and SWS, and is punctuated by a REM sleep period. Each of these sleep stages has very distinguishable electrical properties (frequency and amplitude) observed in electroencephalographic (EEG) recordings (Fig. 14.2). The neurochemical differences between sleep stages are also pronounced. Because each sleep stage has its own physiological signatures, it may be that each serves a unique biological function. Alternatively, sleep stages may work in combination to promote specific functions. Another factor that could point to the importance of one stage of sleep over another is the amount of time spent in each sleep stage. Stage 2 sleep comprises about half of a night of sleep. Slow wave sleep and REM sleep, on the other hand, account for only 20–25% of a night of sleep. Functionally, this could indicate that Stage 2 sleep is the most important sleep stage. However, sleep deprivation for 1 or more days results in several days of "rebound" sleep in animals and humans, in which the amount of REM sleep [16] and SWS [22], but not Stage 2 sleep, increases above pre-deprivation levels as they recover lost sleep. These findings indicate that sleep in mammalian species is not only vital for survival but that specific sleep stages (REM sleep and SWS) may be especially important. This may indicate a unique biological purpose for SWS and REM sleep. Evidence from research in children demonstrates why these stages may be especially important for development. One important property of SWS is that it is the primary time during which human growth hormone (HGH) is secreted. HGH is necessary for physical growth in children, and when HGH secretion is reduced with fragmented slow wave sleep, either due to a sleep disorder (e.g., obstructive sleep apnea) or other situational factors, children's physical growth may be stunted [71]. REM sleep, on the other hand, may play a critical role for brain

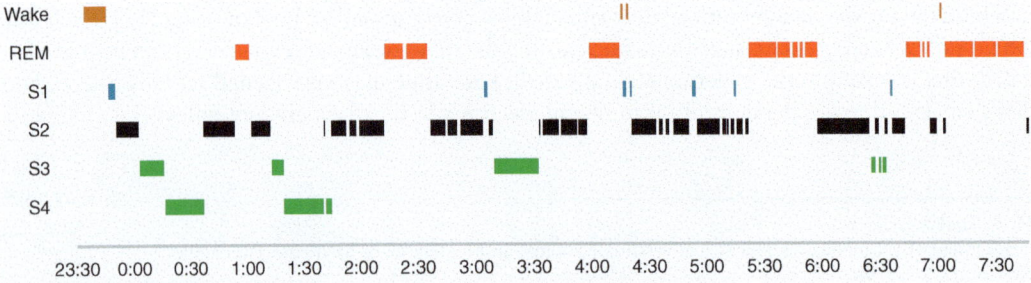

Fig. 14.1 Sleep hypnogram. A night of normal sleep in a young adult. Time of night is represented on the y axis

Brain state	EEG waveform	Frequency range	Neurochemistry Ach	5-HT/NE	Signature events	% of Total sleep time
Active wake	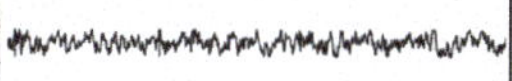	Beta 15–35 Hz	++	++		
Quiet wake	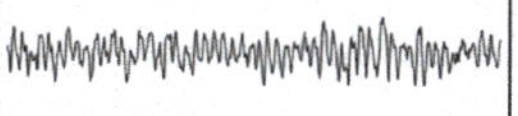	Alpha 8–12 Hz	+	+		
Stage 1	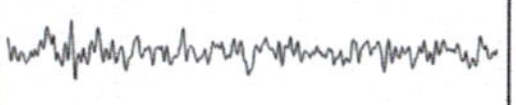	Theta 4–7 Hz	–	–		5%
Stage 2	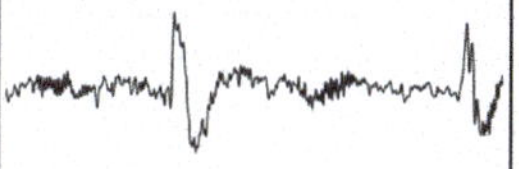	Theta 4–7 Hz	–	–	Spindles / K-complexes 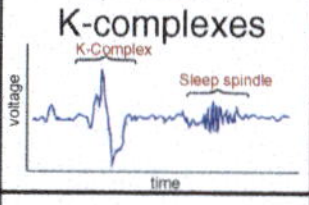	40–50%
Slow wave sleep (SWS)	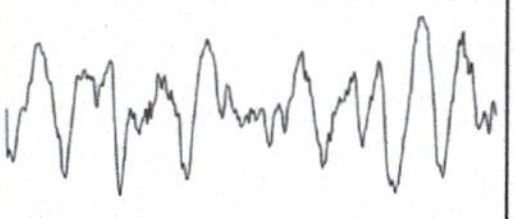	Delta 1–4 Hz	– –	–	Hippocampal sharp wave-ripples 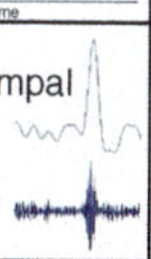	20–25%
REM sleep	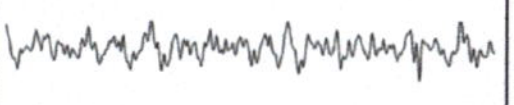	Theta 4–7 hz 'Sawtooth' rhythm	++	– –	Rapid eye movements	20–25%

Fig. 14.2 Stages of sleep. The electrophysiological and neurochemical attributes of sleep are represented in each column. In the "Neurochemistry" column, "++" and "− −" represent waking and nadir levels of a neurotransmitter during the 24-hour day. "Hz" = cycles per second

development [26, 41]. Figure 14.3 shows an abundance of nightly REM sleep obtained during the first year of life, comprising almost 50% of a night of sleep at birth [54]. Disruption of REM sleep during development has been shown to impair normal brain development and memory processing in animal models [44]. While these findings suggest the importance of sleep and particular sleep stages for early development, sleep clearly serves to maintain the health of the organism across the life span, as described below.

Sleep for Restoration and Energy Conservation

The human brain represents about 2% of total body weight, but consumes 20% of the body's oxygen and glucose, which may not be surprising considering the amount of energy the mammalian brain must expend to coordinate the procurement of food, procreation, and the protection of self and territory. It naturally follows that sleep may have evolved to replenish the energy consumed during waking hours. Indeed, to the extent that a healthy sleeper goes to bed feeling fatigued, and wakes up feeling refreshed, it seems more than plausible that sleep must serve a restorative/rejuvenating function. There are two ways of looking at this idea, in terms of energy conservation and energy restoration. Energy conservation relates to the organism's ability to reduce energy expenditures through a corresponding reduction in metabolic processing [5], while restoration relates to the organism's ability to restore body systems back to a homeostatic set point that ensures optimal daytime function [72]. This

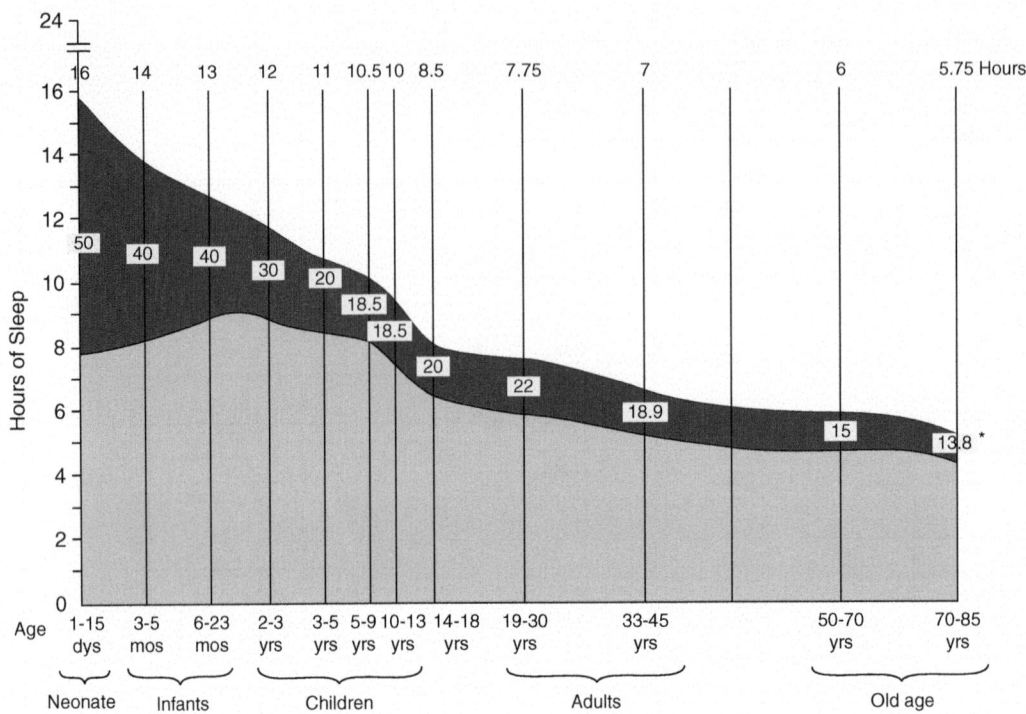

Fig. 14.3 Sleep across the life span. Dark gray, REM sleep; light gray, non-REM sleep. Value in dark gray indicates the percentage time spent in REM sleep with increasing age. (Adapted from: Roffwarg et al. [54])

might entail the rebalancing of neurotransmitters, the recovery and repair of muscle tissue, or a resetting of cognitive functions. It is noteworthy, however, that the conservation and restoration hypotheses are not fully supported by sleep science [51]. For example, about 80 calories an hour are expended during sleep, while 95 calories are expended while sitting awake [70], which equates to 10–15% energy saving over a night of sleep [58], the equivalent of a glass of milk. Regarding neuronal activity during sleep, there are only minimal decreases in neuronal firing rate during non-REM sleep, with increases in firing occurring (sometimes above waking levels) during REM sleep. Brain oxygen and glucose metabolism during REM sleep are similar to those observed while awake but are significantly lower during SWS. However, SWS only represents about 20% of a night of sleep, which tempers the interpretation that energy conservation is the sole function of sleep. On a neuronal level, one recent theory suggests that sleep is fine-tuned for a process termed "synaptic homeostasis": the extent to which synapses have undergone significant experience-dependent changes over the day determines how much the strength of those synapses will be restored during sleep as a means to optimize brain function the following day [62]. This theory has gained traction over the last decade as brain imaging techniques (e.g., high-density EEG imaging) and microscopy have made it easier to view and map electrical and synaptic activity of the sleeping brain. The functional role of such synaptic rebalancing is currently being studied, but it could suggest a role for sleep in restoration at the neuronal level. Lastly, there is recent evidence for the importance of adenosine in sleep regulation. Adenosine levels increase across the day with the accumulation of wakefulness. This increase in adenosine promotes sleepiness, which can be counteracted with caffeine, an adenosine antagonist [63]. Adenosine triphosphate (ATP) levels, which are a direct measure of available energy stores in the brain, are depleted during wake as ATP is dephosphorylated, and adenosine levels increase. Over sleep, however, ATP stores are replenished in preparation for the new day [21], which represents exciting evidence of the potential restorative value of sleep.

Energy conservation/restoration hypotheses derive from the implicit idea that wakefulness is a biologically fatiguing state and that sleep is required to allow for optimal waking function. But, as Allan Rechtschaffen reminds us, "we may need to sleep, not because we have been awake, but because sleep is a biological necessity in its own right" [51]. Additionally, it must be recognized that even if synaptic homeostasis and ATP re-accumulation serve a critical biological function, it is difficult to imagine that they could be the only functions of sleep. Indeed, one reason for this is the aforementioned complexity of sleep. If sleep is simply a restorative/homeostatic brain state, why must we have four distinct sleep stages, with their own neurochemical and physiological signatures? And why do these sleep stages progress in such a well-coordinated way, multiple times over the course of a night (see Fig. 14.1)? This complexity has led many researchers to postulate that a proper theory of sleep function must account for this complexity. As described later in this chapter, this is one reason for the recent surge of interest in the hypothesis that different stages of sleep may serve to strengthen different types of memories acquired during our waking hours. However, given the findings that sleep likely serves a restorative function, we still must address the question of how much sleep is required to optimize this restorative process.

How Much Sleep Do We Need?

Much print, and some science, has been dedicated to the idea that we can decrease sleep time without compromising productivity and overall health [49]. The canonical case is Thomas Edison, who is said to have slept 3–4 hours a night and who demanded that his employees adopt a similar sleep regimen. While some individuals can function optimally with 5 hours of sleep (or less) each night (Fig. 14.4), others require as many as 10 hours of sleep, with healthy young adults typically needing about 8–9 hours of sleep each night to function well. This is because sleep is tightly controlled by circadian and homeostatic influences that defy manipulation/disruption over long periods of time. One example of a failed attempt to cheat the need for sleep has been to adopt a polyphasic sleep regimen, such as Dymaxion sleep. This entails sleeping at strategic times during the day for limited

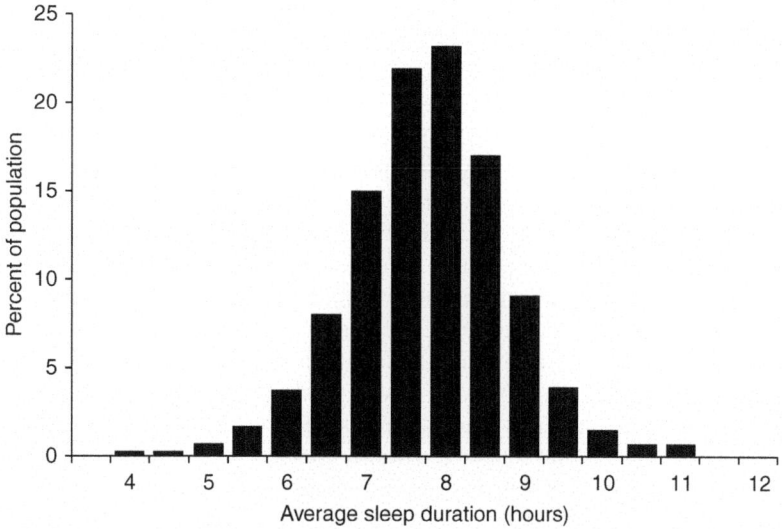

Fig. 14.4 Habitual sleep duration. Hypothetical distribution of sleep duration in young, healthy sleepers. While the average duration lies at about 8 hours, sleep need in healthy sleepers can range widely, from 5 to 11 hours of nightly sleep

durations (e.g., long naps every 4–6 hours) to obtain the benefits of sleep without getting a full night of sleep each day. Because REM sleep and SWS rebound after deprivation, some have tried to ensure that when they do sleep, their total sleep time contains greater amounts of these two stages of sleep. These strategies, however, have never proved successful, simply leaving the individual exposed to the negative consequences of sleep deprivation [23].

Attempts to pharmacologically improve sleep or lengthen sleep times have also met with mixed results. Due to hangover effects and increased risk for addiction, benzodiazepines and barbiturates have fallen out of favor as effective means of enhancing overall sleep quality. The same is true of over-the-counter remedies, such as antihistamines. The newer non-benzodiazepine medications (Z-drugs), such as zolpidem and zaleplon, are better tolerated, shorter-acting, and less addictive than their predecessors. However, their ability to improve objective sleep quality is minimal at best. While modest decreases in the time it takes to fall asleep, and in the number of arousals, have been demonstrated, the major finding has been that it is the individual's *perception* of those arousals and sleep quality that have improved, giving the individual the feeling that they are experiencing healthy sleep [28, 29]. It should also be noted that, while safety profiles for Z-drugs are more favorable than other prescription sleep agents, the propensity for dependence and drug-related adverse events (e.g., falls that occur after awakening during the night while taking these medications) still exist [14, 15]. Even over-the-counter remedies, such as valerian, kava, or chamomile tea, that have mild anxiolytic effects, while not physically harmful, have minimal impact on sleep quality and quantity [4, 34, 69]. After decades of research, the biological state of sleep remains stubbornly resistant to pharmacological manipulation.

Another major factor that dictates how many hours of sleep are optimal for a given individual relates to sleep time across the life span [54] (see Fig. 14.3). Neonates sleep up to 20 hours a day, half of which is composed of REM sleep, which, as mentioned, suggests that REM sleep is likely important for early brain development [20]. Across the life span, two aspects of sleep emerge, especially in mid-later life (>40 y.o.). The first is the gradual decrease in total sleep time. It is not uncommon for older individuals to only get 6 hours of sleep, where they used to get 8–9 hours during their young adult lives. There is a common misperception that this decrease in sleep time is harmful for cognition, executive function, and quality of life. However, there is ample evidence that older individuals perform well in these areas as long as they obtain healthy sleep [19]. As presented in Fig. 14.3, NREM sleep time decreases over time. However, this change largely reflects a reduction in slow wave sleep as we get older. It is not clear what effect SWS loss has on these variables, but there is some evidence that lower SWS amounts in older age may predict age-related memory deficits [6, 43]. Decreased growth hormone expression as a result of decreased SWS may also have an impact on brain health, although findings are scant on this topic [64]. These findings suggest that optimal nightly sleep amounts vary considerably from person to person and that what is likely most important for the health of the individual is to obtain that optimal amount of sleep and to ensure that it occurs during one consolidated block of time, ideally during the night. Fortunately, there are a number of ways to assess whether an individual is getting enough sleep. Well-validated questionnaires such as the Epworth Sleepiness Scale [35] can provide information about how sleepy an individual is in general, which can indicate whether an individual is not getting enough sleep each night (i.e., whether they are sleep restricted (see below)) or suffer from chronic sleep disruption. Measures such as the Pittsburgh Sleep Quality Inventory [10] assess sleep habits and quality of sleep and provide a more accurate assessment about whether an individual may have sleep disorder requiring further evaluation at a sleep disorders laboratory. Another simple and effective way to understand whether someone is obtaining enough sleep would be to find out whether the individual sleeps in on the weekends. Those who adhere to a regular sleep schedule during the week but end up sleeping in 1–2 extra hours on the weekend are very likely not obtaining enough sleep. Once this information is gathered, it becomes much simpler to assess whether the cause is environmental or physiological in nature.

What Happens When We Don't Get Enough Sleep: Sleep Restriction and Sleep Deprivation

Unfortunately, it often the case that modern society actively promotes behaviors that lead to sleep restriction and deprivation [53]. In this section, sleep restriction refers to a chronic curtailing of nightly sleep time, whereas sleep deprivation refers to loss of a sleep bout, as when a student pulls an all-nighter to study for a test. As described in the opening paragraph of this chapter, long-term sleep deprivation can carry dire health consequences. But what are the consequences of seemingly less severe forms of sleep restriction and deprivation? From a public health perspective, we can already answer this question for millions of teenagers and working-age adults who must accept some amount of sleep restriction as a condition of their school schedules and employment. Students whose circadian clock tends to be delayed (i.e., they have a biological tendency to want to sleep later) often have to get up early to go to school [46]. This form of chronic sleep restriction, which results from sleep disorders such as delayed sleep phase syndrome (DSPS), can lead to common problems, such as falling asleep in class, poor attention, and mood dysregulation [3, 42]. However, as we get older, the circadian rhythm tends to advance, resulting in earlier bed times (e.g., 9 pm–4 am), which can also be maladaptive. Fortunately, the circadian rhythm is amenable to manipulation through the use of bright light and/or melatonin [12, 36]. The phase response curve in Fig. 14.5 shows how the application of bright light (>10000 lux) and melatonin during the circadian day have the ability to shift earlier (advance) or later (delay) the circadian rhythm depending on when they are administered. These circadian changes can take place in 2–3 weeks, providing an effective treatment for those whose daytime function has been compromised by a misaligned circadian rhythm.

Regarding sleep deprivation, it is now known that one night of sleep deprivation results in the performance equivalent of an individual with a blood alcohol concentration (BAC) of 0.1, which is above the national legal limit [68]. The effects of sleep deprivation have been well-studied in recent decades [2] and, in addition to impaired reaction times and increased daytime sleepiness, have been linked to

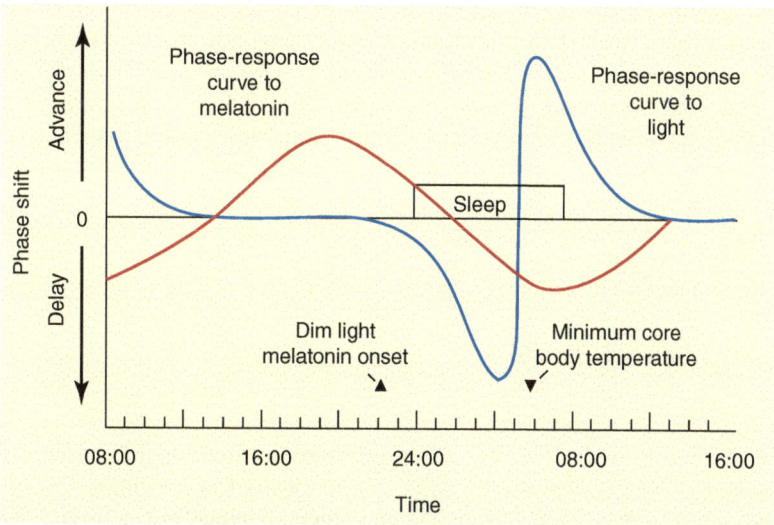

Fig. 14.5 Phase response curve. A shift in circadian phase, either earlier (advanced) or later (delayed) results depending on the timing of administration. Example: bright light administration for 30–45 min at the end of the sleep cycle advances the circadian rhythm, while bright light in the evening tends to delay the circadian rhythm. Red line, melatonin; blue line, bright light. (Adapted from Burgess et al. [9])

altered emotional memory processing [38] and alterations in mood and pain perception [56]. While the negative effects of sleep deprivation are well-documented, individuals still engage in practices that curtail the amount of sleep necessary for optimal daytime function. Most people are aware of some of the situations to avoid to function well during the day, such as not staying up late to study for an exam and not drinking to excess on work nights. However, simple adaptive bedtime practices (sleep hygiene) are often overlooked as meaningful ways to improve sleep [31, 60]. Suggestions for healthy bedtime practices would include:

- Avoid screen time (cell phones and related devices) and watching TV in the bedroom at bedtime.
- Avoid dozing in the evening hours prior to bedtime – remain active during wake to achieve peaceful sleep.
- Create a dark environment that also blocks external noises from car traffic, other family members, etc.
- Use the bedroom for sex and sleep only.
- Drink caffeinated drinks only in the morning.
- Keep a consistent bedtime and wake time.
- Avoid activating medications/beverages after morning hours.

Many individuals see marked improvement in sleep quantity and quality by following simple and consistent bedtime practices.

What Happens When Sleep Is Compromised?

Each of us has a daily sleep need, and when normal sleeping patterns are disrupted, often profound problems result. Individuals with poor or compromised sleep are often referred to a sleep disorders center for a polysomnographic sleep study. The following general examples, and the specific harms described in the next section, highlight the detrimental impact of sleep problems on physical health and daytime function. Obstructive sleep apnea, which is caused by an obstruction of the airway, is characterized by repetitive pauses in breathing during sleep (apneas) that last from 10 to >60 seconds. These apneic events result in brief arousals (almost always unnoticed by the patient) that disrupt the electrical activity of the brain (observed in EEG recordings). These mini-arousals can occur hundreds of times each night and often lead to profound impairment of daytime function, including falling asleep while driving, and even during business meetings, contributing to lost work time and poor work performance. Sleep apnea has been shown to put individuals at increased risk for cardiovascular disease, hypertension, and stroke [18]. The examples below highlight how compromised sleep can become when perpetuated by the direct or secondary effects of certain medical conditions.

Poor Sleep and Physical Health

Diabetes

There is now ample evidence that sleep health is important for maintaining the correct balance between key hormones known to regulate hunger and satiety in humans [55]. Insulin dysregulation is the key feature of diabetes, and it is now known that sleep plays an active role in regulating glucose and insulin levels [37, 65]. However, individuals with sleep disorders such as obstructive sleep apnea, who suffer nightly, often significant, sleep disruption due to apneic events, are at increased risk for insulin resistance [59] and compromised pancreatic function [45, 50]. However, the relationship is bidirectional. One unfortunate symptom of diabetes is nocturia, which causes patients to use the bathroom multiple times a night, further exacerbating their sleep disturbance [24], which worsens their diabetes symptoms. Encouragingly, however, even though sleep fragmentation is known to have significant effects on health, these effects can be reversed. For example, one study found that markers for diabetes risk can be reversed following sleep deprivation simply by allowing participants two nights of recovery sleep [8]. Thus, improving the integrity of sleep patterns can potentially restore an individual to a healthier status.

Obesity

As detailed in the opening paragraph of this chapter, one consequence of sleep deprivation is hyperphagia. As with diabetes, similar negative consequences are observed in the bidirectional relationship between sleep disruption and obesity. Obesity is a major risk factor for obstructive sleep apnea, with increased weight leading to increases in breathing disturbance, largely due to the accumulation of fatty tissue in the airway. One unfortunate consequence of sleep apnea is excessive daytime sleepiness, which is a direct result of increased breathing-related sleep fragmentation. The daytime sleepiness and lethargy that result from OSA impact the desire and ability to remain active during the day, thus increasing obesity and, in turn, sleep apnea. However, sleep disruption also has a major impact on the regulation of key hunger/satiety-related hormones, such as leptin and ghrelin. Leptin, which is stored in adipose tissue, signals to the hypothalamus to stop eating as it accumulates. Individuals who obtain less sleep show lower levels of leptin [61]. Ghrelin, on the other hand, is stored in the lining of the stomach and is responsible for signaling to the hypothalamus to increase feeding behavior. One study showed that individuals who had their sleep restricted for four nights in the lab (4.5 hours of sleep per night) demonstrated increased ghrelin expression and, consequently, increased food intake [7]. These findings clearly demonstrate the importance of sleep in the maintenance of hormonal regulation, and reinforce the well-supported idea that compromised sleep may set in motion a feedback loop that further increases the risk of obesity and sleep disruption.

Immunity

Recent studies also reveal a link between sleep and immune function. Those who experience circadian dysregulation due to shift work (i.e., working during normal sleep hours) will also experience impairments in lymphocyte expression [1, 30] as well as elevated expression of pro-inflammatory cytokines, such as TNF and IL-6 [33]. Increased immune system activation leads to greater systemic inflammation, and compromising the effectiveness of immune function [32] and further disrupting sleep.

Endnote: Sleep and Memory Processing

During normal waking hours, we spend our time engaging in various tasks, learning new information, interacting with people, and responding to problems and challenges as they arise. It is therefore reasonable to hypothesize that the waking brain is optimized for the acquisition of new information and experiences, while the sleeping brain answers these demands by creating a specialized milieu for the further processing and strengthening of those experiences. Much research over the past several decades, but most intensively in the last 20 years, has sought to determine whether sleep is important for information processing [17]. As described above, sleep is characterized by significant neurochemical and electrophysiological changes across the night, as well as significant differences between the individual sleep stages. One reason for the continued excitement about the study of sleep as a brain state well-suited to memory processing is that attributes specific to each sleep stage may be keenly tuned for the processing of different types of memory. Therefore, one of the appeals of this theory of sleep as a potential cognitive enhancer, is that it has the potential to describe why we require distinct stages of non-REM and REM sleep for optimal cognitive function.

Different Sleep Stages for Different Memories

Declarative memories are formed when new factual, spatial, or episodic information is acquired (e.g., when as learning new information in the classroom, memorizing the spatial layout of a town, or remembering episodes from one's life, like one's high school senior prom). These two types of memory are said to be "declarative" because we can verbally or behaviorally express the information when asked to do so. Declarative memories are different from other forms of memory, such as procedural memories (e.g., knowing how to ride a bike or type on a keyboard). As it turns out, there are specific features of individual sleep stages that make them well-suited to the processing of these different types of memory. Stage 2 Sleep: Sleep spindles, for example, are 12–15 Hz bursts of activity that emanate from the thalamus to the cortex uniquely during Stage 2 sleep. A number of studies have shown that increased number and density of sleep spindles (spindles per minute), and amount of time spent in Stage 2 sleep, are both associated with enhanced procedural memory processing, for example, simple typing tasks [67], and other tasks requiring fine motor movements [25]. Slow Wave Sleep (SWS): Declarative memories require the hippocampus for initial learning. Without the hippocampus, the individual loses the ability to form new memories (anterograde amnesia), as befell the patient H.M. when in 1953 his hippocampi were removed to eliminate the locus of his debilitating seizures [13, 57]. Interestingly, there are two properties unique to SWS that make it an ideal candidate brain state for the processing of declarative memories: low brain levels of acetylcholine [27] and the expression of hippocampal sharp-wave ripples [11]. During wake, acetylcholine (ACh) levels are at their highest levels, during which the learning of new information is ongoing. During SWS, however, acetylcholine levels are at their lowest of the 24-hour day, suggesting that SWS may optimize the consolidation of declarative memories. Indeed, studies show that declarative memory is better processed during sleep containing large amounts of SWS [48], and several studies have shown that information learned while awake is "replayed" at a compressed rate during sharp wave-ripple events in SWS [40]. REM sleep: In contrast to SWS, REM sleep is characterized by increased brain activity and metabolism, very low levels of the monoamines (serotonin and norepinephrine), and high levels of ACh relative to other sleep stages. REM sleep is also the sleep stage associated with vivid dreaming with often emotionally laden content. Thus, it is not surprising that REM sleep is associated with the processing of emotional memories, such as memory for emotional images and text [47, 66].

The study of the benefits of sleep for memory processing represents an exciting and novel way of looking at the cognitive benefits of sleep that takes the large body of findings from memory research and maps them onto what is known about the physiology of sleep. In this way, a number of interesting hypotheses can be tested that may help us understand how the complex rhythms and physiology of the sleeping brain serve to optimize, in this case, this vitally important biological function.

Conclusion

The formal scientific study of sleep started with the discovery of rapid eye movement sleep in the early 1950s. However, what remains as the holy grail for many sleep scientists is the identification of a unifying theory of sleep function that can account for all its complexities. While several hypotheses for the function of sleep have been studied over the past several decades, conclusive evidence for a single function or multiple functions of sleep remain elusive. However, what is well known is that the integrity of the nightly sleep cycle is essential for overall cognitive and physiological health. Equally important is mounting evidence of the consequences of poor sleep and lack of sleep that should make clear the central importance of optimizing sleep quantity and quality to enhance cognition, daytime function, brain and physical development, and general well-being. While this chapter has summarized only a fraction of what is known about the nature of sleep, it hopefully establishes a solid introduction for further investigation into health benefits of this fascinating biological state.

References

1. Almeida CM, Malheiro A. Sleep, immunity and shift workers: a review. Sleep Sci. 2016;9(3):164–8.
2. Banks S, Dinges DF. Behavioral and physiological consequences of sleep restriction. J Clin Sleep Med. 2007;3(5):519–28.
3. Baum KT, Desai A, et al. Sleep restriction worsens mood and emotion regulation in adolescents. J Child Psychol Psychiatry. 2014;55(2):180–90.
4. Bent S, Padula A, et al. Valerian for sleep: a systematic review and meta-analysis. Am J Med. 2006;119(12):1005–12.
5. Berger RJ, Phillips NH. Energy conservation and sleep. Behav Brain Res. 1995;69(1–2):65–73.
6. Bliwise DL. Sleep in normal aging and dementia. Sleep. 1993;16(1):40–81.
7. Broussard JL, Kilkus JM, et al. Elevated ghrelin predicts food intake during experimental sleep restriction. Obesity (Silver Spring). 2016a;24(1):132–8.
8. Broussard JL, Wroblewski K, et al. Two nights of recovery sleep reverses the effects of short-term sleep restriction on diabetes risk. Diabetes Care. 2016b;39(3):e40–1.
9. Burgess HJ, Sharkey KM, Eastman CI. Bright light, dark, and melatonin can promote circadian adaptation in night shift workers. Sleep Med Rev. 2002;6:407–20.
10. Buysse DJ, Reynolds CF 3rd, et al. The Pittsburgh Sleep Quality Index: a new instrument for psychiatric practice and research. Psychiatry Res. 1989;28(2):193–213.
11. Buzsaki G. The hippocampo-neocortical dialogue. Cereb Cortex. 1996;6(2):81–92.
12. Cajochen C, Krauchi K, et al. Role of melatonin in the regulation of human circadian rhythms and sleep. J Neuroendocrinol. 2003;15(4):432–7.
13. Corkin S. What's new with the amnesic patient H.M.? Nat Rev Neurosci. 2002;3(2):153–60.
14. Cunnington D. Non-benzodiazepine hypnotics: do they work for insomnia? BMJ. 2012;346:e8699.
15. Daley C, McNiel DE, et al. "I did what?" Zolpidem and the courts. J Am Acad Psychiatry Law. 2011;39(4):535–42.
16. Dement W. The effect of dream deprivation. Science. 1960;131(3415):1705–7.
17. Diekelmann S, Wilhelm I, et al. The whats and whens of sleep-dependent memory consolidation. Sleep Med Rev. 2009;13(5):309–21.
18. Drager LF, McEvoy RD, et al. Sleep apnea and cardiovascular disease: lessons from recent trials and need for team science. Circulation. 2017;136(19):1840–50.
19. Duffy JF, Willson HJ, et al. Healthy older adults better tolerate sleep deprivation than young adults. J Am Geriatr Soc. 2009;57(7):1245–51.
20. Dumoulin Bridi MC, Aton SJ, et al. Rapid eye movement sleep promotes cortical plasticity in the developing brain. Sci Adv. 2015;1(6):e1500105.
21. Dworak M, McCarley RW, et al. Sleep and brain energy levels: ATP changes during sleep. J Neurosci. 2010;30(26):9007–16.
22. Endo T, Schwierin B, et al. Selective and total sleep deprivation: effect on the sleep EEG in the rat. Psychiatry Res. 1997;66(2–3):97–110.
23. Eriksen CA, Gillberg M, et al. Sleepiness and sleep in a simulated "six hours on/six hours off" sea watch system. Chronobiol Int. 2006;23(6):1193–202.
24. Fitzgerald MP, Litman HJ, et al. The association of nocturia with cardiac disease, diabetes, body mass index, age and diuretic use: results from the BACH survey. J Urol. 2007;177(4):1385–9.
25. Fogel SM, Smith CT. The function of the sleep spindle: a physiological index of intelligence and a mechanism for sleep-dependent memory consolidation. Neurosci Biobehav Rev. 2011;35(5):1154–65.
26. Frank MG. Sleep and developmental plasticity not just for kids. Prog Brain Res. 2011;193:221–32.
27. Hasselmo ME. Neuromodulation: acetylcholine and memory consolidation. Trends Cogn Sci. 1999;3(9):351–9.
28. Hedner J, Yaeche R, et al. Zaleplon shortens subjective sleep latency and improves subjective sleep quality in elderly patients with insomnia. The Zaleplon Clinical Investigator Study Group. Int J Geriatr Psychiatry. 2000;15(8):704–12.

29. Huedo-Medina TB, Kirsch I, et al. Effectiveness of non-benzodiazepine hypnotics in treatment of adult insomnia: meta-analysis of data submitted to the Food and Drug Administration. BMJ. 2012;345:e8343.
30. Ibarra-Coronado EG, Pantaleon-Martinez AM, et al. The bidirectional relationship between sleep and immunity against infections. J Immunol Res. 2015;2015:678164.
31. Irish LA, Kline CE, et al. The role of sleep hygiene in promoting public health: a review of empirical evidence. Sleep Med Rev. 2015;22:23–36.
32. Irwin MR. Why sleep is important for health: a psychoneuroimmunology perspective. Annu Rev Psychol. 2015;66:143–72.
33. Irwin MR, Opp MR. Sleep health: reciprocal regulation of sleep and innate immunity. Neuropsychopharmacology. 2017;42(1):129–55.
34. Jacobs BP, Bent S, et al. An internet-based randomized, placebo-controlled trial of kava and valerian for anxiety and insomnia. Medicine (Baltimore). 2005;84(4):197–207.
35. Johns MW. A new method for measuring daytime sleepiness: the Epworth sleepiness scale. Sleep. 1991;14(6):540–5.
36. Khalsa SB, Jewett ME, et al. A phase response curve to single bright light pulses in human subjects. J Physiol. 2003;549(Pt 3):945–52.
37. Knutson KL. Impact of sleep and sleep loss on glucose homeostasis and appetite regulation. Sleep Med Clin. 2007;2(2):187–97.
38. Krause AJ, Simon EB, et al. The sleep-deprived human brain. Nat Rev Neurosci. 2017;18(7):404–18.
39. Kushida CA, Bergmann BM, et al. Sleep deprivation in the rat: IV. Paradoxical sleep deprivation. Sleep. 1989;12(1):22–30.
40. Lee AK, Wilson MA. Memory of sequential experience in the hippocampus during slow wave sleep. Neuron. 2002;36(6):1183–94.
41. Li W, Ma L, et al. REM sleep selectively prunes and maintains new synapses in development and learning. Nat Neurosci. 2017;20(3):427–37.
42. Lo JC, Ong JL, et al. Cognitive performance, sleepiness, and mood in partially sleep deprived adolescents: the need for sleep study. Sleep. 2016;39(3):687–98.
43. Mander BA, Winer JR, et al. Sleep and human aging. Neuron. 2017;94(1):19–36.
44. Marks GA, Shaffery JP, et al. A functional role for REM sleep in brain maturation. Behav Brain Res. 1995;69(1–2):1–11.
45. Morgenstern M, Wang J, et al. Obstructive sleep apnea: an unexpected cause of insulin resistance and diabetes. Endocrinol Metab Clin North Am. 2014;43(1):187–204.
46. Morgenthaler TI, Hashmi S, et al. High school start times and the impact on high school students: what we know, and what we hope to learn. J Clin Sleep Med. 2016;12(12):1681–9.
47. Nishida M, Pearsall J, et al. REM sleep, prefrontal theta, and the consolidation of human emotional memory. Cereb Cortex. 2009;19(5):1158–66.
48. Plihal W, Born J. Effects of early and late nocturnal sleep on declarative and procedural memory. J Cogn Neurosci. 1997;9(4):534–47.
49. Porcu S, Casagrande M, et al. Sleep and alertness during alternating monophasic and polyphasic rest-activity cycles. Int J Neurosci. 1998;95(1–2):43–50.
50. Rajan P, Greenberg H. Obstructive sleep apnea as a risk factor for type 2 diabetes mellitus. Nat Sci Sleep. 2015;7:113–25.
51. Rechtschaffen A. Current perspectives on the function of sleep. Perspect Biol Med. 1998;41(3):359–90.
52. Rechtschaffen A, Bergmann BM, et al. Sleep deprivation in the rat: X. Integration and discussion of the findings. 1989. Sleep. 2002;25(1):68–87.
53. Reynolds AC, Banks S. Total sleep deprivation, chronic sleep restriction and sleep disruption. Prog Brain Res. 2010;185:91–103.
54. Roffwarg HP, Muzio JN, et al. Ontogenetic development of the human sleep-dream cycle. Science. 1966;152(3722):604–19.
55. Schmid SM, Hallschmid M, et al. The metabolic burden of sleep loss. Lancet Diabetes Endocrinol. 2015;3(1):52–62.
56. Schrimpf M, Liegl G, et al. The effect of sleep deprivation on pain perception in healthy subjects: a meta-analysis. Sleep Med. 2015;16(11):1313–20.
57. Scoville WB, Milner B. Loss of recent memory after bilateral hippocampal lesions. J Neurol Neurosurg Psychiatry. 1957;20(1):11–21.
58. Shapiro CM, Goll CC, et al. Heat production during sleep. J Appl Physiol Respir Environ Exerc Physiol. 1984;56(3):671–7.
59. Spiegel K, Knutson K, et al. Sleep loss: a novel risk factor for insulin resistance and type 2 diabetes. J Appl Physiol (1985). 2005;99(5):2008–19.
60. Stepanski EJ, Wyatt JK. Use of sleep hygiene in the treatment of insomnia. Sleep Med Rev. 2003;7(3):215–25.

61. Taheri S, Lin L, et al. Short sleep duration is associated with reduced leptin, elevated ghrelin, and increased body mass index. PLoS Med. 2004;1(3):e62.
62. Tononi G, Cirelli C. Sleep function and synaptic homeostasis. Sleep Med Rev. 2006;10(1):49–62.
63. Urry E, Landolt HP. Adenosine, caffeine, and performance: from cognitive neuroscience of sleep to sleep pharmacogenetics. Curr Top Behav Neurosci. 2015;25:331–66.
64. van Cauter E, Leproult R, et al. Age-related changes in slow wave sleep and REM sleep and relationship with growth hormone and cortisol levels in healthy men. JAMA. 2000;284(7):861–8.
65. van Cauter E, Holmback U, et al. Impact of sleep and sleep loss on neuroendocrine and metabolic function. Horm Res. 2007;67(Suppl 1):2–9.
66. van der Helm E, Walker MP. Sleep and emotional memory processing. Sleep Med Clin. 2011;6(1):31–43.
67. Walker MP, Brakefield T, et al. Practice with sleep makes perfect: sleep-dependent motor skill learning. Neuron. 2002;35(1):205–11.
68. Williamson AM, Feyer AM. Moderate sleep deprivation produces impairments in cognitive and motor performance equivalent to legally prescribed levels of alcohol intoxication. Occup Environ Med. 2000;57(10):649–55.
69. Yurcheshen M, Seehuus M, et al. Updates on nutraceutical sleep therapeutics and investigational research. Evid Based Complement Alternat Med. 2015;2015:105256.
70. Zepelin H. Mammalian sleep. In: Kryger R, Dement WC, editors. Principles and practice of sleep medicine. Philadelphia: W.B. Saunders Company; 2000. p. 82–92.
71. Zhang XM, Shi J, et al. The effect of obstructive sleep apnea syndrome on growth and development in nonobese children: a parallel study of twins. J Pediatr. 2015;166(3):646–50 e641.
72. Zielinski MR, McKenna JT, et al. Functions and mechanisms of sleep. AIMS Neurosci. 2016;3(1):67–104.

Chapter 15
Integrating Mindfulness into a Routine Schedule: The Role of Mobile-Health Mindfulness Applications

Arnold A. P. van Emmerik, Robin Keijzer, and Tim M. Schoenmakers

Keywords Mindfulness · mHealth · eHealth · App · Self-help · Online

---

Key Points
- The number of mindfulness apps is rapidly growing, making mindfulness accessible to a large audience.
- Mindfulness apps and in-session mindfulness courses by teachers with personal experience in mindfulness each possess unique advantages and disadvantages.
- Randomized-controlled studies of mindfulness apps are scarce but showed positive effects in clinical and nonclinical populations and outcome domains.

Introduction

Checking Facebook, receiving and responding to dozens of messages, and checking your email, our smartphones bombard us with large amounts of notifications every day, preventing us from being mindful and contributing to stress [20]. However, smartphones could also play a more positive role, particularly in the area of mobile health. As for mindfulness, there are many mindfulness applications or "apps" for smartphones and tablets, and they hold great promise as a means to integrate mindfulness into a routine schedule. These apps are the logical outcome of two converging developments. Firstly, apps in general are rapidly penetrating many areas of life, including (mental) health. Secondly, mindfulness-based interventions (MBIs) and mindfulness trainings (usually in a face-to-face group format) are becoming increasingly popular and have demonstrated effects in various populations and outcome domains (Chap. 11, which focuses on the traditional face-to-face MBSR/MBCT group formats).

Mindfulness apps have a number of obvious advantages. They are easy to distribute and access, and as a result their reach is much greater than face-to-face formats for teaching mindfulness. Mindfulness apps are very flexible, in the sense that users can choose when and how to use them. Also, they are less costly for users than face-to-face formats and often even free. As to their alleged

---

A. A. P. van Emmerik (✉) · R. Keijzer · T. M. Schoenmakers
Department of Clinical Psychology, University of Amsterdam, Amsterdam, The Netherlands
e-mail: a.a.p.vanemmerik@uva.nl

© Springer Nature Switzerland AG 2020
J. Uribarri, J. A. Vassalotti (eds.), *Nutrition, Fitness, and Mindfulness*, Nutrition and Health,
https://doi.org/10.1007/978-3-030-30892-6_15

dissemination advantages, Wahbeh et al. [23] found a preference for Internet and individual mindfulness formats over group mindfulness formats. Although their study was conducted online and likely biased toward Internet formats for mindfulness training, and people may better be able to appreciate the value of in-session group formats only *after* taking them, these findings underscore the potential of online tools to engage involve people in mindfulness.

In contrast, advantages of face-to-face formats include greater opportunities for participants to motivate each other and to share and discuss individual or common experiences and for teachers to communicate and embody the subtleties and complexities of mindfulness practice. Also, face-to-face formats may convey a certain positive pressure to attend sessions and to establish and maintain a regular mindfulness practice, at least during a training course. As succinctly described by Wahbeh et al. [23], advantages of group formats include "motivation and synergistic learning opportunities" as a result of "meeting other people with similar or other issues which can give a wider perspective on their own situation and allow them to see how others handle their problems," and "encouragement and emotional support for each other instilling a sense of camaraderie." Especially when groups are homogenous in terms of medical complaints or in leading similar lives, they may experience similar challenges in mindfulness and meditation practice, and mutual support may then be very helpful [1]. Disadvantages may include sharing in public which may be "aversive for many people especially those with sensitive diagnoses like posttraumatic stress disorder or depression" and having to "attend at a specific time and day, and travel to a specific location" [23]. Individuals may of course differently weigh these advantages and disadvantages of mindfulness apps and face-to-face formats, and what may be an important advantage for some participants may be unimportant or a disadvantage for others.

When discussing mindfulness apps, one soon runs into the question if it is possible or even ethical to teach mindfulness in other ways than through a teacher with personal experience in mindfulness practice. Proponents of the currently omnipresent mindfulness-based stress reduction (MBSR [11, 12]) and mindfulness-based cognitive therapy (MBCT [16, 17]) formats are firm about the essential role of such a teacher. As Kabat-Zinn paraphrases the stance of Segal, Williams, and Teasdale in his Foreword to their seminal *Mindfulness-Based Cognitive Therapy for Depression* (2013), "having one's own meditation practice as a deep, multidimensional, and textured resource for this curriculum is absolutely essential, not merely recommended," because "there is simply no other way to impart these practices to others and engage with them about their experiences with authenticity and depth without having inhabited them oneself over an extended period of time" (p. xi). From a different angle, Van Dam et al. [21] identified over 20 observational studies or case studies in which adverse effects of meditation were described, such as psychosis, mania, anxiety, panic, depersonalization, and traumatic reexperiencing. These effects may not be very prevalent, but if they occur the presence of an experienced and preferably clinically trained professional may prove to be useful.

We have no doubts about the value and advantages of learning mindfulness from a teacher, or of a personal experience in mindfulness practice of such a teacher, and there is overwhelming scientific and anecdotal support for the positive effects of MBIs delivered by such a teacher. Yet, we believe it is relevant to consider the value of mindfulness training without the presence of a teacher. There are several indications and considerations that suggest a useful role for other modes of teaching and learning mindfulness. First, mindfulness came into existence long before it entered modern Western psychology and has been taught and learned in ways that greatly differ from current practices. For example, Buddhist traditions used different meditation techniques to practice mindfulness, of which Vipassana meditation is most closely related to the Western technique as introduced by Kabat-Zinn. Also, in Buddhism, mindfulness is one step in the so-called Noble Eightfold Path which contains ground rules for "rightful" living and focuses on the liberation of samsara (i.e., rebirth or suffering). Western mindfulness is stripped of such a context and is adjusted to fit better with Western lifestyles and related health problems. What is relevant here is that there is no evidence that points to a minimal or optimal format for teaching mindfulness. Notwithstanding their popularity and demonstrated positive effects, this is also true for MBSR, MBCT, and other teaching formats. Studies of potentially relevant dimensions of MBSR have yielded some interesting but mixed findings. For instance, while the number of class hours seemed unrelated to the effects of MBSR [7], these effects were positively related to the duration of home practice [6].

Second, research demonstrated positive effects of online mindfulness-based interventions. For instance, Spijkerman et al. [19] performed a meta-analysis of 15 randomized-controlled trials of online mindfulness-based interventions in both general and clinical populations. They found a small but significant beneficial impact on depression ($g = 0.29$), anxiety ($g = 0.22$), well-being ($g = 0.23$), and mindfulness ($g = 0.32$) and a moderate effect size on stress ($g = 0.51$). Exploratory subgroup analyses did show significantly larger effect sizes for guided online MBIs than for unguided online MBIs on stress ($g = 0.89$ vs. $g = 0.19$, respectively) and mindfulness ($g = 0.43$ vs. $g = 0.22$, respectively). For depression and anxiety, guidance was not associated with larger improvements. Of note, only one study that was included in the meta-analysis ([13]; see below) examined a mindfulness app; the other unguided MBIs were web browser-based.

In addition, Cavanagh et al. [5] conducted a meta-analysis of 15 randomized-controlled trials (four of which were also included in Spijkerman et al.'s meta-analysis) of guided and unguided self-help mindfulness and acceptance-based interventions. They found small to medium effects of the joint guided and unguided interventions on mindfulness and acceptance, depression, and anxiety. They also report that "post-hoc tests suggest larger effects for guided mindfulness and acceptance-based self-help than for unguided self-help" (p. 127), but unfortunately provide no data about the magnitude or significance of the difference in effects. Also, their meta-analysis included only four studies of self-help MBIs (as opposed to acceptance-based or combined mindfulness and acceptance-based interventions) and no studies of MBIs that were delivered via apps. As the authors conclude however, their findings suggest that mindfulness "can be learnt by self-help" (p. 126) "through interventions that require little or no therapist resource" (p. 128). Furthermore, while not denying that "the quality of the teaching of such interventions is not a key ingredient, nor that subtle inner qualities of the teacher facilitate change" (p. 128), their findings "challenge the widely held view that face-to-face teaching of such interventions is an *essential* ingredient to achieving successful outcomes for participants" (p. 128, italics added).

Third, the position that mindfulness can only be taught by a teacher with personal experience in mindfulness practice leaves unanswered the question of the type and extent of personal experience that is required. As with the format and duration of MBIs, there is simply no evidence that points to a minimal or optimal type and extent of personal mindfulness experience that is required for teaching mindfulness.

In sum, the above meta-analyses show that online (but not necessarily unguided; [19]) and unguided (but not necessarily online; [5]) MBIs are effective means to teach mindfulness, though perhaps not as effective as in-session classes with a mindfulness teacher present. Likely, as apps and other digital means will get more and more intelligent, they will also become more able at simulating the guidance of a real trainer or do even more. For example, Hudlicka [10] performed a small-scale pilot study of a virtual MBSR coach in a web-based interface. The coach gave customized feedback and support in an interactive manner. This appeared to be more effective than a self-administered MBSR training without such a coach. Another example is a virtual meditation coach which provides feedback during meditation based on users' breathing [18].

Taken together, there is great value in existing mindfulness formats such as MBSR or MBCT, and these empirically supported interventions are not something lightly to be tampered with. At the same time, they are just one way of teaching mindfulness. Mindfulness apps are another, and each has its own unique possibilities and limitations. The remainder of this chapter therefore reviews the research literature on the effects of mindfulness apps and proposes a number of future directions for the further study of mindfulness apps.

Effects of Mindfulness Apps on Health

While the number and use of mindfulness apps are rapidly increasing, methodologically rigid research of their effects is lagging behind [14, 15]. Furthermore, the few published studies have examined apps that greatly vary in content and have included varying clinical and nonclinical populations and outcomes. Unfortunately, no studies to date have directly tested the effects of mindfulness apps on positive nutrition, fitness, or other health behaviors. The same is true for chronic diseases related to such health behaviors, such as prediabetes and diabetes, cardiovascular disease, or chronic kidney disease. Below, we review the available randomized-controlled studies of the effects of mindfulness apps on mindfulness and other outcomes.

Ly et al. [13] compared an 8-week mindfulness course delivered by an app to a behavioral activation program of similar duration in patients with major depressive disorder. They found large, comparable reductions of depression after both interventions which lasted for at least 6 months but noted that the lack of a no-intervention control condition does not rule out spontaneous recovery and other alternative explanations of participants' improvements. Furthermore, participants were instructed to write weekly reflections on "their work and thoughts on the current treatment week" and "received personal feedback on their reflection from their therapist" (p. 6–7). Hence, the self-help mindfulness app was complemented with a limited amount of therapeutic attention.

Economides et al. [8] investigated the effects of "Take 10," i.e., the first 10 introductory 10-minute meditation sessions of the highly popular Headspace mindfulness app. Take 10 was compared to a control condition that comprised a similar number of psychoeducational sessions on mindfulness of equal duration. Ingeniously, the experimental and control sessions were administered through the same app using the same voice and were presented to participants as well-being programs. As a result, this is probably the most rigidly controlled study to date, in terms of isolating the purportedly active elements of this mindfulness app. Compared to psychoeducation alone, Take 10 demonstrated positive effects on affect ($d = 0.47$), irritability ($d = 0.44$), and stress resulting from external pressure or event load ($d = 0.45$). No differential effect was found for stress associated with personal vulnerability to stress, as measured with the Stress Overload Scale [2, 3]. In an earlier comparison of Take 10 to a neutral but active control task (the Catch Notes app), Howells et al. [9] found significant improvements of positive affect and depression, but not of satisfaction with life, social-psychological prosperity, and negative affect. Unfortunately, none of these studies collected follow-up data, and the long-term stability of these positive effects is therefore unclear. Finally, Bennike et al. [4] randomly assigned healthy participants either to 30 days of mindfulness meditation training with the Headspace app or to a control intervention consisting of 30 days of brain training with Lumosity (see www.luminosity.com). They measured effects on mind wandering and trait mindfulness. Only the Headspace group showed significant decreases in mind wandering and significant increases in trait mindfulness.

Van Emmerik et al. [22] conducted a randomized waiting-list controlled trial of the "VGZ Mindfulness Coach," a mindfulness app that was developed by a large Dutch health-care insurance company. The VGZ Mindfulness Coach offers 40 mindfulness exercises and background information about mindfulness without any form of therapeutic guidance. It showed large ($d = 0.77$) and statistically significant increases of mindfulness after 8 weeks. Also, there were large decreases of general psychiatric symptoms ($d = -0.68$) and moderate increases of psychological, social, and environmental quality of life ($d = 0.38, 0.38$, and 0.36, respectively). Except for social quality of life, these gains were maintained for at least 3 months.

Conclusion and Future Directions

The few published randomized-controlled studies that we discussed above suggest that mindfulness apps can bring about positive effects on a range of outcomes. At the same time, it is clear that there is a strong need for further randomized and adequately controlled studies of the effects of mindfulness apps, especially given the growing popularity of these apps. Specifically, we suggest that future research address the following issues.

First, and especially relevant in view of the focus of this book, research is needed that specifically tests the effects of mindfulness apps on positive nutrition, fitness, or other health behaviors and in turn on the actual health conditions associated with these health behaviors.

Second, the effects of mindfulness apps on trait mindfulness are not routinely assessed or correlated with health effects. Therefore, the assumption that increases in trait mindfulness mediate positive health effects of these apps is still untested. Of note, two randomized-controlled studies that included mindfulness measures [4] (Van Emmerik et al. [22]) did find positive effects on mindfulness but did not test mediation effects of increased mindfulness on health outcomes.

Third, perhaps mindfulness apps may turn out to have most value not as an alternative but as an adjunct to in-session or guided online formats for teaching mindfulness. Studies of blended formats are therefore needed. A case in point, we are currently examining if mindfulness apps can support participants of MBSR to maintain a regular mindfulness practice after the course has ended.

Fourth, many studies of online MBIs are dominated by female participants. For instance, in a recent meta-analysis, the percentage of female participants in the included studies ranges from 43% to 90% [19]. In our own study [22], 96% of the participants were female. It would be interesting to explore why this is the case and to what extent it constitutes a problem in generalizing findings from MBI studies (and perhaps mindfulness research at large) to male populations.

In conclusion, we believe that mindfulness apps are here to stay. Their disadvantages and limitations should not be ignored, but neither should their advantages and possibilities. Instead, *in the spirit of mindfulness*, we advocate an open, curious, and nonjudgmental stance toward the opportunities they offer for making the world a little bit more mindful.

References

1. Allen NB, Chambers R, Knight W, Blashki G, Ciechomski L, Hassed C, et al. Mindfulness-based psychothera-pies: a review of conceptual foundations, empirical evidence and practical considerations. Aust N Z J Psychiatry. 2006;40(4):285–94.
2. Amirkhan JH. Stress overload: a new approach to the assessment of stress. Am J Community Psychol. 2012;49(1–2):55–71.
3. Amirkhan JH, Urizar GG, Clark S. Criterion validation of a stress measure: the stress overload scale. Psychol Assess. 2015;27(3):985–96.
4. Bennike IH, Wieghorst A, Kirk U. Online-based mindfulness training reduces behavioral markers of mind wandering. J Cogn Enhanc. 2017;1(2):172–81.
5. Cavanagh K, Strauss C, Forder L, Jones F. Can mindfulness and acceptance be learnt by self-help? A systematic review and meta-analysis of mindfulness and acceptance-based self-help interventions. Clin Psychol Rev. 2014;34:118–29.
6. Carmody J, Baer RA. Relationships between mindfulness practice and levels of mindfulness, medical and psychological symptoms and well-being in a mindfulness-based stress reduction program. J Behav Med. 2008;31(1):23–33.
7. Carmody J, Baer RA. How long does a mindfulness-based stress reduction program need to be? A review of class contact hours and effect sizes for psychological distress. J Clin Psychol. 2009;65(6):627–38.
8. Economides M, Martman J, Bell MJ, Sanderson B. Improvements in stress, affect, and irritability following brief use of a mindfulness-based smartphone app: a randomized controlled trial. Mindfulness. 2018;9(5):1584–93.
9. Howells A, Ivtzan I, Eiroa-Orosa FJ. Putting the 'app' in happiness: a randomised controlled trial of a smartphone-based mindfulness intervention to enhance wellbeing. J Happiness Stud. 2014;17(1):163–85.
10. Hudlicka E. Virtual training and coaching of health behavior: example from mindfulness meditation training. Patient Educ Couns. 2013;92(2):160–6.
11. Kabat-Zinn J. Full catastrophe living; using the wisdom of your body and mind to face stress, pain and illness. London: Piatkus; 1996.
12. Kabat-Zinn J. Full catastrophe living; how to cope with stress, pain and illness using mindfulness meditation. London: Little, Brown Book Group; 2013.
13. Ly KH, Trüschel A, Jarl L, Magnusson S, Windahl T, Johansson R, et al. Behavioural activation versus mindfulness-based guided self-help treatment administered through a smartphone application: a randomised controlled trial. BMJ Open. 2014;4(1):e003440.

14. Mani M, Kavanagh DJ, Hides L, Stoyanov SR. Review and evaluation of mindfulness-based iphone apps. JMIR Mhealth Uhealth. 2015;3(3):e82.
15. Plaza I, Demarzo MM, Herrera-Mercadal P, García-Campayo J. Mindfulness-based mobile applications: literature review and analysis of current features. JMIR Mhealth Uhealth. 2013;1(2):e24.
16. Segal ZV, Williams JMG, Teasdale JD. Mindfulness-based cognitive therapy for depression: a new approach to preventing relapse. New York: Guilford Publications; 2002.
17. Segal Z, Williams M, Teasdale J. Mindfulness-based cognitive therapy for depression. New York: The Guilford Press; 2013.
18. Shamekhi A, Bickmore T. Breathe with me: a virtual meditation coach, vol. 9238, p. 279–82. Presented at the International Conference on Intelligent Virtual Agents, Springer International Publishing; 2015.
19. Spijkerman MPJ, Pots WTM, Bohlmeijer ET. Effectiveness of online mindfulness-based interventions in improving mental health: a review and meta-analysis of randomised controlled trials. Clin Psychol Rev. 2016;45:102–14.
20. Thomée S, Härenstam A, Hagberg M. Mobile phone use and stress, sleep disturbances, and symptoms of depression among young adults-a prospective cohort study. BMC Public Health. 2011;11(1):66.
21. Van Dam NT, Van Vugt MK, Vago DR, Vago DR, Schmalzl L, Saron CD, et al. Mind the hype: a critical evaluation and prescriptive agenda for research on mindfulness and meditation. Perspect Psychol Sci. 2017;9:174569161770958.
22. Van Emmerik AAP, Berings F, Lancee J. Efficacy of a mindfulness-based mobile application: a randomized waiting-list controlled trial. Mindfulness. 2018;9:187–98.
23. Wahbeh H, Svalina MN, Oken BS. Group, one-on-one, or internet? Preferences for mindfulness meditation delivery format and their predictors. Open Med J. 2014;1:66–74.

Part IV
Use of This Integrated Approach in Different Populations

Chapter 16

Health Promotion and Chronic Disease Prevention with eHealth Technology in the General Population

Samantha R. Paige

Keywords Chronic disease prevention · Health promotion · eHealth literacy · Social media · Patient-provider communication

---

Key Points
- People continue to use eHealth programs despite limited evidence for their effectiveness in preventing chronic disease.
- Health literacy and numeracy are foundational elements of eHealth literacy that are driven by situational and sociocultural factors, both of which are critical in assessing patients' skills and motivation to use eHealth.
- Proactively and openly discussing the sociocultural motivations, use, and skills related to eHealth with patients may have a positive effect on the patient-practitioner relationship and behaviors protective against chronic disease.
- eHealth literacy varies by age, race/ethnicity, and rurality, drawing attention to the need for tailored and culturally- adapted interventions.

Introduction

Electronic health (eHealth) technologies and applications (or programs) have revolutionized how health promotion clinicians deliver chronic disease prevention education [46]. eHealth technologies broadly include smartphones, tablets, and wearable devices, whereas eHealth programs include social media, downloadable apps, and electronic health records. eHealth is deeply ingrained in the healthcare experience. Nearly 90% of the US population has access to the Internet [54] and nearly 80% have used it for health-related purposes [23]. Advantages of eHealth include the opportunity to monitor, track, and inform healthcare and data management, and to interact with other online patients and practitioners in the comfort and convenience of their own homes [62]. To augment chronic disease prevention efforts clinicians must be aware of ways to leverage eHealth to promote behaviors that are protective for leading causes of death globally.

S. R. Paige (✉)
Department of STEM Translational Communication Center, University of Florida, Gainesville, FL, USA
e-mail: paigesr190@ufl.edu

© Springer Nature Switzerland AG 2020
J. Uribarri, J. A. Vassalotti (eds.), *Nutrition, Fitness, and Mindfulness*, Nutrition and Health, https://doi.org/10.1007/978-3-030-30892-6_16

This chapter outlines the potential of eHealth to facilitate health promotion and chronic disease prevention in the general population. First, I present the current state of evidence for eHealth programs in promoting mindfulness, physical activity, and healthy eating. Next, I discuss the role of health promotion clinicians and educators in facilitating conversations with patients about eHealth programs to supplement chronic disease prevention. This includes gauging the skills and health-related needs of patients in negotiating the best eHealth approach for them. Finally, I conclude the chapter by synthesizing literature on eHealth use and skills among patient groups who are at the greatest risk for chronic disease.

Evidence for eHealth Promotion Programs

Table 16.1 summarizes the evidence of eHealth programs for physical activity, healthy eating, and mindfulness.

Applications for Physical Activity and Nutrition

Although inconsistent [35, 73], research has demonstrated that eHealth programs have the capacity to promote physical activity and healthy eating [20] and to support physiological health parameters central to preventing chronic disease [60]. These programs are considered most effective if they incorporate theoretical underpinnings to facilitate customized goal setting, self-monitoring, and social support or accountability through interactions with other online users [33, 45, 60]. Content analyses report that eHealth programs incorporate these theoretically driven and evidence-based behavior change techniques [5, 40, 75]. Their representation, however, is generally substandard and insufficient to promote sustained behavior change within publicly available eHealth programs [4, 8]. Despite limited evidence-based features and subsequent recommendations to caution eHealth program use in practice, patients continue to use these programs and report positive outcomes related to physical activity and nutrition [60, 71]. Therefore, the use and efficacy of these programs is likely due to the relevancy and quality of the content that is valued by the user.

Applications for Mindfulness

Apple iTunes, one of the largest international technology conglomerates, named "Calm" (meditation and sleep stories) the 2017 App of the Year for the United States, Australia, Ireland, New

Table 16.1 Summary of eHealth efficacy and content quality

eHealth program	Intervention evidence for efficacy	Content quality
Applications (structured apps)		
Physical activity	Positive	Unacceptable[a]
Nutrition/diet	Positive	Unacceptable[a]
Mindfulness	N/A	Acceptable
Social media (unstructured)		
Physical activity	N/A[b]	Poor[c]
Nutrition/diet	N/A[b]	Poor[c]
Mindfulness	N/A	N/A

[a]Unacceptable = Some use of behavior change techniques, but not enough to sustain behavior change
[b]Positive association between social media use and behavior but no interventional efficacy evidence
[c]Poor = Evidence-based behavior change techniques are generally excluded

Zealand, and the United Kingdom [3]. This attention gives great acclamation to mindfulness as a health practice and its delivery through eHealth programs. Two recent reviews of mindfulness eHealth programs on iTunes and Google Play found that the vast majority of these apps are misclassified as "mindfulness" [38, 55]. Apps that appropriately used the term "mindfulness," however, applied features that leveraged behavioral accountability through meditation and sleep tracking as well as social network development. These studies demonstrate that there is evidence that these apps contain high-quality information delivery, including visual aesthetics and engagement. While recent randomized controlled trials have identified positive short-term effects (e.g., reduced stress, improved quality of life) upon the use of mindfulness eHealth programs [30, 66], their efficacy to have a longitudinal effect on chronic disease physiologic indicators (e.g., cholesterol, blood pressure) is less known.

Mindfulness is an active lifestyle adjustment, requiring regular attention and practice. Despite high rates of eHealth use, mindfulness eHealth programs are often meppel downloaded but not used on a regular basis [55]. Nearly half of all eHealth app users stop using the programs because of hidden costs (despite the app being free when downloaded), burden of entering data daily, and ultimately a loss of interest [34]. To promote regular use, Plaza and colleagues [55] encourage practitioners to recommend mindfulness apps that monitor user progress and foster social influence and interactivity. However, clinical trials are needed to measure which app features are most efficacious and encourage regular use.

Social Media for Physical Activity, Nutrition, and Mindfulness

Social media are publicly available and predominantly user-generated programs that can be leveraged for health promotion. Despite the increasing popularity since 2006, there is limited formal evidence for the efficacy of using social media to promote physical activity, nutrition, or mindfulness. A study supplementing a physical activity intervention with a Facebook self-monitoring group yielded similar results as the control group without a Facebook membership [12]. Content analyses of social media platforms report that most nutrition and physical activity posts exclude elements of evidence-based behavior change theory identified in the literature as critical for behavior change [51, 72]. This is not surprising as users freely create user-generated content without formal training in health promotion or message design, blurring the lines of information and source credibility. One important affordance of social media, however, is to facilitate social support and collaborative networks to promote protective health behaviors, given that the users feel comfortable sharing their personal information.

Acceptance and Uptake of eHealth for Chronic Disease Prevention

eHealth programs remain in high demand despite inconsistent or inconclusive evidence. Over 20% of Internet users report using an eHealth app [11], and about 80% report accessing health information on social media [22]. According to Carroll et al. [11], downloading an app is an active step toward behavior change. People who are most likely to download an eHealth app are younger, are college educated, reside in urban regions, and feel motivated to engage in physical activity and healthy eating. There is limited evidence that race, ethnicity, or income is associated with app uptake. Similarly, Smith and Anderson [64] report that social media uptake is generally equal by gender and race/ethnicity. Although there is an upward trend in geographic region, adults who live in rural regions and are over the age of 65 report lower Internet and social media adoption as compared to their younger counterparts in more urban and suburban regions of the nation.

Clinicians must acknowledge that patients are not empty vessels waiting to be filled by static and factual information at the clinic. Rather, they are actively acquiring and assimilating knowledge from eHealth programs whether intentionally or unintentionally, to inform their healthcare beliefs and values. When not used haphazardly, eHealth has great potential to reach at-risk subgroups of the population and facilitate health education and social collaborations to help achieve their health informational needs and behavioral goals to prevent chronic disease. Health promotion clinicians and educators should use eHealth programs as a *supplement* (not a substitute) to a multi-faceted approach to optimize behavioral and health outcomes [60]. As such, eHealth programs should be leveraged as a public health tool and openly discussed in the patient-practitioner context rather than avoided due to their questionable or undetermined quality.

Patient-Practitioner Communication About eHealth Promotion

The emergence of eHealth has allowed patients to take an active role in decision-making at various points of their healthcare experience. Patients use eHealth before a healthcare appointment to learn about their symptoms and prepare questions, in order to make the best of their brief time with the clinician [7]. Nearly 80% of patients refer to the Internet following a healthcare appointment to seek clarification and second opinions from users on online discussion forums, especially if their interaction with the professional led to dissatisfaction or worry [36]. The Internet also provides temporary healthcare assistance when patients, especially those who are uninsured or low-income, cannot obtain immediate access to a clinician [1].

Clinicians' reactions to patient disclosure about eHealth information seeking and usage have significant effects on the patient-professional relationship and patients' health behaviors. Clinicians remain the most trusted and valued source of health information, so patients are generally willing to disregard information learned from the Internet if their clinician disagrees with the content [7, 69]. Patients expect their clinicians to positively acknowledge their attempts, contextualize the content to justify why it does or does not apply to their unique situation, and ultimately verify its credibility and outline any limitations [7, 63]. Clinicians who violate this expectation and patronize patients for using eHealth can significantly damage the relationship. Bylund et al. [10] found that patients reported greater satisfaction, validation, and reduced worry when clinicians acknowledged patients' efforts to use eHealth in an attempt to prepare for their appointment. The opposite was true when clinicians dismissed or negatively acknowledged patients' attempts. This is relevant to chronic disease prevention, as positive communication results in greater prevention efforts and adherence [68].

Patients who are at the greatest risk for chronic disease use eHealth programs; however, they are unlikely to initiate a discussion with their clinician about the experience and information learned. Middle-age white adults who are educated and in good health most often initiate discussions about eHealth information with their clinician [69]. Patients who do not initiate these conversations are likely embarrassed or concerned that their clinician may not approve or care about their interest [63]. These concerns are magnified when patients have limited confidence in their ability to evaluate the credibility or applicability of the information found online [48]. Despite patient acknowledgment of their limitations in using eHealth and the high degree of trust in healthcare professionals [28], patients are still unlikely to initiate conversations with their clinician to gain clarity of information obtained on the Internet [17].

Clinicians must be proactive in discussing patients' eHealth use to cultivate a patient-practitioner relationship conducive to shared learning and decision-making. Over 80% of patients who use the Internet report learning new health information, and over half (52%) believe this information is accurate [29]. Understanding patients' eHealth information preferences and expectations presents a teachable moment, wherein clinicians can critically discuss the benefits and drawbacks of online information. Clinicians can encourage patients to use empirically supported resources that are relevant to their current situation and are also consistent with their eHealth needs and abilities.

eHealth Skills and Chronic Disease Prevention

Health Literacy and Numeracy

Only 12% of the US population has proficient health literacy and 9% in numeracy [13]. Health literacy is defined as the knowledge and skills to access, understand, apprise, and apply health information in diverse healthcare contexts across the lifespan [65]. Numeracy (i.e., quantitative literacy or health numeracy) is an element of health literacy, as it incorporates skills related to understanding and applying numbers through a process of quantitative reasoning in order to function productively in the healthcare context [58]. This type of quantitative reasoning includes performing basic calculations, interpreting results of graphs and charts, as well as comprehending scientific results of empirical research [25]. Limited numeracy affects both patients and clinicians, which contributes to avoidance and limited confidence to communicate risk and numeric expressions [58].

Health literacy and numeracy are important for mobilizing chronic disease prevention. Low health literacy is associated with limited use of preventive healthcare services [61], and health literacy proficiency is associated with the engagement in health promoting behaviors protective against chronic disease [6, 65]. Similarly, patients with higher numeracy are more likely to engage in proactive prevention and maintenance behaviors, such as blood pressure monitoring [56]. Currently, however, the direct effect of numeracy and informed decision-making is less known [56, 58].

Similar to the highly socio-contextual features of health literacy [65], numeric uncertainty and simultaneous affective response derived from low numeracy is what likely ultimately leads patients to over- or underestimate their risk for a condition [58]. Mulder and colleagues [43] report that the negative effects of low numeracy in interpreting nutrition labels can be alleviated when a patient has a high degree of motivation or involvement in food preparation. In youth and adolescent populations, learning numeracy skills while participating in structured exercise programs results in meeting physical activity guidelines [52, 67]. Further, high-quality patient-practitioner communication can overcome perceived literacy limitations that prevent cancer screening behaviors [15]. As a cognitive and social skill set, attention to the dynamic and social elements that form patient health literacy is critical to promote chronic disease prevention.

eHealth Literacy

Widespread adoption of the Internet and its available social networks offers a low-cost opportunity to enhance the literacy of healthcare consumers worldwide [32]. Health literacy provides an indication of eHealth use and proficiency. Patients with high functional health literacy are more likely than their low health literate counterparts to adopt and perceive nutrition and physical activity eHealth apps as useful and easy to use [37]. Differences exist in how patients at varying levels of health literacy attend to and recall health information. Meppelink and Bol [39], for example, found that attention to health-related illustrations resulted in greater recall among individuals with low health literacy. Among individuals with high health literacy, attention to text-based messages yielded greater recall. Beyond basic health-related reading and writing proficiency, skills related to navigating the offline healthcare system have a positive but weak association with eHealth proficiency, including accessing, evaluating, and acting upon online health information [21]. These results confirm the importance of considering patients' health literacy regarding eHealth but also illustrate there are additional skills beyond basic literacy that are important to optimize the eHealth experience.

By definition, eHealth literacy comprises the skills to understand, exchange, evaluate, and apply online health information in the face of adversity stemming from dynamic contextual factors [50]. A reciprocal relationship exists between eHealth literacy as an antecedent and a consequence of patient empowerment and healthcare engagement [50, 53]. Considering patients' eHealth literacy is a critical consideration for chronic disease prevention. Greater eHealth literacy is associated with enhanced patient-professional communication [44], cancer-related screenings [41], and physical activity and healthy eating [42]. Operational behaviors include functional (understand), communicative (exchange), critical (evaluate), and translational (apply) eHealth literacies (see Table 16.2 and Fig. 16.1).

Table 16.2 eHealth literacy dimensions

Dimension	Definition/description
Functional	"Basic skills reading and writing (typing) about health to effectively function on the Internet" ([48], p. 10)
Communicative	"The ability to collaborate, adapt, and control communication about health with users on social online environments with multimedia" ([48], p. 10). This extends beyond the technical skills of communication within an online environment or the function of simply crafting a text-based message with a virtual keyboard. Rather, this is the ability to manage the essence of online conversations among diverse sources (e.g., experts, providers, uninformed peers, informed peers) in order to obtain or exchange health information
Critical	"The ability to evaluate the credibility, relevance, and risks of sharing and receiving health information on the Internet" ([48], p. 10). Skill set needed for patients to critically evaluate the credibility, safety, and relevance of online health information according to its content (e.g., language), the source (e.g., experts, informed peers, uninformed peers), and the platform from which it is presented (e.g., app, social media, PHR)
Translational	"The ability to apply health knowledge gained from the Internet across diverse ecological contexts" ([48], p. 10). Translational literacy is the highest cognitive level of the eHealth literacy, meaning it is informed and built upon from all previous eHealth literacy dimensions (i.e., critical, communicative, functional)

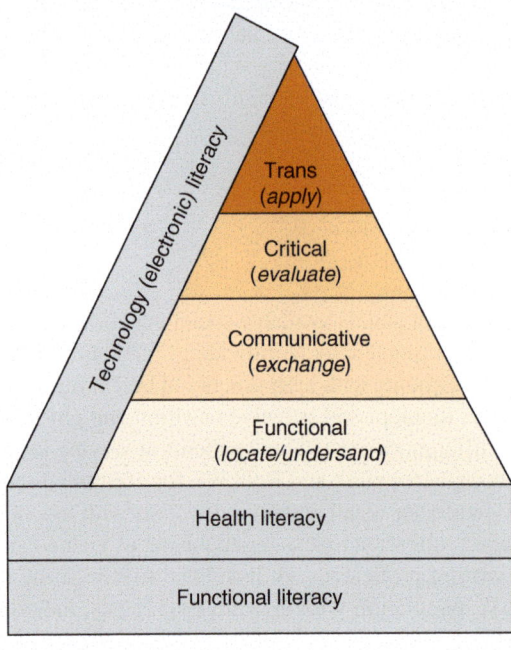

Fig. 16.1 Hierarchical intrapersonal eHealth skill set [50]

To navigate and benefit from eHealth, users call upon the cognitive and social skills of eHealth literacy to overcome adversities posed by online experiences [50]. Much like offline transactions of patient education and inquiry, there are physical (e.g., screen and keyboard functioning), semantic (e.g., community acronyms, scientific jargon), physiological (e.g., pain), and psychological (e.g., uncertainty, emotion) factors that challenge the eHealth experience [50]. These factors are often influenced by sociocultural determinants and influential in healthcare decision-making. Creating user-centered and literacy-sensitive programs are interventions that alleviate these factors [9]. However, semantic and psychological factors, which are less often considered, also influence the eHealth experience, influencing the desired type and quality of content [50]. Eliciting information about patients' eHealth needs, understanding perceived eHealth affordances, and examining how users overcome this constellation of factors will be critical in optimizing the eHealth experience and "matching" eHealth programs to patients.

eHealth Literacy Among Patients at Risk for Chronic Disease

Age

eHealth literacy is generally lower among older adults, as compared to their younger counterparts. Members of the Baby Boomer and Silent generations (born 1928–1964) have less eHealth awareness and lower confidence in their skills to access and engage with eHealth resources, as compared to Millennials (born 1981–1996) and members of Generation X (born 1965–1980; [48]). Age-related differences are attributed to biopsychosocial factors, which have a reciprocal effect on engaging in protective health behaviors. Clinicians must consider patients' eHealth acceptability, cognitive and physical state, and their desire to use social systems (both online or offline) to facilitate the eHealth experience.

Generational Factors

The acceptability and proficiency of eHealth is likely driven by generational differences. Generation X created the Internet and technology, whereas Millennials grew up with technology as a central tool to shape their personal and social identity. This is contrary to Baby Boomers and members of the Silent Generation, who had already established these critical identities and learned how to navigate life and healthcare in the absence of technology. Given the centrality of technology to their lives and everyday functioning, digital natives (i.e., Millennials, some members of Generation X) are roughly considered experts at assimilating technological features and translating information from online to offline settings. Baby Boomers and members of the Silent Generation, however, report lower adoption of technology and accepting it as a tool to navigate their health and the healthcare system [18]. Older adults tend to have limited trust in the Internet, especially when it comes to eHealth and confidence in its ability to securely protect their personal health information [76]. This effect is compounded when they lack the confidence and proficiency to easily navigate eHealth programs [47, 49]. As such, security concerns coupled with infrequent use of eHealth programs are significant forces that drive generational differences in eHealth literacy.

Biological Factors

The aging process alters the structural and physiologic functioning of the brain. According to Harada et al. [26], crystallized intelligence remains stable in normal cognitive aging, with most declining changes occurring in the form of fluid intelligence. Crystallized intelligence includes core knowledge, skills, and abilities that are developed over time, whereas fluid intelligence involves critical thinking, problem solving, processing speed (cognitive and motor), and reasoning in unfamiliar contexts. Generally, older adults have deeper crystallized intelligence than younger adults, primarily because they have had more life experiences to develop and apply these core skills. In the context of eHealth, however, crystallized intelligence is likely not an inherent strength among older adults, especially those in the Baby Boomer and Silent generations. Rather, younger adults possess greater core knowledge, skills, and abilities surrounding eHealth, given the diffusion of technology during their formative years. This has significant potential to contribute to older adults' declining cognitive and physical proficiency to navigate eHealth programs, adapt technological features and techniques, and collaborate with other online users to learn new information that can be assimilated to offline behaviors protective of chronic disease. Consistent with evidence supporting that cognitive building can help to alleviate the negative effects of aging [26], greater practice using eHealth and age-tailored interventions can enhance the skills of those at risk for low eHealth literacy [70].

Social Factors

eHealth skills can be strengthened across the lifespan with systems in place to facilitate social support. Hayat et al. [27] found that patients across the lifespan with compromised eHealth literacy reported positive health outcomes, especially if they were able to connect with homogeneous online users. Among adults over the age of 50, there is evidence that perceived trust in generic support groups declines with age but trust in Facebook increases [47]. This may be attributed to the close-knit ties of "friends" on Facebook. Among a sample of college students, reliance on social media for health-related information was associated with a high degree of eHealth literacy [49]. In this study, the relationship between social media use and eHealth literacy was strengthened if students reported heterogeneous social ties that provided novel information, but not emotional or relational support. Therefore, the type and degree of desired online social support varies across the lifespan to influence eHealth literacy.

Race/Ethnicity

African American (67%) and Hispanic adults (73%) are more likely than white adults (58%) to use smartphones to access health information [2]. Although there is no statistically significant difference in racial/ethnic adoption of eHealth apps [11], there is evidence that African Americans are more likely to use eHealth-related tracking services if they use online media (e.g., social media), access information to help another person, and have health insurance [16]. This is consistent with the finding of Rosenbaum et al. [59] that African Americans, although underrepresented in the literature, are more likely to participate in weight loss and management programs if the intervention includes a smartphone element. Further reports indicate that these active eHealth patients are more likely to participate if they have high eHealth literacy [31]. Although seminal research found no evidence for racial/ethnic differences in eHealth literacy [44], more recent research by Paige et al. [47] found that US Black/African Americans have a higher degree of eHealth literacy than white adults. Given the high degree of eHealth use and proficiency, smartphones remain an important technology to deliver culturally adapted and credible information and address healthcare disparities in chronic disease prevention, especially among at-risk racial/ethnic minorities [24]. African Americans with a high degree of eHealth literacy are more likely to trust health information from YouTube and online religious organizations and government entities than their white counterparts [47]. Attention must be paid to developing culturally adapted messages and interventions delivered through smartphones to both patients and caregivers from these accepted information sources.

Rurality

To date, there is limited knowledge about the eHealth literacy of patients who reside in rural locations [14]. Redmond [57] found that rural freshman college students were less skilled in their eHealth awareness and seeking skills, as compared to their non-rural counterparts. Interestingly, the self-reported ability of both rural and non-rural college students to evaluate and apply information learned was quite similar. Nearly a decade later, Witten and Humphry [74] reported that rural Hawaiian adults had access and confidence in eHealth resource awareness but felt challenged in their ability to interpret and apply the information learned from electronic sources. The narrowing digital divide in rural communities means it will be important for clinicians to consider the unique attributes of this unique subgroup, including eHealth acceptability and the sociocultural influence on desired health information (e.g., complementary medicine versus traditional medicine).

Conclusion

eHealth technologies and programs are critical tools to alleviate the burden of chronic disease in the general population. Structured and unstructured eHealth programs are used by the public and often result in positive behavior change, despite limitations in their quality and integrated evidence-based elements of behavior change theory. A reasonable explanation is that patients are aware of their information and behavior change needs and they have the skills (eHealth literacy) to adapt and appropriate functions of eHealth to meet those individual needs. As the quality of eHealth programs continue to improve and evidence for their efficacy continues to grow, clinicians must be proactive and facilitate open discussions about how eHealth can be supplemented within preventative healthcare plans. There is limited policy and support for clinicians to formally measure health literacy and eHealth literacy at each appointment to determine the appropriateness of eHealth [19]. Therefore, a more patient-centric approach would be to encourage clinicians to elicit conversations about patients' eHealth skills, motivations, and informational needs related to chronic disease prevention. Open discussions about eHealth skills and information needs can cultivate productive patient-provider relationships leading to culturally adapted and tailored approaches for chronic disease prevention.

References

1. Amante DJ, Hogan TP, Pagoto SL, English TM, Lapane KL. Access to care and use of the internet to search for health information: results from the US national health interview survey. J Med Internet Res. 2015;17(4). https://doi.org/10.2196/jmir.4126.
2. Anderson M. Racial and ethnic differences in how people use mobile technology. 2015, April 30. Retrieved from http://www.pewresearch.org/fact-tank/2015/04/30/racial-and-ethnic-differences-in-how-people-use-mobile-technology/.
3. Apple. Best of 2017. 2018. Retrieved 18 Sept 2018, from https://developer.apple.com/app-store/best-of-2017/apps-of-the-year/.
4. Azar KMJ, Lesser LI, Laing BY, Stephens J, Aurora MS, Burke LE, Palaniappan LP. Mobile applications for weight management: theory-based content analysis. Am J Prev Med. 2013;45(5):583–9. https://doi.org/10.1016/j.amepre.2013.07.005.
5. Bardus M, van Beurden SB, Smith JR, Abraham C. A review and content analysis of engagement, functionality, aesthetics, information quality, and change techniques in the most popular commercial apps for weight management. Int J Behav Nutr Phys Act. 2016;13:35. https://doi.org/10.1186/s12966-016-0359-9.
6. Berkman NC, Sheridan SL, Donahue KE, Halpern DJ, Crott K. Low health literacy and health outcomes: an updated systematic review. Ann Intern Med. 2011;155:97–107. https://doi.org/10.7326/0003-4819-155-2-201107190-00005.

7. Bowes P, Stevenson F, Ahluwalia S, Murray E. "I need her to be a doctor": patients' experiences of presenting health information from the internet in GP consultations. Br J Gen Pract. 2012;62(604):e732–8. https://doi.org/10.3399/bjgp12X658250.

8. Breton ER, Fuemmeler BF, Abroms LC. Weight loss-there is an app for that! But does it adhere to evidence-informed practices? Transl Behav Med. 2011;1(4):523–9. https://doi.org/10.1007/s13142-011-0076-5.

9. Brown W, Yen PY, Rojas M, Schnall R. Assessment of the health IT usability evaluation model (Health-ITUEM) for evaluating mobile health (mHealth) technology. J Biomed Inform. 2013;46(6):1080–7.

10. Bylund CL, Gueguen JA, Sabee CM, Imes RS, Li Y, Sanford AA. Provider-patient dialogue about internet health information: an exploration of strategies to improve the provider-patient relationship. Patient Educ Couns. 2007;66(3):346–52. https://doi.org/10.1016/j.pec.2007.01.009.

11. Carroll JK, Moorhead A, Bond R, LeBlanc WG, Petrella RJ, Fiscella K. Who uses mobile phone health apps and does use matter? A secondary data analytics approach. J Med Internet Res. 2017;19(4). https://doi.org/10.2196/jmir.5604.

12. Cavallo DN, Tate DF, Ries AV, Brown JD, DeVellis RF, Ammerman AS. A social media-based physical activity intervention. Am J Prev Med. 2012;43(5):527–32.

13. Centers for Disease Control and Prevention. Understanding literacy and numeracy. 2016, December 19. https://www.cdc.gov/healthliteracy/learn/UnderstandingLiteracy.html.

14. Chesser AK, Keene Woods N, Smothers K, Rogers N. Health literacy and older adults. Gerontol Geriatr Med. 2016;2. https://doi.org/10.1177/2333721416630492.

15. Ciampa PJ, Osborn CY, Peterson NB, Rothman RL. Patient numeracy, perceptions of provider communication and colorectal cancer screening utilization. J Health Commun. 2010;15(3):157–68. https://doi.org/10.1080/10810730.2010.522699.

16. Chisolm DJ, Sarkar M. E-health use in African American internet users: can new tools address old disparities? Telemed J E Health. 2015;21(3):163–9. https://doi.org/10.1089/tmj.2014.0107.

17. Chung JE. Patient–provider discussion of online health information: results from the 2007 health information national trends survey (HINTS). J Health Commun. 2013;18(6):627–48. https://doi.org/10.1080/10810730.2012.743628.

18. Chung JE, Park N, Wang H, Fulk J, McLaughlin M. Age differences in perceptions of online community participation among non-users: an extension of the technology acceptance model. Comput Hum Behav. 2010;26:1674–84.

19. Collins SA, Currie LM, Bakken S, Vawdrey DK, Stone PW. Health literacy screening instruments for eHealth applications: a systematic review. J Biomed Inform. 2012;45(3):598–607. https://doi.org/10.1016/j.jbi.2012.04.001.

20. Coughlin SS, Whitehead M, Sheats JQ, Mastromonico J, Hardy D, Smith SA. Smartphone applications for promoting healthy diet and nutrition: a literature review. Jacobs J Food Nutr. 2015;2(3):021.

21. Del Giudice P, Bravo G, Poletto M, De Odorico A, Conte A, Brunelli L, Arnoldo L, Brusaferro S. Correlation between eHealth literacy and health literacy using the eHealth literacy scale and real-life experiences in the health sector as a proxy measure of functional health literacy: a cross-sectional web-based survey. J Med Internet Res. 2018;20(10):e281. https://doi.org/10.2196/jmir.9401.

22. Fox S. Health topics. 2011, February 1. Retrieved from http://www.pewinternet.org/2011/02/01/health-information-is-a-popular-pursuit-online/.

23. Fox S. The social life of health information. 2014, January 15. Retrieved 7 May 2018, from http://www.pewresearch.org/fact-tank/2014/01/15/the-social-life-of-health-information/.

24. Gibbons MC, Leisher L, Slamon RE, Bass S, Kandadai V, Beck JR. Exploring the potential of Web 2.0 to address health disparities. J Health Comm. 2011;16:77–89.

25. Golbeck AL, Ahlers-Schmidt CR, Paschal AM, Dismuke SE. A definition and operational framework for health numeracy. Am J Prev Med. 2005;29(4):375–6.

26. Harada CN, Natelson Love MC, Triebel KL. Normal cognitive aging. Clin Geriatr Med. 2013;29(4):737–52. https://doi.org/10.1016/j.cger.2013.07.002.

27. Hayat T, Brainin E, Neter E. With some help from my network: supplementing eHealth literacy with social ties. J Med Internet Res. 2017;19(3):e98. https://doi.org/10.2196/jmir.6472.

28. Hesse BW, Nelson DE, Kreps GL, Croyle RT, Arora NK, Rimer BK, Viswanath K. Trust and sources of health information. Arch Intern Med. 2005;165:2618–24.

29. Houston TK, Allison JJ. Users of internet health information: differences by health status., users of internet health information: differences by health status. J Med Internet Res. 2002;4(2):E7. https://doi.org/10.2196/jmir.4.2.e7.

30. Huberty J, Green J, Glissman C, Larkey L, Puzia M, Lee C. Efficacy of the mindfulness meditation mobile app "Calm" to reduce stress among college students: Randomized controlled trial. JMIR mHealth uHealth. 2019;7(6):e14273. https://doi.org/10.2196/14273.

31. James DC, Harville C. eHealth literacy, online help-seeking behavior, and willingness to participate in mHealth chronic disease research among African Americans, Florida, 2014–2015. Prev Chronic Dis. 2016;13:160210. https://doi.org/10.5888/pcd13.160210.

32. Jiang S, Beaudoin CE. Health literacy and the Internet: an exploratory study on the 2013 HINTS survey. Comput Hum Behav. 2016;58:240–8.

33. Kebede M, Steenbock B, Helmer SM, Sill J, Mollers T, Pischke CR. Identifying evidence-informed physical activity apps: content analysis. JMIR Mhealth Uhealth. 2018;6(12):e10314. https://doi.org/10.2196/10314.

34. Krebs P, Duncan DT. Health app use among US mobile phone owners: a national survey. JMIR Mhealth Uhealth. 2015;3(4):e101. https://doi.org/10.2196/mhealth.4924.

35. LaPlante C, Peng W. A systematic review of eHealth interventions for physical activity: an analysis of study design, intervention characteristics, and outcomes. Telemed J E Health. 2011;17(7):509–23. https://doi.org/10.1089/tmj.2011.0013.

36. Li N, Orrange S, Kravitz RL, Bell RA. Reasons for and predictors of patients' online health information seeking following a medical appointment. Fam Pract. 2014;31(5):550–6.

37. Mackert M, Mabry-Flynn A, Champlin S, Donovan EE, Pounders K. Health literacy and health information technology adoption: the potential for a new digital divide. J Med Internet Res. 2016;18(10):e264. https://doi.org/10.2196/jmir.6349.

38. Mani M, Kavanagh DJ, Hides L, Stoyanov SR. Review and evaluation of mindfulness-based iPhone apps. JMIR Mhealth Uhealth. 2015;3(3):e82. https://doi.org/10.2196/mhealth.4328.

39. Meppelink C, Bol N. Exploring the role of health literacy on attention to and recall of text-illustrated health information. Journal of Computers in Human Behavior. 2015;48(C):87–93. https://doi.org/10.1016/j.chb.2015.01/027.

40. Middelweerd A, Mollee JS, van der Wal CN, Brug J, te Velde SJ. Apps to promote physical activity among adults: a review and content analysis. Int J Behav Nutr Phys Act. 2014;11:97. https://doi.org/10.1186/s12966-014-0097-9.

41. Mitsutake S, Shibata A, Ishii K, Oka K. Association of eHealth literacy with colorectal cancer knowledge and screening practice among internet users in Japan. J Med Internet Res. 2012;14(6). https://doi.org/10.2196/jmir.1927.

42. Mitsutake S, Shibata A, Ishii K, Oka K. Associations of eHealth literacy with health behavior among adult Internet users. J Med Internet Res. 2016;18(7):e192. https://doi.org/10.2196/jmir.5413.

43. Mudlers MDGH, Cornielle O, Klein O. Label reading, numeracy, and food and nutrition involvement. Appetite. 2018;128:214–22. https://doi.org/10.1016/j.appet.2018.06.003.

44. Neter E, Brainin E. eHealth literacy: extending the digital divide to the realm of health information. J Med Internet Res. 2012;14(1):e19. https://doi.org/10.2196/jmir.1619.

45. Norman GJ, Zabinski MF, Adams MA, Rosenberg DE, Yaroch AL, Atienza AA. A review of eHealth interventions for physical activity and dietary behavior change. Am J Prev Med. 2007;33(4):336–45. https://doi.org/10.1016/j.amepre.2007.05.007.

46. Ossebaard HC, Van Gemert-Pijnen L. eHealth and quality in health care: implementation time. Int J Qual Health Care. 2016;28(3):415–9. https://doi.org/10.1093/intqhc/mzw032.

47. Paige SR, Krieger JL, Stellefson ML. The influence of eHealth literacy on perceived trust in online health communication channels and sources. J Health Commun. 2017;22(1):53–65. https://doi.org/10.1080/10810730.2016.1250846.

48. Paige SR, Miller MD, Krieger JL, Stellefson M, Cheong J. eHealth literacy across the lifespan: a measurement invariance study. J Med Internet Res. 2018. https://doi.org/10.2196/10434.

49. Paige SR, Stellefson M, Chaney BH, Chaney JD, Alber JM, Chappell C, Barry AE. Examining the relationship between online social capital and eHealth literacy: implications for Instagram use for chronic disease prevention among college students. Am J Health Educ. 2017;48(4):264–77. https://doi.org/10.1080/19325037.2017.1316693.

50. Paige SR, Stellefson M, Krieger JL, Anderson-Lewis C, Cheong J, Stopka C. Proposing a transactional model of electronic health (eHealth) literacy: concept analysis. J Med Internet Res. 2018;20(10):e10175. https://doi.org/10.2196/10175.

51. Patha S, Hayhurt C, Ray N, Hilton H, Hine C, Payne H, West J. Health behavior change theories in physical activity pins on Pinterest: a content analysis. Health Educ Care. 2017;2(1):1–7. https://doi.org/10.15761/HEC.1000115.

52. Peters E, Hibbard J, Slovic P, Dieckmann N. Numeracy skill and the communication, comprehension, and use of risk-benefit information. Health Aff. 2007;26(3):741–8. https://doi.org/10.1377/hlthaff.26.3.741.

53. Petrič G, Atanasova S, Kamin T. Ill literates or illiterates? Investigating the eHealth literacy of users of online health communities. J Med Internet Res. 2017;19(10):e331. https://doi.org/10.2196/jmir.7372.

54. Pew Research Center. Internet/broadband fact sheet. 2018, February 5. Retrieved 15 Mar 2018, from http://www.pewinternet.org/fact-sheet/internet-broadband/.

55. Plaza I, Demarzo MMP, Herrera-Mercadal P, Garcia-Campayo J. Mindfulness-based mobile applications: Literature review and analysis of current features. JMIR mHealth uHealth. 2013;1(2):e24. https://doi.org/10.2196/mhealth.2733.

56. Rao VN, Tuttle LA, Sheridan SL, Lin FC, Shimbo D, Diaz KM, Hinderliter AL, Viera AJ. The effect of numeracy level on completeness of home blood pressure monitoring. J Clin Hypertens. 2015;17(1):39–45. https://doi.org/10.1111/jch.12443.

57. Redmond TL. Electronic (digital) health information competency: A comparative analysis of knowledge and skills of rural and non-rural freshman college students. Mount Pleasant, MI: Central Michigan University; 2007.

58. Reyna VF, Nelson WL, Han PK, Dieckmann NF. How numeracy influences risk comprehension and medical decision making. Psychol Bull. 2009;135(6):943–73. https://doi.org/10.1037/a0017327.
59. Rosenbaum DL, Piers AD, Schumacher LM, Kase CA, Butryn ML. Racial and ethnic minority enrollment in randomized controlled trials of behavioural weight loss utilizing technology: a systematic review. Obes Rev. 2017;18(7):808–17. https://doi.org/10.1111/obr.12545.
60. Schoeppe S, Alley S, van Lippevelde W, Bray NA, Williams SL, Duncan MJ, Vandelanotte C. Efficacy of interventions that use apps to improve diet, physical activity and sedentary behaviour: a systematic review. Int J Behav Nutr Phys Act. 2016;13(127). https://doi.org/10.1186/s12966-016-0454-y.
61. Scott TL, Gazmararian JA, Williams MV, Baker DW. Health literacy and preventive health care use among Medicare enrollees in a managed care organization. Med Care. 2002;40(5):395–404.
62. Shaw T, McGregor D, Brunner M, Keep M, Janssen A, Barnet S. What is eHealth (6)? Development of a conceptual model for eHealth: qualitative study with key informants. J Med Internet Res. 2017;19(10):e324. https://doi.org/10.2196/jmir.8106.
63. Silver MP. Patient perspectives on online health information and communication with doctors: a qualitative study of patients 50 years old and over. J Med Internet Res. 2015;17(1). https://doi.org/10.2196/jmir.3588.
64. Smith A, Anderson M. Social media use in 2018. 2018, March 1. Retrieved 12 Sept 2018, from http://www.pewinternet.org/2018/03/01/social-media-use-in-2018/.
65. Sorensen K, Van den Broucke S, Fullam J, Doyle G, Pelikan J, Slonska Z, Brand H, HLS-EU. Health literacy and public health: a systematic review and integration of definitions and models. BMC Public Health. 2012;12:80. https://doi.org/10.1186/1471-2458-12-80.
66. van Emmerik AAP, Berings F, Lancee J. Efficacy of a mindfulness-based mobile application: A randomized waiting-list controlled trial. Mindfulness. 2018;9(1):187–198. https://doi.org/10.1007/s12671-017-0761-7.
67. Vetter M, O'Connor H, O'Dwyer N, Orr R. Learning "Math on the Move": effectiveness of a combined numeracy and physical activity program for primary school children. J Phys Act Health. 2018;15(7):492–8. https://doi.org/10.1123/jpah.2017-0234.
68. Villani J, Mortensen K. Patient-provider communication and timely receipt of preventive services. Prev Med. 2013;57(5):658–63. https://doi.org/10.1016/j.ypmed.2013.08.034.
69. Volkman JE, Luger TM, Harvey KL, Hogan TP, Shimada SL, Amante D, et al. The National Cancer Institute's Health Information National Trends Survey [HINTS]: a national cross-sectional analysis of talking to your doctor and other healthcare providers for health information. BMC Fam Pract. 2014;15(1):111. https://doi.org/10.1186/1471-2296-15-111.
70. Watkins I, Xie B. eHealth literacy interventions for older adults: a systematic review of the literature. J Med Internet Res. 2014;16(11). https://doi.org/10.2196/jmir.3318.
71. West JH, Belvedere LM, Andreasen R, Frandsen C, Hall PC, Crookston BT. Controlling your "App"etite: how diet and nutrition-related mobile apps lead to behavior change. JMIR Mhealth Uhealth. 2017;5(7). https://doi.org/10.2196/mhealth.7410.
72. Wilkinson JL, Strickling K, Payne HE, Jensen KC, West JH. Evaluation of diet-related infographics on Pinterest for use of behavior change theories: a content analysis. JMIR Mhealth Uhealth. 2016;4(4). https://doi.org/10.2196/mhealth.6367.
73. Williams G, Hamm MP, Shulhan J, Vandermeer B, Hartling L. Social media interventions for diet and exercise behaviours: a systematic review and meta-analysis of randomised controlled trials. BMJ Open. 2014;4(2):e003926. https://doi.org/10.1136/bmjopen-2013-003926.
74. Witten NA, Humphry J. The electronic health literacy and utilization of technology for health in a remote Hawaiian community: Lana'i. Hawai'i J Med Public Health. 2018;77(3):51–9.
75. Yang CH, Maher JP, Conroy DE. Implementation of behavior change techniques in mobile applications for physical activity. Am J Prev Med. 2015;48(4):452–5. https://doi.org/10.1016/j.amepre.2014.10.010.
76. Zulman DM, Kirch M, Zheng K, An LC. Trust in the internet as a health resource among older adults: analysis of data from a nationally representative survey. J Med Internet Res. 2011;13(1):e19. https://doi.org/10.2196/jmir.1552.

Chapter 17
Integrative Approach in Cardiovascular Disease

Devinder Singh Dhindsa, Jia Shen, Pratik B. Sandesara, and Laurence S. Sperling

Keywords Cardiovascular disease · Prevention · Meditation · Mindfulness · Physical activity Cardiac rehabilitation · Nutrition

Key Points
- Cardiovascular disease (CVD) remains the major cause of morbidity and mortality in the developed world.
- Due to the economic impact of CVD, low-cost interventions are of particular interest.
- Physical activity is an underutilized, but critical, component of primary and secondary prevention of CVD.
- Meditation and mindfulness may have a role in prevention of CVD, though there is inconclusive evidence at this time.
- Dietary patterns have been found to significantly influence cardiometabolic risk factors.

Introduction

Cardiovascular disease (CVD) remains the leading cause of morbidity and mortality in the developed world [1]. In addition to the human cost of the disease, the economic cost of treating CVD is substantial. More than $200 billion are spent annually in the United States on treating patients with CVD, which is expected to increase to over $800 billion by 2030 [2]. The impact and cost of cardiovascular disease on our healthcare system has generated interest in finding low-cost interventions to address the epidemic. The aim of this chapter is to discuss the low-cost interventions such as physical activity, dietary interventions, and mindfulness/meditation.

D. S. Dhindsa · P. B. Sandesara · L. S. Sperling (✉)
Division of Cardiology, Department of Medicine, Emory University School of Medicine, Emory Clinical Cardiovascular Research Institute, Atlanta, GA, USA
e-mail: lsperli@emory.edu

J. Shen
Division of Cardiology, University of California San Diego, San Diego, CA, USA

© Springer Nature Switzerland AG 2020
J. Uribarri, J. A. Vassalotti (eds.), *Nutrition, Fitness, and Mindfulness*, Nutrition and Health, https://doi.org/10.1007/978-3-030-30892-6_17

Physical Activity and Fitness

Physical inactivity (PA) is widely recognized as an independent risk factor for cardiovascular disease (CVD) and associated with an estimated 6% of the coronary artery disease (CAD) burden worldwide [3]. Physical activity and fitness, on the other hand, are associated with a 25% reduction in all-cause mortality in CAD patients and 20–30% in the general population [4]. Despite the well-known cardiovascular benefits of exercise, 50.3% of men and 53.3% of women in the United States fail to meet general aerobic physical activity guidelines for adults (>30 minutes of moderate-intensity physical activity on most days of the week) [5]. Prevention of CVD entails primordial (prevention of risk factors), primary (treatment of risk factors), and secondary (prevention of recurrent cardiovascular events), which can be modulated by environmental (e.g., air pollution) and psychosocial stressors, lifestyle changes, and cardioprotective medications. Exercise-based cardiac rehabilitation (CR), which incorporates a structured exercise program, is the cornerstone for secondary prevention of CVD and is also associated with improvement in risk factors (e.g., blood pressure, lipids, rate of smoking) [6].

Benefits of Exercise

The cardioprotective effects of regular PA and improved cardiorespiratory fitness are achieved by multiple direct and indirect mechanisms. These include improvements in multiple CVD risk factors together with anti-atherogenic, anti-inflammatory, psychological, anti-ischemic, antithrombotic, and antiarrhythmic effects [6–8]. Cardiorespiratory fitness (CRF) is a powerful independent predictor of mortality in patients with CVD [7]. In patients with CAD, each 1 MET (1 MET = 3.5 ml of oxygen uptake/kg of body weight/minute) increase in exercise capacity is associated with an 8–35% reduction in mortality and is comparable to the mortality benefit achieved from cardioprotective medications, such as statins, beta blockers, low-dose aspirin, and angiotensin-converting enzyme inhibitors after MI [9]. For the least fit, least active, high-risk cohort (bottom 20%; <5 METs) with CVD, referral to structured exercise-based CR programs may be the key to improving cardiovascular health and outcomes.

Exercise training in patients with CVD leads to improved exercise capacity. Aerobic training increases the peak oxygen uptake (VO2max) and reduces the submaximal heart rate, systolic blood pressure, rate-pressure product (RPP), and subsequently decreases the myocardial oxygen requirement. As a result, the angina threshold (or exercise time to onset of ischemia) is increased. The magnitude of increase in VO2max varies with the severity of underlying disease and is often less in patients with CVD compared to healthy individuals, but the greatest potential for improvement is in the most deconditioned individuals. On average, CR patients usually have an 11–36% increase in VO2max with exercise training [8]. Improvements in the efficiency of oxygen delivery to tissues, myocardial oxygen supply, and HR recovery are also seen with exercise training. For patients with CVD, exercise training is associated with low risk of cardiovascular events in the supervised rehabilitation setting. Studies in the CR population show that the risk of cardiac arrest and death is approximately 1 in 115,000 and 1 in 750,000 patient hours of participation, respectively [7].

Exercise Prescription

The recommended intensity of exercise is usually determined by the baseline exercise testing. As an alternative to exercise testing, the maximum heart rate (HR) can be calculated using the following formula: maximum HR = 208 − (0.7 × age) [10]. HR reserve is the maximal HR minus the resting HR. In patients with CVD, the minimum or threshold intensity for improving cardiorespiratory fitness (VO2max) is about 45% of the oxygen uptake reserve. This corresponds to approximately 70% of the maximum HR achieved during symptom-limiting exercise testing [11]. Gradually, this should be increased to 50–80% of peak exercise capacity with HR reserve or oxygen uptake reserve [7]. The intensity should be reduced by approximately 10 beats below the ischemic threshold (HR at which typical angina occurs) for patients who are symptomatic. Adjunctively, the Borg Rating of Perceived Exertion (RPE) scale can also be used to determine the intensity of exercise [12]. Patients who are unable to attend supervised exercise training sessions should continue to exercise independently due to the cardiovascular benefits. In this case, the exercise intensity can be safely determined by using the "talk test," where patients are instructed to exercise at the highest intensity possible while able to have a comfortable conversation [7].

Moderate Versus High-Intensity Interval Training

Recent studies have compared the effectiveness of moderate-intensity continuous exercise training versus high-intensity interval training on changes in aerobic capacity and measures of CV function in coronary patients with and without postinfarction heart failure who were being optimally medically managed. Wisloff and colleagues randomized 27 patients with stable postinfarction heart failure (HF) to either moderate continuous training (70% of peak heart rate) or high-intensity aerobic interval training (95% of peak heart rate) 3 times per week for 12 weeks or to a control group that received standard advice regarding PA [13]. Improvements in cardiorespiratory fitness (46% vs 14%, p < 0.001), left ventricular remodeling, and brachial artery flow-mediated dilation (endothelial function) were greater with high-intensity aerobic interval training than moderate continuous training. Interval training seems more effective than continuous exercise for the improvement of aerobic capacity in CVD, but additional long-term studies assessing safety, compliance, and morbidity and mortality following interval training are needed [14].

Resistance Training

Resistance training should be incorporated into most exercise training programs. The increase in muscle mass, strength, and endurance improve the ability to perform activities of daily living in patients with CVD. These exercises should target major muscle groups (e.g., chest press, leg press, abdominal crunch/curl-up, biceps curl, etc.) to reduce the demands of daily activities, such as carrying and lifting objects. The training regimen should include a single set of 8–10 different exercises at a load that allows 8–15 repetitions [7]. In patients with heart disease, the Valsalva maneuver (forced expiration against a closed glottis) during resistance training can cause symptoms of myocardial ischemia due to increase in blood pressure and myocardial work. Patients may experience lightheadedness or dizziness if cardiac output is reduced [15]. Therefore, resistance training should be avoided in patients with unstable CAD, decompensated HF, severe aortic stenosis, hypertrophic cardiomyopathy, and retinopathy (risk of vitreous hemorrhage and retinal detachment) [15]. In addition, resistance training involving the upper body should be delayed for 8–12 weeks in patients with coronary artery bypass grafting (CABG) surgery and sternotomy to allow healing of the sternal wound [15].

Summary

Although data support PA as a proven preventive and therapeutic CV intervention, incorporating exercise into a comprehensive care plan remains largely neglected in contemporary medicine. Improving utilization of exercise in the face of increasingly busy lifestyles, especially the use of CR for secondary prevention, should be a priority. Our approach to CVD prevention and management must evolve to encompass pharmacological, interventional, and lifestyle modifications in the treatment armamentarium.

Meditation and Mindfulness

Another low-cost intervention that has generated considerable attention is meditation and mindfulness, an approach that has existed for thousands of years in a number of Eastern traditions [16]. According to the National Health Interview Survey (NHIS), 8.0% of US adult respondents stated they practice some form of meditation, although higher rates were claimed in those with chronic diseases, including CVD [17]. 17% of patients with chronic CVD indicated that they participated in mind-body therapies, and 94% of those that participated subjectively felt that these therapies were helpful [18]. In a population of Canadian patients with acute coronary syndrome (ACS), 35% stated they had participated in mind-body therapy at some point in their life, with 25% of respondents indicating they were currently practicing mind-body therapy [19].

There are a number of definitions of meditation and mindfulness. Meditation can be defined as "a family of mental practices that are designed to improve concentration, increase awareness of the present moment, and familiarize a person with the nature of their own mind" [20]. Similarly, a consensus definition of mindfulness is divided into two components, "The first component involves the self-regulation of attention so that it is maintained on immediate experience, thereby allowing for increased recognition of mental events in the present moment. The second component involves adopting a particular orientation toward one's experiences in the present moment, an orientation that is characterized by curiosity, openness, and acceptance" [21]. Traditions of mindfulness and meditation are developed to help participants of these practices maintain control of their attention, enhance awareness of self, and regulate emotions. The potential impact of this practice on health, particularly cardiovascular disease and its risk factors, is the subject of this section.

Meditation/Mindfulness for Primary Prevention of CVD

To date there has not been adequate data related to meditation and mindfulness on the primary prevention of cardiovascular mortality or the end points of nonfatal myocardial infarction (MI) or stroke. Two small studies, with 73 and 109 patients, showed that in those randomized to transcendental meditation training, improved survival was seen over the course of their follow-up, as compared to those randomized to the control group [22, 23]. In a post hoc analysis of the same two trials, a 23% reduction in all-cause mortality and 30% reduction in cardiovascular mortality were observed [2]. These results are striking if valid and accordingly need to be reproduced in a large, multicenter randomized controlled trial. There are more data on the effect of mindfulness and meditation on addressing traditional and nontraditional CVD risk factors.

Impact of Meditation and Mindfulness on CVD Risk Factors

Stress, Anxiety, and Depression

Stress, anxiety, and depression have been recognized as nontraditional risk factors for CVD [24–27]. In a meta-analysis of 18 randomized control trials, moderate-to-large reductions in depression symptoms within groups participating in mindful meditation were demonstrated [28]. Another meta-analysis of studies focusing on participants with a current depressive or anxiety episode found significant benefits on depressive symptom severity for mindfulness training relative to controls [29]. Mindfulness meditation programs showed a modest improvement in stress/distress in patients in a meta-analysis of randomized control trials by the Agency for Healthcare Research and Quality [30]. In patients with CVD, those who participated in mindfulness meditation had significantly lower levels of perceived stress and anger [31]. In addition, perceived decreases in mental stress have correlated with decreases in biomarkers of stress in those undergoing mindfulness meditation (i.e., salivary cortisol, salivary amylase, interleukin-6), although the impact of these findings on clinical outcomes require further investigation [32–35].

Hypertension

Mindfulness meditation has been studied for blood pressure reduction, with largely mixed results. The Hypertension Analysis of Stress Reduction Using Mindfulness Meditation and Yoga (HARMONY) trial did not find any benefit in patients randomized to an 8-week mindfulness-based stress reduction program as compared to the control [36]. In contrast, a small study of 20 older, low-income, African-Americans showed that in those randomized to a mindfulness meditation program, a 22 mmHg lower systolic blood pressure (SBP) (p = 0.020), as well as a 17 mmHg reduction in diastolic blood pressure (p = 0.003) was seen [37]. A limitation of this trial was the small sample size, though the results were dramatic. Several other studies have shown more modest results. 201 black patients with angiographic evidence of CVD randomized to a transcendental meditation program were shown to have a 4.9 mmHg lower SBP than those randomized to health education alone [38]. However, a 2007 Agency for Healthcare Research and Quality report consisting of numerous meta-analyses found no significant benefit between a number of meditation techniques as compared to health education [39]. A 2015 meta-analysis of 12 randomized controlled trials of African-American patients found a mean reduction of systolic/diastolic BP of 4/2 mmHg, respectively, when compared to controls [40]. Clearly, the ability to generalize the findings of the effect of mindfulness and meditation on hypertension is limited by the lack of the reproducibility of results and requires further investigation.

Tobacco Use

The efficacy of mindfulness meditation has shown some benefit in tobacco cessation. In a study of 27 smokers randomized to mindfulness meditation or relaxation training, a 60% reduction in smoking was seen in those in the mindfulness meditation arm, with no change in smoking seen in the relaxation training group. This correlated with functional MRI studies showing increased activity in the anterior cingulate and prefrontal cortex in the meditation group, indicating higher activity in the areas responsible for self-control [41]. A meta-analysis of four RCTs of mindfulness training as compared to control showed 25% of patients participating in mindfulness training were able to remain abstinent from smoking for more than 4 months, as compared to 14% of the control groups (tobacco cessation counselling alone) [42].

Medication Nonadherence

There have been no studies of the effect of mindfulness meditation on adherence to medications in a CVD population specifically [43]. However, studies in other chronic diseases, specifically HIV, have shown some promising results regarding adherence. In a pilot randomized controlled trial of 72 HIV-infected youth randomized to mindfulness meditation or control, those in the intervention group were 44% more likely to have gone from high viral load to low viral load, a finding that is thought likely due to improved antiretroviral therapy adherence [44]. Further randomized controlled trials are needed, particularly in a population of patients with CVD, to determine the efficacy of mindfulness and meditation on improving medication adherence.

Summary

Meditation and mindfulness may play a role in reducing CVD morbidity and mortality, though at present this is inconclusive given insufficient data. Meditation and mindfulness do represent a low-cost intervention that may have some benefit in mitigating some of the risk factors for CVD. Accordingly, the American Heart Association Scientific Statement has indicated "Meditation may be considered as a reasonable adjunct to guideline-directed cardiovascular risk reduction by those interested in this lifestyle modification, with the understanding that the benefits of such intervention remain to be better established" [20].

The mainstay of cardiovascular prevention is the implementation of proven guideline-directed approaches for primary prevention and addressing CVD risk factors. Further research is needed regarding the benefit of mindfulness and meditation, with emphasis on randomized control trials with adequate power and long-term follow-up to evaluate cardiovascular outcomes and mortality. Currently available data consists of small trials with short-term follow-up, with limited data on CVD and CV mortality. Current recommendations are that these interventions may be used as a low-harm adjunct to proven behavioral approaches and therapies for CVD prevention.

Nutrition and Cardiovascular Disease

Dietary patterns influence cardiometabolic risk factors including adiposity, blood pressure, glucose-insulin homeostasis, lipids, endothelial function, inflammation, cardiac function, thrombosis, and vascular adhesion (Fig. 17.1). High body mass index is the second and third leading cause of morbidity and mortality in the United States [46] as consumption of high-calorie diets is resulting in an epidemic of obesity and insulin resistance. Healthy dietary practices, at all stages of life, are integral to the prevention and treatment of CVD [47]. Observational and randomized studies on diet and health

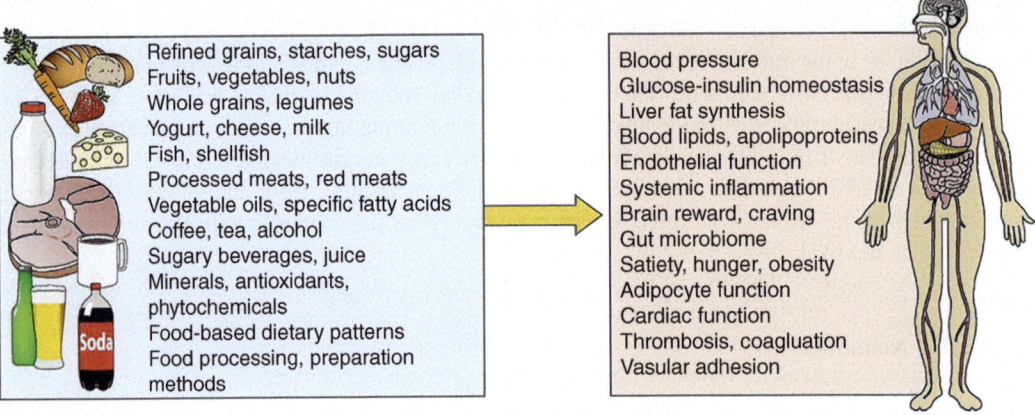

Fig. 17.1 Diet and cardiometabolic risk – pathways and mechanisms. Each of these dietary factors influences many or even all of these pathways. (Used with permission from Mozaffarian [45])

outcomes are challenging due to difficulties in measuring dietary intake and adherence over periods of time needed to see an effect on cardiovascular health [48]. As a result, current dietary recommendations are based on a combination of observational studies and interventional trial evidence supplemented by findings from mechanistic studies [47]. Dietary recommendations have evolved from nutrient-based to food-based dietary patterns which are more easily translatable when counseling patients [49]. In this section we review the current evidence and recommendations for nutritional interventions in the prevention and treatment of cardiometabolic disease.

Excess Caloric Intake

Excess caloric intake, usually in the form of saturated fatty acids, added sugars, sodium-laden foods, and refined grains, results in accumulation of fat and weight gain. Selection of a nutrient-dense dietary pattern that leads to maintenance of a healthy body weight is crucial for maintaining cardiometabolic health. Currently, the US Department of Health recommends adult women and men consume between 1600–2400 and 2000–3000 calories per day, respectively, depending on activity level [50]. Caloric restriction leads to significant improvements in inflammation and insulin sensitivity resulting in decreased atherosclerosis [51]. Unfortunately, significant sustained weight loss through dieting can be difficult to maintain. Evidence suggests that low-carbohydrate and Mediterranean diets are superior to low-fat diets in maintaining weight loss [52].

Dietary Patterns and Food Groups

Dietary patterns represent the overall combination of foods habitually consumed, which produce synergistic effects on cardiovascular health. The dietary patterns with the most evidence of cardiovascular benefit are the Dietary Approaches to Stop Hypertension (DASH), Mediterranean, and American Heart Association (AHA) patterns. Importantly, they share several fundamental characteristics. These include the high consumption of minimally processed food from plant sources such as fruits, nuts/seeds, vegetables (excluding corn and white potatoes), legumes, and whole grains and, in addition, a focus on low-to-moderate consumption of dairy, eggs, poultry, and seafood, as well as minimal consumption of red meats, processed meats, foods rich in refined grains, starches, and added sugars (Table 17.1). These diets are higher in fiber, vitamins, antioxidants, minerals, phenolics, and unsaturated fats and lower in carbohydrates, salt, and saturated fats.

The consumption of minimally processed, plant-derived foods such as fruits, non-starchy vegetables, beans/legumes, and nuts/seeds has been consistently associated with improved cardiometabolic outcomes [53, 54]. Observed long-term benefits are supported by controlled trials using dietary patterns rich in these food groups [55]. Various phytochemicals and micronutrients such as folate, potassium, fiber, and flavonoids are hypothesized to be responsible for the observed benefits. Potatoes are a widely consumed starchy vegetable and are rich in fiber and vitamins C and B6. However, their consumption results in a high-glucose load and has been associated with greater weight gain, type 2 diabetes, and CVD [56]. As a result, potato consumption is excluded from recommendations to increase vegetable intake.

The consumption of whole grains is associated with a substantially lower risk of CVD and mortality [57]. Whole grains consist of an endosperm (starch) encased by bran and germ layers rich in fiber, protein, B vitamins, flavonoids, antioxidants, and phytochemicals. When whole grains are intact (e.g., quinoa) or partially intact (e.g., stone ground oats), the bran protects the starchy endosperm from rapid oral and gastric digestion resulting in greater satiety and a lower glycemic response [58].

Table 17.1 Dietary Principles for Cardiometabolic Health[a, b] [45]

Food group	Goal	One serving equals	Examples
Consume more			
Fruits	3 servings/day	1 medium-sized fruit ½ cup of fresh, frozen, dried or unsweetened canned fruit ½ cup of 100% fruit juice	Blueberries, strawberries, apple, orange, banana, grapes, avocado, mango, and tomato. Whole fruits are preferable to 100% juice which should be limited to ≤1 serving/day
Vegetables (including legumes, excluding potatoes)	3 servings/day	2 cups of raw leafy vegetables 1 cup of cut raw/cooked vegetables 1 cup of 100% vegetable juice ½ cup of cooked beans	Focus on spinach, kale, and other green leafy plants, broccoli, carrots, onions, peppers, peas, beans, and lentils. Minimize starchy vegetables, especially corn and potatoes
Whole grains[c]	3 servings/day	1 slice of bread 1 cup of cereal ½ cup of cooked rice, pasta, or cereal	Oats, quinoa, bulgur, couscous, barley, whole-grain breads, cereals, and brown rice
Nut, seeds	4 servings/week	1 ounce (24 almonds, 18 cashews, 15 pecans or walnut halves)	Almonds, walnuts, hazelnuts, cashews, pecans, sunflower seeds, and sesame seeds
Fish, shellfish	≥2 servings/week	3.5 ounces (100 g)	Prefer oily fish such as salmon, tuna, mackerel, trout, herring, and sardines
Dairy products (especially yogurt and cheese)	2–3 servings/day	1 cup of skim milk or yogurt 1 ounce of cheese	Yogurt, cheese, or low-fat/skim milk
Vegetable oils (especially phenolic and unsaturated fat-rich oils)	2–6 servings/day	1 teaspoon of oil 1 tablespoon of vegetable spread	Prefer extra virgin olive oil, soybean, and canola oil. Consider safflower and peanut oil and margarine spreads
Eggs	1 egg or 2 egg whites per day		
Consume less			
Refined grains, starches, and added sugars[c]	No more than 1–2 servings/day	1 slice bread ½ cup of rice or cereal 1 sweet or dessert	White bread, white rice, most breakfast cereals, crackers, granola bars, sweets, bakery desserts, and added sugars
Processed meats	No more than 1 serving/week	1.75 ounces (50 g)	Preserved (sodium, nitrates) meats such as bacon, sausage, hot dogs, pepperoni, salami, and low-fat deli meats (turkey, chicken, ham)
Unprocessed red meats	No more than 1–2 servings/week	3.5 ounces (100 g)	Fresh/frozen beef, lamb, or pork
Trans fat	Avoid	Any food containing partially hydrogenated vegetable oil	Certain stick margarines, commercially prepared baked foods, snack foods, and deep fried foods
Other nutrient considerations			
Fiber	Consume 28–30 g/day	Whole grains, fruits, vegetables, legumes, nuts, and seeds	
Saturated fat	<7–8% of daily caloric intake	Soft margarines or meat; avoid butter, cream, beef tallow, lard, and tropical oils (palm and coconut oil)	

Table 17.1 (continued)

Food group	Goal	One serving equals	Examples
Sodium	<2000 mg/day <1500 mg/day if hypertensive	Often used as a preservative. Common hidden sources include bread, chicken, cheese, processed meats, soups, and canned foods	
Alcohol	No more than 2 drinks/day men and 1–1.5 drinks/day women	12 ounces of beer 8 ounces of malt liquor 5 ounces of wine 1.5 ounces of distilled spirits	
Sugar-sweetened beverages	Avoid	8-ounce beverage 1 small sweet pastry or dessert	Soda, fruit drinks, sports drinks, energy drinks, and iced teas
Coffee (black)	3–4 cups daily	8-ounce cup	n/a

[a]Based on a 2000 kcal/diet. Servings should be adjusted accordingly for lower or higher energy consumption
[b]Adapted from Mozaffarian [45]
[c]When selecting whole grains, use and consider the ratio of carbohydrate to dietary fiber. Food with ratios <10:1 (or >1 g of fiber for every 10 g of carbohydrate) are preferable. Minimally processed whole grains are preferable to finely milled whole grains

Refined and highly processed grains (e.g., white bread or pasta) should be consumed in moderation or avoided. A ratio of total carbohydrate to dietary fiber of <10:1 can be useful when trying to identify healthier grain choices [59].

Nuts and legumes are rich sources of plant proteins, fatty acids, fiber, antioxidant vitamins, minerals, and phytochemicals [53]. Frequent nut consumption is associated with decreased inflammatory markers, increased resistance to cholesterol oxidation, and decreased LDL-C and increased HDL-C [60]. In high-risk individuals the consumption of a Mediterranean dietary pattern supplemented with olive oil or nuts significantly reduced cardiovascular events by 30% compared to a control reduced-saturated fat diet [55]. A meta-analysis of 25 observational studies found that 4 servings per week of nuts was inversely associated with fatal CVD [HR = 0.76 (95% CI: 0.69–0.84)] and nonfatal CVD [HR = 0.78 (95% CI: 0.67–0.92)] [53].

Fish are a rich source of polyunsaturated omega-3 fatty acids (PUFA). Deep saltwater fish, such as salmon, mackerel, and tuna, are generally fattier and contain higher concentrations of omega-3 free fatty acids than other fish. Omega-3 fatty acids improve cholesterol profiles, endothelial function, blood pressure, and reduce inflammation, thrombosis, and myocardial oxygen demand [61]. In comparison with little or no consumption, moderate consumption of fish (2–4 servings/week) is associated with lower risk of fatal CVD (HR = 0.79 (95% CI: 0.67–0.92)]; however, this benefit was not seen with higher consumption [62]. The effects of fish consumption on other vascular conditions such as stroke and heart failure have been inconclusive [61]. The bioconcentration of organic pollutants, such as methylmercury and dioxins, in larger wild-caught predatory fish may reduce some of the cardiovascular benefits of their consumption [63]. The danger is greatest in the neurocognitive development of the fetus. Pregnant and nursing women should follow US Food and Drug Administration guidance to eat 2–3 servings/week of a variety of fish lower in mercury [64].

Dairy products represent a diverse class of foods with complex effects on cardiometabolic health that may be a result of their differing amounts of calcium, vitamin D, fat, fermentation, and probiotic composition in milk, cheese, and yogurt products [45]. The consumption of dairy, especially yogurt, is weakly associated with decreased systolic and diastolic blood pressure, abdominal obesity, and cardiovascular events [65, 66]. Current evidence supports moderate consumption of yogurt and possibly cheese, with the choice between low fat and whole fat being up to personal preference [45].

Meat is a rich source of protein and fat but contains no fiber and few antioxidant nutrients; its energy displaces that from plant foods, which contain an abundance of essential nutrients and antioxidants [67].

The consumption of processed meats (i.e., hamburgers, hot dogs, cold cuts) has been shown to increase the risk of CVD in a linear fashion [68]. This is thought to be due to the high concentrations of sodium and nitrites, which are used as preservatives in processed meats. The consumption of red meats (i.e., beef, lamb, pork) is associated with an increased risk for type 2 diabetes and cardiovascular disease [68, 69]. In comparison the consumption of eggs and poultry has not been consistently shown to negatively impact cardiometabolic health [70, 71]. The substitution of processed and red meats with other sources of protein such as fish, poultry, and eggs is associated with a lower incidence of cardiovascular disease and mortality [69, 72]. These recommendations are summarized in Table 17.1.

Beverages

Numerous studies have shown that higher consumption of sugar-sweetened beverages (SSB), such as sodas, energy drinks, and artificial juices, is associated with an increased prevalence of obesity, type 2 diabetes, and cardiovascular disease [73, 74]. These associations are likely attributable to a high glycemic/insulin response in combination with low satiation resulting in increased adiposity [75]. The consumption of black coffee has a J-shaped relationship with CVD – with the consumption of 3–4 cups daily associated with lowest risk [76]. Similarly, alcohol also demonstrates a J-shaped relationship with cardiovascular disease, with both abstainers and heavy drinkers having increased risk compared to moderate drinkers [77, 78]. The exact nadir of risk varies by age, sex, and ethnicity but is lowest in individuals who consume 1–2 drinks per day [78]. In addition, the pattern of drinking is important: benefits are seen with moderate use across multiple days per week, not with high levels on a few days [79]. The consumption of alcohol is not benign and is associated with an increased risk of cancers, liver disease, cardiomyopathy, and accidents [80]. Alcohol intake should not be encouraged solely as a means to reduce CVD risk; rather patients who already drink should be advised to do so in moderation.

Sodium

Dietary sodium raises blood pressure in a dose-dependent fashion with stronger effects among the elderly, those with preexisting hypertension, and blacks [81]. High sodium intake is associated with increased risk of stroke, CVD, and mortality [82]. Overall, the sum of the evidence suggests that optimal levels of sodium intake are <2 g/day with possible additional benefit down to <1.5 g/day in patients with hypertension, HF, or chronic kidney disease [81, 83]. In North America, ~75% of dietary sodium comes from packaged foods and restaurants, with minor contributions from home cooking or table salt [84]. Patients should be warned to avoid these "hidden" sources of dietary sodium, such as the AHA's salty six common foods, including breads and rolls, sandwiches, cold cuts and cured meats, pizza, soup, and burritos and tacos.

Summary

Dietary patterns have been found to significantly influence cardiometabolic risk factors (Fig. 17.1). Recommendations should focus on specific foods or dietary patterns instead of focusing on single isolated nutrients. Selection of a nutrient-dense dietary pattern that leads to maintenance of a healthy body weight is crucial for maintaining cardiometabolic health. Dietary patterns that are rich in fruits,

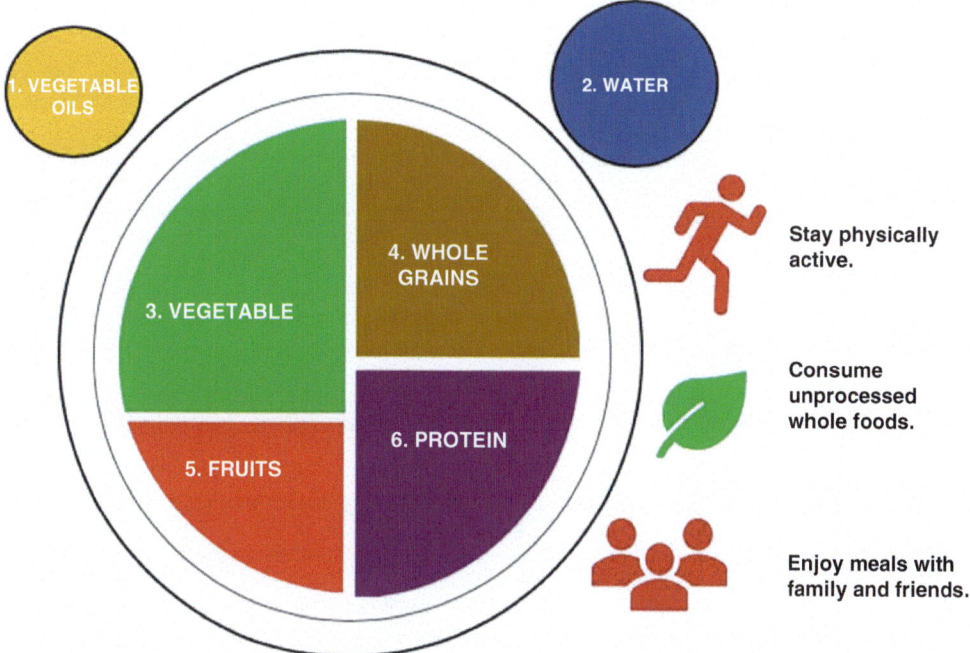

1. Vegetable Oils: Minimal use of healthy plant-based oils, such as olive and canola oils. Avoid saturated fats, such as butter, and tropical oils such as coconut and palm oil.

2. Water: Drink 1-2 L of water daily. Drink tea or black coffee. Limit milk and juice to 1 serving/day. Avoid sugar-sweetened beverages, such as soda and energy drinks. Limit alcohol to 2 servings/day in men and 1.5 servings/day in women.

3. Vegetables: Approximately half of your plate should consist of non-starchy vegetables, such as spinach, kale, peppers, carrots, and broccoli. The greater the variety the better. Limit/avoid the consumption of starchy vegetables, such as potatoes and corn.

4. Whole Grains: Approximately one quarter of your plate should consist of whole grains, such as quinoa, farro, oats, or brown rice. Avoid refined "white" grains such as white bread or rice.

5. Fruits: Approximately one fifth of your plate should consist of a variety of fruits, such as apples, oranges, and berries. These make an excellent dessert.

6. Protein: Approximately one quarter of your plate should consist of a protein such as fish, poultry, soy, or nuts. Limit red meats and avoid processed meats, such as bacon, hot dogs, or cold cuts.

Fig. 17.2 Heart-healthy plate

vegetables, nuts, whole grains, and fish; encourage moderate consumption of dairy, poultry, and eggs; and have minimal consumption or avoidance of red meats, processed foods, refined grains, and sugars demonstrate the greatest cardiometabolic health benefits. These recommendations are summarized in Fig. 17.2.

Conclusion

Approximately 90% of cardiovascular risk can be mediated via control of modifiable risk factors [85]. The interventions listed above represent low-cost, low-risk interventions that add to the therapeutic armamentarium for clinicians and patients. Implementation of programs and strategies to support the adoption of these interventions in those at risk is an important component of cardiovascular disease prevention going forward.

References

1. World Health Organization. Global health observatory data repository. Cardiovascular diseases, deaths per 100,000. Data by country. 2016. Available at: http://apps.who.int/gho/data/node.main.A865CARDIOVASCULAR?lang=en. Accessed 22 Aug 2018.
2. Heidenreich PA, Trogdon JG, Khavjou OA, Butler J, Dracup K, Ezekowitz MD, Finkelstein EA, Hong Y, Johnston SC, Khera A, Lloyd-Jones DM, Nelson SA, Nichol G, Orenstein D, Wilson PW, Woo YJ, on behalf of the American Heart Association Advocacy Coordinating Committee; Stroke Council; Council on Cardiovascular Radiology and Intervention; Council on Clinical Cardiology; Council on Epidemiology and Prevention; Council on Arteriosclerosis; Thrombosis and Vascular Biology; Council on Cardiopulmonary; Critical Care; Perioperative and Resuscitation; Council on Cardiovascular Nursing; Council on the Kidney in Cardiovascular Disease; Council on Cardiovascular Surgery and Anesthesia, and Interdisciplinary Council on Quality of Care and Outcomes Research. Forecasting the future of cardiovascular disease in the United States: a policy statement from the American Heart Association. Circulation. 2011;123(8):933–44.
3. Lee IM, Shiroma EJ, Lobelo F, Puska P, Blair SN, Katzmarzyk PT. Effect of physical inactivity on major non-communicable diseases worldwide: an analysis of burden of disease and life expectancy. Lancet (London, England). 2012;380(9838):219–29.
4. Iestra JA, Kromhout D, van der Schouw YT, Grobbee DE, Boshuizen HC, van Staveren WA. Effect size estimates of lifestyle and dietary changes on all-cause mortality in coronary artery disease patients: a systematic review. Circulation. 2005;112(6):924–34.
5. Centers for Disease Control and Prevention. Prevalence of regular physical activity among adults--United States, 2001 and 2005. MMWR Morb Mortal Wkly Rep. 2007;56:1209–12.
6. Sandesara PB, Lambert CT, Gordon NF, Fletcher GF, Franklin BA, Wenger NK, et al. Cardiac rehabilitation and risk reduction: time to "rebrand and reinvigorate". J Am Coll Cardiol. 2015;65(4):389–95.
7. Fletcher GF, Ades PA, Kligfield P, Arena R, Balady GJ, Bittner VA, et al. Exercise standards for testing and training: a scientific statement from the American Heart Association. Circulation. 2013;128(8):873–934.
8. Leon AS, Franklin BA, Costa F, Balady GJ, Berra KA, Stewart KJ, et al. Cardiac rehabilitation and secondary prevention of coronary heart disease: an American Heart Association scientific statement from the Council on Clinical Cardiology (Subcommittee on Exercise, Cardiac Rehabilitation, and Prevention) and the Council on Nutrition, Physical Activity, and Metabolism (Subcommittee on Physical Activity), in collaboration with the American Association of Cardiovascular and Pulmonary Rehabilitation. Circulation. 2005;111(3):369–76.
9. Boden WE, Franklin BA, Wenger NK. Physical activity and structured exercise for patients with stable ischemic heart disease. JAMA. 2013;309(2):143–4.
10. Roy S, McCroy J. Validation of maximal heart rate prediction equations based on sex and physical activity status. Int J Exerc Sci. 2015;8:318–30.
11. Swain DP, Brawner CA, American College of Sports Medicine. ACSM's resource manual for guidelines for exercise testing and prescription. Philadelphia: Lippincott Williams & Wilkins; 2012.
12. Borg GA. Psychophysical bases of perceived exertion. Med Sci Sports Exerc. 1982;14:377–81.
13. Wisloff U, Stoylen A, Loennechen JP, Bruvold M, Rognmo O, Haram PM, et al. Superior cardiovascular effect of aerobic interval training versus moderate continuous training in heart failure patients: a randomized study. Circulation. 2007;115(24):3086–94.
14. Elliott AD, Rajopadhyaya K, Bentley DJ, Beltrame JF, Aromataris EC. Interval training versus continuous exercise in patients with coronary artery disease: a meta-analysis. Heart Lung Circ. 2015;24(2):149–57.
15. Williams MA, Haskell WL, Ades PA, Amsterdam EA, Bittner V, Franklin BA, et al. Resistance exercise in individuals with and without cardiovascular disease: 2007 update: a scientific statement from the American Heart Association Council on Clinical Cardiology and Council on Nutrition, Physical Activity, and Metabolism. Circulation. 2007;116(5):572–84.
16. Gawler I, Bedson P. Meditation. An in-depth guide. Jeremy P. Tarcher/Penguin: New York; 2011. Accessed 29 Aug 2018.
17. National Center for Complementary and Integrative Health. Use of complementary health approaches in the U.S. National Health Interview Survey. National Center for Complementary and Integrative Health. National Institute of Medicine; 2012. Available at: https://nccih.nih.gov/research/statistics/NHIS/2012/mind-body/meditation. Accessed 22 Sept 2018.
18. Yeh GY, Davis RB, Phillips RS. Use of complementary therapies in patients with cardiovascular disease. Am J Cardiol. 2006;98:673–68.
19. Leung YW, Tamim H, Stewart DE, Arthur HM, Grace SL. The prevalence and correlates of mind-body therapy practices in patients with acute coronary syndrome. Complement Ther Med. 2008;16(5):254–61.
20. Levine GN, Lange RA, Bairey-Merz CN, Davidson RJ, Jamerson K, Mehta PK, et al. Meditation and cardiovascular risk reduction. a scientific statement from the American Heart Association. J Am Heart Assoc. 2017;6(10):e002218.

21. Bishop SR, Lau M, Shapiro S, et al. Mindfulness: a proposed operational definition. Clin Psychol-Sci Pract. 2004;11(3):230–41.
22. Alexander CN, Langer EJ, Newman RI, Chandler HM, Davies JL. Transcendental meditation, mindfulness, and longevity: an experimental study with the elderly. J Pers Soc Psychol. 1989;57(6):950–64.
23. Barnes J, Schneider RH, Alexander CN, Rainforth M, Staggers F, Salerno J. Impact of transcendental meditation on mortality in older African Americans with hypertension—eight-year follow-up. J Soc Behav Pers. 2005;17:201–16.
24. Celano CM. Anxiety disorders and cardiovascular disease. Curr Psychiatry Rep. 2016;18(11):101.
25. Dimsdale JE. Psychological stress and cardiovascular disease. J Am Coll Cardiol. 2008;51(13):1237–46.
26. Hare DL, Toukhsati SR, Johansson P, Jaarsma T. Depression and cardiovascular disease: a clinical review. Eur Heart J. 2014;35(21):1365–72.
27. Roest AM, Martens EJ, de Jonge P, Denollet J. Anxiety and risk of incident coronary heart disease: a meta-analysis. J Am Coll Cardiol. 2010;56(1):38–46.
28. Jain FA, Walsh RN, Eisendrath SJ, Christensen S, Cahn BR. Critical analysis of the efficacy of meditation therapies for acute and subacute phase treatment of depressive disorders: a systematic review. Psychosomatics. 2015;56(2):140–52.
29. Strauss C, Cavanagh K, Oliver A, Pettman D. Mindfulness-based interventions for people diagnosed with a current episode of an anxiety or depressive disorder: a meta-analysis of randomised controlled trials. PLoS One. 2014;9(4):e96110.
30. Goyal M, Singh SS, Sibinga EM, Gould NF, Rowland-Seymour A, Sharma R, Berger Z, Sleicher D, Maron DD, Shihab HM, Ranasinghe PD, Linn S, Saha S, Bass EB, Haythornthwaite JA. Meditation programs for psychological stress and well-being. Comparative effectiveness review no. 124. Agency for Healthcare Research and Quality: Rockville; 2014.
31. Momeni J, Omidi A, Raygan F, Akbari H. The effects of mindfulness-based stress reduction on cardiac patients blood pressure, perceived stress, and anger: a single-blind randomized controlled trial. J Am Soc Hypertens: JASH. 2016;10(10):763–71.
32. Carlson LE, Doll R, Stephen J, Faris P, Tamagawa R, Drysdale E, et al. Randomized controlled trial of mindfulness-based cancer recovery versus supportive expressive group therapy for distressed survivors of breast cancer. J Clin Oncol. 2013;31(25):3119–26.
33. Lipschitz DL, Kuhn R, Kinney AY, Donaldson GW, Nakamura Y. Reduction in salivary alpha-amylase levels following a mind-body intervention in cancer survivors--an exploratory study. Psychoneuroendocrinology. 2013;38(9):1521–31.
34. Pace TW, Negi LT, Adame DD, Cole SP, Sivilli TI, Brown TD, et al. Effect of compassion meditation on neuroendocrine, innate immune and behavioral responses to psychosocial stress. Psychoneuroendocrinology. 2009;34(1):87–98.
35. Rosenkranz MA, Davidson RJ, Maccoon DG, Sheridan JF, Kalin NH, Lutz A. A comparison of mindfulness-based stress reduction and an active control in modulation of neurogenic inflammation. Brain Behav Immun. 2013;27(1):174–84.
36. Blom K, Baker B, How M, Dai M, Irvine J, Abbey S, et al. Hypertension analysis of stress reduction using mindfulness meditation and yoga: results from the HARMONY randomized controlled trial. Am J Hypertens. 2014;27(1):122–9.
37. Palta P, Page G, Piferi RL, Gill JM, Hayat MJ, Connolly AB, et al. Evaluation of a mindfulness-based intervention program to decrease blood pressure in low-income African-American older adults. J Urban Health: Bull N Y Acad Med. 2012;89(2):308–16.
38. Schneider RH, Grim CE, Rainforth MV, Kotchen T, Nidich SI, Gaylord-King C, et al. Stress reduction in the secondary prevention of cardiovascular disease: randomized, controlled trial of transcendental meditation and health education in blacks. Circ Cardiovasc Qual Outcomes. 2012;5(6):750–8.
39. Ospina MB, Bond K, Karkhaneh M, Tjosvold L, Vandermeer B, Liang Y. Meditation practices for health: state of the research. Rockville: Agency for Healthcare Research and Quality Evidence Report/Technology; Assessment Number 155; 2007.
40. Bai Z, Chang J, Chen C, Li P, Yang K, Chi I. Investigating the effect of transcendental meditation on blood pressure: a systematic review and meta-analysis. J Hum Hypertens. 2015;29(11):653–62.
41. Tang YY, Tang R, Posner MI. Brief meditation training induces smoking reduction. Proc Natl Acad Sci U S A. 2013;110(34):13971–5.
42. Oikonomou MT, Arvanitis M, Sokolove RL. Mindfulness training for smoking cessation: a meta-analysis of randomized-controlled trials. J Health Psychol. 2017;22(14):1841–50.
43. Salmoirago-Blotcher E, Carey MP. Can mindfulness training improve medication adherence? Integrative review of the current evidence and proposed conceptual model. Explore: J Sci Heal. 2018;14(1):59–65.
44. Sibinga EMS, Perry-Parrish C, Thorpe K, Mika M, Ellen JM. A small mixed-method RCT of mindfulness instruction for urban youth. Explore: J Sci Heal. 2014;10(3):180–6.

45. Mozaffarian D. Dietary and policy priorities for cardiovascular disease, diabetes, and obesity. A comprehensive review. Circulation. 2016;133(2):187–225.

46. Mokdad AH, Ballestros K, Echko M, Glenn S, Olsen HE, Mullany E, et al. The state of US health, 1990–2016: burden of diseases, injuries, and risk factors among US states. JAMA. 2018;319(14):1444–72.

47. Eckel RH, Jakicic JM, Ard JD, de Jesus JM, Houston Miller N, Hubbard VS, et al. 2013 AHA/ACC guideline on lifestyle management to reduce cardiovascular risk: a report of the American College of Cardiology/American Heart Association task force on practice guidelines. Circulation. 2014;129(25 Suppl 2):S76–99.

48. Yu E, Malik VS, Hu FB. Cardiovascular disease prevention by diet modification: JACC health promotion series. J Am Coll Cardiol. 2018;72(8):914–26.

49. Jacobs DR Jr, Tapsell LC. Food, not nutrients, is the fundamental unit in nutrition. Nutr Rev. 2007;65(10):439–50.

50. Department of Health and Human Services; U S Department of Agriculture. Dietary guidelines for Americans 2015–2020. La Vergne: Skyhorse Publishing Inc.; 2017.

51. Fontana L, Meyer TE, Klein S, Holloszy JO. Long-term calorie restriction is highly effective in reducing the risk for atherosclerosis in humans. Proc Natl Acad Sci U S A. 2004;101(17):6659–63.

52. Shai I, Schwarzfuchs D, Henkin Y, Shahar DR, Witkow S, Greenberg I, et al. Weight loss with a low-carbohydrate, Mediterranean, or low-fat diet. N Engl J Med. 2008;359(3):229–41.

53. Afshin A, Micha R, Khatibzadeh S, Mozaffarian D. Consumption of nuts and legumes and risk of incident ischemic heart disease, stroke, and diabetes: a systematic review and meta-analysis. Am J Clin Nutr. 2014;100(1):278–88.

54. Gan Y, Tong X, Li L, Cao S, Yin X, Gao C, et al. Consumption of fruit and vegetable and risk of coronary heart disease: a meta-analysis of prospective cohort studies. Int J Cardiol. 2015;183:129–37.

55. Estruch R, Ros E, Salas-Salvadó J, Covas MI, Corella D, Arós F, Gómez-Gracia E, Ruiz-Gutiérrez V, Fiol M, Lapetra J, Lamuela-Raventos RM, Serra-Majem L, Pintó X, Basora J, Muñoz MA, Sorlí JV, Martínez JA, Fitó M, Gea A, Hernán MA, Martínez-González MA, PREDIMED Study Investigators. Primary prevention of cardiovascular disease with a Mediterranean diet supplemented with extra-virgin olive oil or nuts. N Engl J Med. 2018;378(25):e34.

56. Borch D, Juul-Hindsgaul N, Veller M, Astrup A, Jaskolowski J, Raben A. Potatoes and risk of obesity, type 2 diabetes, and cardiovascular disease in apparently healthy adults: a systematic review of clinical intervention and observational studies. Am J Clin Nutr. 2016;104(2):489–98.

57. Aune D, Keum N, Giovannucci E, Fadnes LT, Boffetta P, Greenwood DC, et al. Whole grain consumption and risk of cardiovascular disease, cancer, and all cause and cause specific mortality: systematic review and dose-response meta-analysis of prospective studies. BMJ (Clinical Research ed). 2016;353:i2716.

58. Holt SH, Brand-Miller JC, Stitt PA. The effects of equal-energy portions of different breads on blood glucose levels, feelings of fullness and subsequent food intake. J Am Diet Assoc. 2001;101(7):767–73.

59. Mozaffarian RS, Lee RM, Kennedy MA, Ludwig DS, Mozaffarian D, Gortmaker SL. Identifying whole grain foods: a comparison of different approaches for selecting more healthful whole grain products. Public Health Nutr. 2013;16(12):2255–64.

60. Shen J, Wilmot KA, Ghasemzadeh N, Molloy DL, Burkman G, Mekonnen G, et al. Mediterranean dietary patterns and cardiovascular health. Annu Rev Nutr. 2015;35:425–49.

61. Mozaffarian D, Wu JHY. Omega-3 fatty acids and cardiovascular disease: effects on risk factors, molecular pathways, and clinical events. J Am Coll Cardiol. 2011;58(20):2047–67.

62. Zheng J, Huang T, Yu Y, Hu X, Yang B, Li D. Fish consumption and CHD mortality: an updated meta-analysis of seventeen cohort studies. Public Health Nutr. 2012;15(4):725–37.

63. Bergkvist C, Berglund M, Glynn A, Wolk A, Akesson A. Dietary exposure to polychlorinated biphenyls and risk of myocardial infarction – a population-based prospective cohort study. Int J Cardiol. 2015;183:242–8.

64. US Food and Drug Administration UEPA. Advice on what pregnant women and parents should know about eating fish. Rockville: US Food and Drug Administration UEPA; 2017.

65. Guo J, Astrup A, Lovegrove JA, Gijsbers L, Givens DI, Soedamah-Muthu SS. Milk and dairy consumption and risk of cardiovascular diseases and all-cause mortality: dose-response meta-analysis of prospective cohort studies. Eur J Epidemiol. 2017;32(4):269–87.

66. Toledo E, Delgado-Rodriguez M, Estruch R, Salas-Salvado J, Corella D, Gomez-Gracia E, et al. Low-fat dairy products and blood pressure: follow-up of 2290 older persons at high cardiovascular risk participating in the PREDIMED study. Br J Nutr. 2009;101(1):59–67.

67. Carlsen MH, Halvorsen BL, Holte K, Bohn SK, Dragland S, Sampson L, et al. The total antioxidant content of more than 3100 foods, beverages, spices, herbs and supplements used worldwide. Nutr J. 2010;9:3.

68. Micha R, Michas G, Mozaffarian D. Unprocessed red and processed meats and risk of coronary artery disease and type 2 diabetes – an updated review of the evidence. Curr Atheroscler Rep. 2012;14(6):515–24.

69. Pan A, Sun Q, Bernstein AM, Schulze MB, Manson JE, Stampfer MJ, et al. Red meat consumption and mortality: results from 2 prospective cohort studies. Arch Intern Med. 2012;172(7):555–63.

70. Abete I, Romaguera D, Vieira AR, Lopez de Munain A, Norat T. Association between total, processed, red and white meat consumption and all-cause, CVD and IHD mortality: a meta-analysis of cohort studies. Br J Nutr. 2014;112(5):762–75.
71. Shin JY, Xun P, Nakamura Y, He K. Egg consumption in relation to risk of cardiovascular disease and diabetes: a systematic review and meta-analysis. Am J Clin Nutr. 2013;98(1):146–59.
72. Bernstein AM, Sun Q, Hu FB, Stampfer MJ, Manson JE, Willett WC. Major dietary protein sources and risk of coronary heart disease in women. Circulation. 2010;122(9):876–83.
73. Malik VS, Popkin BM, Bray GA, Després J-P, Hu FB. Sugar sweetened beverages, obesity, type 2 diabetes and cardiovascular disease risk. Circulation. 2010;121(11):1356–64.
74. Xi B, Huang Y, Reilly KH, Li S, Zheng R, Barrio-Lopez MT, et al. Sugar-sweetened beverages and risk of hypertension and CVD: a dose-response meta-analysis. Br J Nutr. 2015;113(5):709–17.
75. Malik VS, Schulze MB, Hu FB. Intake of sugar-sweetened beverages and weight gain: a systematic review. Am J Clin Nutr. 2006;84(2):274–88.
76. Ding M, Bhupathiraju SN, Satija A, van Dam RM, Hu FB. Long-term coffee consumption and risk of cardiovascular disease: a systematic review and a dose-response meta-analysis of prospective cohort studies. Circulation. 2014;129(6):643–59.
77. Ronksley PE, Brien SE, Turner BJ, Mukamal KJ, Ghali WA. Association of alcohol consumption with selected cardiovascular disease outcomes: a systematic review and meta-analysis. BMJ (Clinical Research ed). 2011;342:d671.
78. Zhao J, Stockwell T, Roemer A, Naimi T, Chikritzhs T. Alcohol consumption and mortality from coronary heart disease: an updated meta-analysis of cohort studies. J Stud Alcohol Drugs. 2017;78(3):375–86.
79. Bagnardi V, Zatonski W, Scotti L, La Vecchia C, Corrao G. Does drinking pattern modify the effect of alcohol on the risk of coronary heart disease? Evidence from a meta-analysis. J Epidemiol Community Health. 2008;62(7):615–9.
80. Danaei G, Ding EL, Mozaffarian D, Taylor B, Rehm J, Murray CJ, et al. The preventable causes of death in the United States: comparative risk assessment of dietary, lifestyle, and metabolic risk factors. PLoS Med. 2009;6(4):e1000058.
81. Mozaffarian D, Fahimi S, Singh GM, Micha R, Khatibzadeh S, Engell RE, et al. Global sodium consumption and death from cardiovascular causes. N Engl J Med. 2014;371(7):624–34.
82. Poggio R, Gutierrez L, Matta MG, Elorriaga N, Irazola V, Rubinstein A. Daily sodium consumption and CVD mortality in the general population: systematic review and meta-analysis of prospective studies. Public Health Nutr. 2015;18(4):695–704.
83. Aburto NJ, Ziolkovska A, Hooper L, Elliott P, Cappuccio FP, Meerpohl JJ. Effect of lower sodium intake on health: systematic review and meta-analyses. BMJ (Clinical Research ed). 2013;346:f1326.
84. Brown IJ, Tzoulaki I, Candeias V, Elliott P. Salt intakes around the world: implications for public health. Int J Epidemiol. 2009;38(3):791–813.
85. Yusuf S, Hawken S, Ounpuu S. Effect of potentially modifiable risk factors associated with myocardial infarction in 52 countries (the INTERHEART study): case-control study. J Cardiopulm Rehabil Prev. 2005;25(1):56–7.

Chapter 18
Integrative Approach in Chronic Kidney Disease

Ahmed Arslan Yousuf Awan, Samaya Javed Anumudu, Edlyn Bustamante Alghafir, and Sankar Dass Navaneethan

Keywords Nutrition in chronic kidney disease · Pre-dialysis care · Social support · Technology

Key Points
- Nutrition in CKD

  - Protein
  - Sodium
  - Phosphorus
  - Potassium
  - Role of dietician and nutritionist

- Exercise in CKD
- Social Support
- Pre-dialysis Care

  - Timing of referral to nephrologist
  - Quality of life
  - Depression

- Technology in CKD

A. A. Y. Awan
Department of Medicine, Division of Nephrology, Baylor College of Medicine, Houston, TX, USA

S. J. Anumudu
Department of Nephrology, Baylor College of Medicine, Houston, TX, USA

E. B. Alghafir
Department of Clinical Nutrition, Ben Taub Hospital (Harris Health System), Houston, TX, USA

S. D. Navaneethan (✉)
Department of Medicine, Section of Nephrology, Baylor College of Medicine, Houston, TX, USA
e-mail: Sankar.Navaneethan@bcm.edu

© Springer Nature Switzerland AG 2020
J. Uribarri, J. A. Vassalotti (eds.), *Nutrition, Fitness, and Mindfulness*, Nutrition and Health,
https://doi.org/10.1007/978-3-030-30892-6_18

Introduction

Chronic kidney disease (CKD) is a multidimensional chronic medical condition defined as an abnormality of kidney structure or function, present for more than 3 months, with a detrimental impact on overall health. CKD has emerged as a global public health problem [18]. According to the Centers for Disease Control and Prevention, in 2017, 30 million people or approximately 15% of the US adults were estimated to have CKD with higher prevalence among women and blacks [33]. CKD is classified based on the etiology (diabetic vs. nondiabetic), how well the kidney filters blood (glomerular filtration rate [GFR] category), and the amount of albumin (or protein) excretion in urine. While a significant proportion of patients with CKD die of cardiovascular disease, end-stage kidney disease (ESKD) requiring dialysis or kidney transplantation is a significant problem with a substantial economic burden for health-care systems [36, 47]. Worldwide, the leading causes of CKD are diabetes and hypertension. However, other risk factors include obesity, glomerulonephritis, cystic kidney disease, chronic interstitial nephritis, and various causes of acute kidney injury (AKI). Often, individuals with CKD are not aware of underlying kidney disease and are referred late to nephrologists. The multifaceted nature of CKD requires a holistic and integrative approach to treatment and management by both patients and clinicians (from various specialties) by not only medications but also nutrition, fitness, and promoting an overall sense of well-being.

Nutrition in CKD

Protein Intake

Experimental studies conducted three decades ago suggested the relationship of high-protein intake with glomerulosclerosis and tubulointerstitial injury and proposed that protein restriction improved the pattern of injury [16, 46]. This was later confirmed in patients with diabetic nephropathy, nephrotic syndrome, and non-proteinuric diabetes [6, 7, 19, 25]. The proposed mechanism of injury is dilatation of afferent arteriole by high-protein diet leading to glomerular hyperfiltration [42]. However, in recent years, the focus has shifted to a concept known as net endogenous acid production (NEAP), which describes a balance between the generation of acid from sulfur-containing amino acids in diet and alkalinity from potassium salts of organic acids [40]. In other words, not all proteins are created equal when it comes to adversely affecting the patients with CKD. The net decline in GFR is dependent on NEAP and is ameliorated by alkali therapy. Proteins from plant sources (fruits and vegetables) have beneficial effects by generating bicarbonate load and reducing NEAP. Increasing alkali load by intake of fruits and vegetables is comparable to [13], or slightly better than [14], oral sodium bicarbonate or sodium citrate therapy in reducing progression of CKD. Conversely, high consumption of red and processed meat is associated with increased risk of CKD progression and mortality.

Protein intake of 0.6–0.8 g/kg edema-free, lean body weight is recommended for patients with CKD while trying to maintain adequate calorie intake of 30–35 kcal/kg body weight. This goal should be liberalized if there are clinical signs of protein-energy wasting (PEW), and in general, high-protein intake (>1.3 g/kg) should be avoided. Clinicians can monitor compliance with dietary protein restriction using the formula described by Maroni et al. [30], utilizing the fact that dietary proteins are excreted either as urea or non-urea nitrogen (NUN) after degradation. NUN averages about 0.031 g N/kg body weight/day and can be added to measured 24-hour urinary urea nitrogen to assess total nitrogen intake. As protein is 16% nitrogen, total nitrogen intake can be converted to protein intake by dividing it by 0.16. These calculations assume steady-state nitrogen balance and require a steady level of blood urea nitrogen and patients' body weight applicable usually to clinically stable outpatients.

Clinicians have always expressed concern that low-protein diet may lead to hypoalbuminemia that increases the risk of mortality in this patient population. However, patients with CKD who are fed restricted amount of protein reduce their oxidation of amino acids and degradation of proteins, leading to a neutral nitrogen balance. This is true even in patients with nephrotic syndrome, where restricting dietary protein intake paradoxically leads to a small but significant decrease in proteinuria and an increase in serum albumin levels [11, 21]. Recommended protein intake for patients with nephrotic syndrome is 0.8 g protein/kg body weight (plus 1 g per g of proteinuria). However, a low-protein diet is not recommended for proteinuria of >15 g or in the presence of catabolic milieu (vasculitis, gluco-corticoids, etc.). Table 18.1 provides recommendations from various societies regarding dietary intake of protein.

Limited data exist on the role of very low-protein diet to delay dialysis. Brunori et al. [3] conducted a study in Italy including elderly (>70 years) patients with GFR of 5–7 ml/min/1.73m^2 BSA without uremia and randomized them to dialysis vs. very low-protein diet (0.3 g/kg body weight) supplemented with keto-analogues, amino acids, and multivitamins (sVLPD). Patients were started on dialysis if they developed uremic symptoms, significant electrolyte abnormalities, fluid overload, or evidence of malnutrition. The study was designed to evaluate possible non-inferiority in mortality in the diet group compared with dialysis group. Results suggested that sVLPD is safe when postponing dialysis treatment by a median of 10.7 months (range: 1–54 months). More importantly, there were

Table 18.1 Nutritional guidelines from various societies for adults with non-dialysis-dependent CKD

Nutrient	KDIGO 2012	KDOQI 2007	ADA (for diabetic kidney disease) 2014	NICE UK guidelines (updates 2014)
Protein intake	Avoid high-protein intake >1.3 g/kg/day in adults with CKD at risk of progression 0.8 g/kg/day in adults with GFR <30 ml/min/1.73m^2	For GFR <25 ml/min/1.73 m^2, 0.6 g/kg/d should be considered However, if unable to tolerate or cannot meet energy requirements, 0.75 g/kg/d may be prescribed	Specific target not provided. Recommends "usual" (not high) protein intake	Do not offer low-protein diets (dietary protein intake of less than 0.6–0.8 g/kg/day) to people with CKD
Sodium intake	Less than 2 g per day of sodium (5 g of sodium chloride)	Reduction of intake to 2.3 g/d as recommended by DASH diet	Reduce sodium to less than 2.3 g/d as recommended for the general population	Offer dietary advice about salt intake appropriate to the severity of CKD
Potassium intake	No specific target but "recommend that individuals with CKD receive expert dietary advice and information in the context of an education program, tailored to the severity of CKD and the need to intervene on salt, phosphate, potassium, and protein intake where indicated"	No specific recommendation but recommends nutritional counseling	No specific target provided	Offer dietary advice about potassium intake appropriate to the severity of CKD
Phosphorus intake	No specific target but recommendation as above	No specific target but recommends nutritional counseling	No specific target provided	Offer dietary advice about phosphate intake appropriate to the severity of CKD.

KDIGO Kidney Disease: Improving Global Outcomes, *KDOQI* Kidney Disease Outcomes Quality Initiative, *ADA* American Diabetes Association fewer hospital admissions and reduced length of stay in the dietary restriction arm, due to reduced complications related to vascular access. Notably, people with diabetes and patients with left ventricular ejection fraction <30% were excluded from the study. Walser et al. have previously shown that renal replacement therapy can be delayed using 0.3 g/kg/day protein diet in patients with GFR of less than 10 ml/min (<15 ml/min in people with diabetes) for a median duration of 353 days [48]. Although these studies have relatively small sample sizes and such stringent dietary restriction may not be easy to implement in all patients with significantly reduced GFR, it certainly is a viable option for elderly patients who do not wish to start dialysis.

Sodium Intake in CKD

Patients with CKD are usually "salt sensitive" (a term used to describe the inability to regulate blood pressure and extracellular fluid volume status in the face of salt load) and benefit greatly from restricting dietary salt intake. Reduced salt intake not only reduces systolic blood pressure and positively affects volume status of the patient but also reduces the proteinuria and may augment the beneficial effects of diuretics and renin-angiotensin-aldosterone system blockade in patients with nephrotic syndrome [26, 31]. However, it is not established beyond doubt that a low-sodium diet slows the progression of CKD [43]. Observational studies in the general population and those with CKD reported a J-shaped relationship between dietary salt intake and adverse outcomes, with sodium intake less than 2–3 g and more than 5 g being associated with worse CV outcomes [9, 32, 45]. Kidney disease improving global outcomes (KDIGO) guidelines recommend lowering salt intake to less than 2 g per day of sodium (corresponding to 5 g of sodium chloride) in adults unless contraindicated. Keeping in mind that there is no proven benefit of the generally recommended target of less than 2.3 g/d [17], the compliance may be reduced due to issues with palatability, and low-sodium intake may lead to inadequate calorie intake (especially in the USA) in this patient population; a target of less than 4 g (3 g for patients with fluid overload problems) may be more practical and has also been advocated [20]. Dietary salt restriction is only possible if patients are willing to prepare meals at home using fresh ingredients due to the high sodium content of foods bought at fast-food restaurants and from processed or tinned food products.

Phosphorus Intake in CKD

There has been consistent observational evidence from epidemiologic studies linking hyperphosphatemia with poor clinical outcomes, especially for cardiovascular events and mortality as well as CKD mineral and bone disorders. However, substantial evidence confirming that reduction in serum phosphate levels improves patient outcomes is lacking. Both dietary and pharmacologic interventions are currently employed to reduce serum phosphorus levels in CKD. Accordingly, the recommendation is to reduce daily phosphorus intake to no more than 800 mg/day. Table 18.2 lists foods that contain high amounts of phosphorus. Besides these apparent sources, phosphorus is a hidden but integral component of most processed and packaged foods and may not be listed on the nutritional labels. Clinicians should also be aware that phosphorus is also present in some of the medications commonly prescribed to kidney patients, like amlodipine and lisinopril, and quantity may vary depending on the manufacturer [44]. Patient education regarding various sources of exogenous phosphorus is the cornerstone of dietary management of CKD and plays a significant role in reducing pill burden of phosphate binders and avoiding complications of secondary hyperparathyroidism. The type of phosphate consumed also affects serum phosphate levels, with higher levels after

Table 18.2 Foods containing high levels of phosphorous and potassium

Foods containing high levels of phosphorous	Foods containing high levels of potassium
Cheese (Swiss, Cheddar, American)	Spinach
Milk, yogurt	Brussels sprout
Custard, pudding, ice cream	Potato (higher content if eaten with peel)
Carbonated drinks (Coke, Pepsi, Dr. Pepper)	Broccoli
Chocolate	Beans and lentils
Dried fruit	Artichokes
Peanuts	Tomatoes
Almonds	Bananas
Cashews	Avocados
Peanut butter	Cantaloupe
Salmon, lobster, crab	Mango
Liver	Orange
Beef	Juices of high potassium fruits and vegetables
Brown rice	Milk, yogurt, cheese
Pumpkin seeds, sunflower seeds	Salt substitutes

consumption of dairy products compared to the similar amount of phosphate ingested with meat or grains. In contrast, less than 50% of organic phosphate derived from plant sources (nuts, legumes, cereals, etc.) is absorbed.

Potassium Intake in CKD

Hyperkalemia is a common complication in CKD (especially among those with advanced CKD), and both hypo- and hyperkalemia are associated with increased risk for death in this population. The recommended potassium intake for patients with CKD is less than 2 g/day, although consensus is lacking. Table 18.2 lists foods containing high potassium content.

Role of the Renal Registered Dietitian Nutritionist

Patients with CKD are faced with an uphill task of following myriad dietary restrictions while trying to maintain adequate caloric intake and avoiding protein-energy wasting (PEW). This task is even more complex among those with comorbidities such as hypertension, diabetes, or congestive heart failure. A dedicated renal dietitian can help them navigate this maze and answer the question that CKD patients invariably pose to their physicians: "What's left that I can eat?" Renal dietitians can suggest various sample meal plans (see Table 18.3) and tailor them according to patients' ethnic background (American, Hispanic, Asian Indian, etc.) and personal preferences while trying to avoid the risk of excluding vital nutrients. Dietitians are not only skilled at recommending nutritional changes but also monitoring and implementing them by following the outcomes expected from dietary manipulations. Frequent visits with a renal dietitian are required to reinforce various recommendations, follow progress, and establish a partnership where the patient starts taking charge of their health with support and encouragement from the dietitian. An assessment of patients' food and nutrition knowledge deficit and a detailed nutritional history is vital before any recommendations for dietary restrictions are made. Food diaries can be used as a tool for monitoring the progress. To make it less cumbersome for the patient, some dietitians use a stepwise approach, where protein restriction is

Table 18.3 Sample dietary plan for a 70 kg patient with CKD stage 4–5 not on dialysis (56 g of protein, almost 2100 kcals)

Meal pattern:
4 oz. of meat, fish, poultry, or egg for high biological value protein
½ cup milk/yogurt
3 portions of low potassium fruit
3 portions of low potassium vegetables
6 portions of low potassium/phosphorus bread/cereals/starches

Breakfast	Lunch	Dinner
Homemade parfait: ½ cup plan or vanilla yogurt ½ cup mixed berries 1 cup of corn or rice dry cereal	Chicken wrap: 2 oz. cooked chicken 2 flour tortillas 1 cup of raw spinach ½ cup sliced cucumbers ¼ cup shredded carrots 1 Tb mayonnaise 1 clementine/tangerine Homemade lemonade/clear color soda/ tea	Turkey sandwich: 2 oz. cooked turkey breast 2 slices of toasted white bread 1-cup of shredded lettuce or cabbage ½ cup of sliced bell pepper and red onion 1 Tb mayonnaise 1 apple Homemade lemonade/clear color soda/tea
Half cup of dry cereal (rice/corn preferably) 1 cup rice milk ½ cup strawberries 1 slice of bagel 1 Tb cream cheese 1 TB of jam (apricot/strawberry/grape)	Mediterranean sandwich: 2 oz. cooked beef ½ small pita bread 1 cup grilled eggplant, zucchini, and onions 1 cup shredded lettuce 1 Tb olive oil mixed with dry herbs 1 peach Homemade lemonade/clear color soda/ tea	Salmon dinner: 2 oz. of cooked salmon (seasoned with TB of olive oil and lemon) 1 cup of white rice cooked with peas, and carrots 1 cup of green beans (seasoned with olive oil, lemon, smashed garlic, and black pepper) ½ cup fruit cocktail Homemade lemonade/clear color soda/tea
1 English muffin 1 Tb kefir cheese ½ cup of berries 1 cup of coffee with cream and sugar	Egg salad: 2 boiled eggs ½ cup of shredded lettuce (iceberg, arugula, Bibb, Boston, red leaf, or green leaf lettuces) ½ cup of sliced red onions and bell peppers ½ cup of sweet corn 12 unsalted crackers ½ cup of grapes Homemade lemonade/clear color soda/tea	Tuna dinner: 2 oz. fresh tuna 1 cup of asparagus 1 cup of pasta (seasoned with olive oil, fresh smashed garlic, and Italian herbs) ½ cup pineapple chunks Homemade lemonade/clear color soda/tea

discussed and implemented during the initial visit, and sodium, potassium, and phosphorus restriction is deferred to later visits when protein intake is near target. In the USA, dietitians are approved providers of medical nutrition therapy for patients with GFR of less than 50 mL/min/1.73 m², as well as patients who have diabetes. The Centers for Medicare and Medicaid Services allows 3 hours of medical nutrition therapy in the first year (can be achieved over multiple visits) and 2 hours in second year and beyond.

Exercise in CKD

KDIGO guidelines recommend moderate physical activity for 30 minutes five times per week in patients with CKD [22]. Similar to the non-CKD population, there is a significant association between physical inactivity and increased morbidity in patients with CKD [1, 35]. Physical activity can improve neuromuscular functioning and muscle mass, exercise tolerance, and cardiorespiratory fitness besides improving control of hypertension and diabetes. However, observational data show that

Table 18.4 Barriers and facilitators to exercise and physical activity

Barriers	Facilitators
Sickness or fatigue	Support from family and friends
Shortness of breath	CKD-specific exercise classes
Lack of motivation	Desire to feel better
Lack of time	Exercising with others
Lack of access to exercise facilities	Enjoying how exercise feels
Lack of encouragement and support	Feeling healthy
Lack of knowledge about the benefits of physical activity	Belief in one's ability to be physically active
	Wanting to manage weight

physical activity declines with the progression of CKD, especially in elderly patient population and is associated with increased risk of death [41].

Exercise is a specific form of physical activity that is structured, repetitive, and intended to maintain or improve physical fitness [5]. Multiple barriers and facilitators of exercise have been identified and can be addressed in a multidisciplinary fashion (Table 18.4) [51]. Although there is a dearth of evidence-based exercise programs in patients with CKD, a simple prescription of home-based, moderate-intensity aerobic exercise like brisk walking or cycling for 30 minutes to 1 hour, 3–5 times a week has been shown to improve physical functioning and reduce cardiovascular risk [15]. Resistance exercise can promote anabolic triggers including serum IGF-1, testosterone, and human growth hormone, which has the potential to prevent or slow muscle wasting. However, professional supervision is recommended for patients undergoing resistance training to prevent injury. Among dialysis patients, physical activity is limited, and recent clinical trial evidence suggests that simple, personalized, home-based, low-intensity exercise program managed by dialysis staff may improve physical performance and quality of life [29]. From a medical standpoint, treatment of anemia is a modifiable risk factor for decreased exercise tolerance and fatigue. Therefore, treating anemia can help patients' exercise capacity and willingness to participate in physical activity.

Social Support and Role of Renal Social Worker

As evident from the discussion above, management of CKD requires a significant change in a patient's lifestyle, dietary habits, and daily routine and has the potential to impact social interactions and personal relationships. Thus, it is challenging for a person to be compliant with dietary and medication regimens and keep up their motivation to stay healthy without vigorous support from family and friends. It wouldn't be an exaggeration to say that "it takes a village" to take good care of a patient with CKD and to keep them an active and functioning member of the society. This becomes even more important with the progression of CKD and when it comes time to start renal replacement therapy in the form of dialysis or transplant [8]. A multidisciplinary approach, including physicians, dietitians, nurses, health-care technicians, and renal social workers, is required to facilitate patients' transition to the optimum renal replacement therapy and to help them deal with the strain this endeavor places on their schedules, employment, personal relations, finances, and appearances. Renal social worker has a pivotal role to play in the care of patients with CKD [4]. They can provide psychosocial perspective to the health-care team and help them better understand the perspectives of patients coming from diverse cultural, religious, and socioeconomic backgrounds. The renal social worker can also be a patient advocate and help them navigate and secure health-care insurance based on their employment status, work history, and income category. Social workers are also trained to recognize early signs of depression and mental health issues in patients with CKD (as described later) and can offer useful insights into a patients' noncompliance with treatments and follow-up [39].

Pre-End-Stage Kidney Disease (ESKD) Care

Timely referral to nephrologists by primary care physicians has been shown to improve long-term outcomes for patients with CKD. According to the National Kidney Foundation-Kidney Disease Outcomes Quality Initiative (NKF-KDOQI) clinical practice guideline for CKD, patients should be referred to a nephrologist when they have CKD stage 4 with their GFR less than 30 mL/min/1.73 m [34] among other indications. Late nephrology referral is an independent risk factor for early death on dialysis [50]. Additionally, early pre-ESKD care for patients by nephrologists is associated with greater likelihood of access to the kidney transplantation wait list, initiating hemodialysis with the use of arteriovenous fistula or graft, and selecting home dialysis as modality of choice [10, 49].

As a result of a timely referral, nephrologists can build rapport with their patients and help manage their related comorbidities to delay progression to ESKD, improve quality of life, and reduce hospitalizations and emergent-start dialysis. They can educate patients approaching ESKD on possible kidney transplantation and various dialysis modalities, including home dialysis vs. in-center dialysis by discussions during office visits and also through participation in CKD education classes. Clinicians can also work closely with dietitians and use online resources to educate and guide patients on their respective dietary modifications.

In addition to providing medical care, clinicians can aid patients by trying to improve their quality of life and tailoring therapy to their respective long-term goals. For example, if a patient wishes to continue working and needs a flexible schedule when initiating dialysis, peritoneal and/or home dialysis may be a better option as opposed to thrice weekly in-center hemodialysis. Likewise, if patients wish to pursue palliative care instead of starting dialysis, clinicians can collaborate with the palliative care team to help ensure the best supportive care for their patients while honoring their wishes and personal preferences.

Depression in CKD

Depressive symptoms have been associated with increased mortality among patients with CKD and ESKD [23, 24]. In a meta-analysis of cohort studies examining the association between depression and death in people with CKD, depression was associated with an increased risk of mortality [38]. Likewise, in a systematic review and meta-analysis of observational studies examining the prevalence of depression in CKD, Palmer et al. noted approximately one-quarter of adults with CKD are depressed when assessed by clinical interview. When questionnaire-based tools are used to identify depressive symptoms, prevalence is estimated to be higher in patients on dialysis. Furthermore, approximately one-quarter of patients with CKD stages 1–5 or kidney transplant recipients are thought to have depressive symptomatology when questionnaires are used for assessment [37]. According to the KDOQI clinical practice guidelines, every dialysis patient should be seen by a social worker at dialysis initiation and biannually to assess their psychological state, focusing on the presence of depression, anxiety, and hostility. If present, patients should be treated [12]. Psychopharmacological and psychosocial interventions are often used to help with depressive symptoms in patients with CKD/ESKD. Treatment options range from counseling and referral to psychiatrists to use of antidepressant medications and cognitive behavioral intervention (CBI). Lerma et al. demonstrated the beneficial effects of 5 weeks of CBI for reducing depression and anxiety symptoms and improving the overall quality of life in ESKD patients on hemodialysis [27]. Insight into the various psychosocial factors affecting individuals with CKD can lead to improved screening by providers and timely referral to mental health experts to improve long-term outcomes for this population.

Use of Technology in CKD

With growing reliance on technology and the use of the internet in everyday life, care of patients with CKD has also been transformed. Incorporation of technology and associated resources for patient care is slowly improving and has tremendous growth potential. Both patients and health-care workers can use available technology via smartphones, smartwatches, laptops, and other devices to improve access to care, delivery of information, and educational support.

Telehealth is defined by the US Department of Health and Human Services as "the use of electronic information and telecommunications technologies to support and promote long-distance clinical health care, patient and professional health-related education, public health and health administration" (https://www.healthit.gov/topic/health-it-initiatives/telemedicine-and-telehealth). Examples of such technologies include the use of the internet, video conferencing, media streaming, text messaging, and wireless communications—all of which can be used by providers to help improve CKD related care and education, especially for patients in remote areas who do not have quick access to clinicians. Online health-care system portals have drastically improved physician-patient communication, with expedited refill requests for medications and access to their test results electronically at home or on the go.

Mobile health (mHealth) is an essential and popular telehealth-related application that provides health-care information through mobile devices (https://www.healthit.gov/topic/health-it-initiatives/telemedicine-and-telehealth). Individuals can access various applications on their mobile devices to help track their fitness and nutrition, which would be helpful for patients monitoring their weight and electrolyte intake closely, store their personal health information that they can share with their health-care professionals, and help interpret their health information. Furthermore, clinicians can use various "apps" and various trusted websites in their day-to-day practice for patient care. For example, there are several calculators for clinician reference that can be accessed through different apps including some that help calculates individual patients' risk of CKD progression and those that help interpret acid-base disturbances. "My food coach" app developed by the National Kidney Foundation helps patients to understand the complex nutritional requirement of CKD patients. Table 18.5 lists some useful online resources and applications for CKD patients and practitioners who take care of them.

The use of social media (e.g., Twitter) in medical education is a growing trend that can help improve clinician engagement and expand collaboration among physicians but can also be associated with controversy. It can be an excellent venue for clinicians to obtain helpful and up-to-date clinical information and network with other health-care professionals which can benefit their patients and research. However, given the vast amount of information available online, clinicians should be careful of their resources and rely on evidence-based medicine for verification and should always respect and protect patient confidentiality.

Table 18.5 Online resources for patients and health-care professionals

My food coach application by the National Kidney Foundation	Helps understand and manage nutritional requirements in CKD
H2Overload application by the National Kidney Foundation	Helps manage fluid intake/balance, weight, and blood pressure
CRN pocket guide application by the National Kidney Foundation	Pocket guide for nutritional assessment of patients with kidney disease
www.kidney.org/nutrition	National Kidney Foundation website for information on diet and kidney disease
www.niddk.nih.gov/health-information/kidney-disease	National Institute of Diabetes and Digestive and Kidney Diseases website for kidney disease information
www.nutrition.va.gov/kidney.asp	US Department of Veterans Affairs website for medical nutrition therapy (MNT) related to CKD

While incorporation of technology into medical practice offers many benefits, it does come with limitations, especially for those with limited access to and literacy for technology including computers and smartphones. Therefore, clinicians need to evaluate each patient individually for their needs and face-to-face communication and education remains vital [2].

Conclusions

CKD is a complex chronic disease that begins as damage to kidney structure and function but with progression affects all the organ systems of the body and numerous aspects of a patient's life. Just as the scope of this disease is broad so is the management that requires constant input from a multidisciplinary health-care team as well as significant support of patients' family and friends. The multidisciplinary care could also be cost-effective [28]. Prompt recognition of CKD by primary care physicians is essential to institute early dietary and lifestyle interventions, and referral to nephrologists as kidney function declines. Health-care teams must recognize the individual needs of each patient and tailor therapy according to patients' educational, cultural, and socioeconomic background. There are various aspects to the treatment of patients with CKD and interventions should be introduced in a stepwise fashion, to avoid overwhelming the patient. Due to the chronic, unrelenting nature of the disease and tough lifestyle modifications, some noncompliance from the patients should be expected, and the health-care team should not get frustrated in their efforts to counsel the patient and express compassion. With an integrative approach to CKD, we can successfully attempt to slow down the progression of disease and buy our patients precious years off renal replacement therapy and when its time, transition them to renal replacement therapy in an optimal manner, so they can continue to stay active members of their family and productive members of the society.

Bibliography and Further Reading

1. Beddhu S, Baird BC, Zitterkoph J, Neilson J, Greene T. Physical activity and mortality in chronic kidney disease (NHANES III). Clin J Am Soc Nephrol. 2009;4:1901–6.
2. Bonner A, Gillespie K, Campbell KL, Corones-Watkins K, Hayes B, Harvie B, Kelly JT, Havas K. Evaluating the prevalence and opportunity for technology use in chronic kidney disease patients: a cross-sectional study. BMC Nephrol. 2018;19:28.
3. Brunori G, Viola BF, Parrinello G, De Biase V, Como G, Franco V, Garibotto G, Zubani R, Cancarini GC. Efficacy and safety of a very-low-protein diet when postponing dialysis in the elderly: a prospective randomized multicenter controlled study. Am J Kidney Dis. 2007;49:569–80.
4. Callahan MB. Begin with the end in mind: the value of outcome-driven nephrology social work. Adv Chronic Kidney Dis. 2007;14:409–14.
5. Caspersen CJ, Powell KE, Christenson GM. Physical activity, exercise, and physical fitness: definitions and distinctions for health-related research. Public Health Rep. 1985;100:126–31.
6. D'amico G, Gentile MG. Effect of dietary manipulation on the lipid abnormalities and urinary protein loss in nephrotic patients. Miner Electrolyte Metab. 1992;18:203–6.
7. D'amico G, Gentile MG, Manna G, Fellin G, Ciceri R, Cofano F, Petrini C, Lavarda F, Perolini S, Porrini M. Effect of vegetarian soy diet on hyperlipidaemia in nephrotic syndrome. Lancet. 1992;339:1131–4.
8. Dobrof J, Dolinko A, Lichtiger E, Uribarri J, Epstein I. Dialysis patient characteristics and outcomes: the complexity of social work practice with the end stage renal disease population. Soc Work Health Care. 2001;33:105–28.
9. Garofalo C, Borrelli S, Provenzano M, De Stefano T, Vita C, Chiodini P, Minutolo R, De Nicola L, Conte G. Dietary salt restriction in chronic kidney disease: a meta-analysis of randomized clinical trials. Nutrients. 2018;10:732.
10. Gillespie BW, Morgenstern H, Hedgeman E, Tilea A, Scholz N, Shearon T, Burrows NR, Shahinian VB, Yee J, Plantinga L, Powe NR, Mcclellan W, Robinson B, Williams DE, Saran R. Nephrology care prior to end-stage renal disease and outcomes among new ESRD patients in the USA. Clin Kidney J. 2015;8:772–80.

11. Giordano M, De Feo P, Lucidi P, Depascale E, Giordano G, Cirillo D, Dardo G, Signorelli SS, Castellino P. Effects of dietary protein restriction on fibrinogen and albumin metabolism in nephrotic patients. Kidney Int. 2001;60:235–42.

12. Goh ZS, Griva K. Anxiety and depression in patients with end-stage renal disease: impact and management challenges – a narrative review. Int J Nephrol Renovasc Dis. 2018;11:93–102.

13. Goraya N, Simoni J, Jo C, Wesson DE. Dietary acid reduction with fruits and vegetables or bicarbonate attenuates kidney injury in patients with a moderately reduced glomerular filtration rate due to hypertensive nephropathy. Kidney Int. 2012;81:86–93.

14. Goraya N, Simoni J, Jo CH, Wesson DE. A comparison of treating metabolic acidosis in CKD stage 4 hypertensive Kidney disease with fruits and vegetables or sodium bicarbonate. Clin J Am Soc Nephrol. 2013;8:371–81.

15. Heiwe S, Jacobson SH. Exercise training in adults with CKD: a systematic review and meta-analysis. Am J Kidney Dis. 2014;64:383–93.

16. Hostetter TH, Meyer TW, Rennke HG, Brenner BM. Chronic effects of dietary protein in the rat with intact and reduced renal mass. Kidney Int. 1986;30:509–17.

17. Jain N, Reilly RF. Effects of dietary interventions on incidence and progression of CKD. Nat Rev Nephrol. 2014;10:712–24.

18. Jha V, Garcia-Garcia G, Iseki K, Li Z, Naicker S, Plattner B, Saran R, Wang AY, Yang CW. Chronic kidney disease: global dimension and perspectives. Lancet. 2013;382:260–72.

19. Jibani MM, Bloodworth LL, Foden E, Griffiths KD, Galpin OP. Predominantly vegetarian diet in patients with incipient and early clinical diabetic nephropathy: effects on albumin excretion rate and nutritional status. Diabet Med. 1991;8:949–53.

20. Kalantar-Zadeh K, Fouque D. Nutritional management of chronic kidney disease. N Engl J Med. 2017;377:1765–76.

21. Kaysen GA, Gambertoglio J, Jimenez I, Jones H, Hutchison FN. Effect of dietary protein intake on albumin homeostasis in nephrotic patients. Kidney Int. 1986;29:572–7.

22. KDIGO 2012. KDIGO 2012 clinical practice guideline for the evaluation and management of chronic kidney disease. Kidney Int. 2013;3(suppl):1–150.

23. Kellerman QD, Christensen AJ, Baldwin AS, Lawton WJ. Association between depressive symptoms and mortality risk in chronic kidney disease. Health Psychol. 2010;29:594–600.

24. Kimmel PL, Peterson RA, Weihs KL, Simmens SJ, Alleyne S, Cruz I, Veis JH. Multiple measurements of depression predict mortality in a longitudinal study of chronic hemodialysis outpatients. Kidney Int. 2000;57:2093–8.

25. Kontessis PA, Bossinakou I, Sarika L, Iliopoulou E, Papantoniou A, Trevisan R, Roussi D, Stipsanelli K, Grigorakis S, Souvatzoglou A. Renal, metabolic, and hormonal responses to proteins of different origin in normotensive, non-proteinuric type I diabetic patients. Diabetes Care. 1995;18:1233.

26. Kwakernaak AJ, Krikken JA, Binnenmars SH, Visser FW, Hemmelder MH, Woittiez AJ, Groen H, Laverman GD, Navis G, Holland Nephrology Study (HONEST) Group. Effects of sodium restriction and hydrochlorothiazide on RAAS blockade efficacy in diabetic nephropathy: a randomised clinical trial. Lancet Diabetes Endocrinol. 2014;2:385–95.

27. Lerma A, Perez-Grovas H, Bermudez L, Peralta-Pedrero ML, Robles-Garcia R, Lerma C. Brief cognitive behavioural intervention for depression and anxiety symptoms improves quality of life in chronic haemodialysis patients. Psychol Psychother. 2017;90:105–23.

28. Lin E, Chertow GM, Yan B, Malcolm E, Goldhaber-Fiebert JD. Cost-effectiveness of multidisciplinary care in mild to moderate chronic kidney disease in the United States: a modeling study. PLoS Med. 2018;15:E1002532.

29. Manfredini F, Mallamaci F, D'arrigo G, Baggetta R, Bolignano D, Torino C, Lamberti N, Bertoli S, Ciurlino D, Rocca-Rey L, Barilla A, Battaglia Y, Rapana RM, Zuccala A, Bonanno G, Fatuzzo P, Rapisarda F, Rastelli S, Fabrizi F, Messa P, De Paola L, Lombardi L, Cupisti A, Fuiano G, Lucisano G, Summaria C, Felisatti M, Pozzato E, Malagoni AM, Castellino P, Aucella F, Abd Elhafeez S, Provenzano PF, Tripepi G, Catizone L, Zoccali C. Exercise in patients on dialysis: a multicenter, randomized clinical trial. J Am Soc Nephrol. 2017;28:1259–68.

30. Maroni BJ, Steinman TI, Mitch WE. A method for estimating nitrogen intake of patients with chronic renal failure. Kidney Int. 1985;27:58–65.

31. McMahon EJ, Bauer JD, Hawley CM, Isbel NM, Stowasser M, Johnson DW, Campbell KL. A randomized trial of dietary sodium restriction in CKD. J Am Soc Nephrol. 2013;24:2096–103.

32. Mills KT, Chen J, Yang W, Appel LJ, Kusek JW, Alper A, Delafontaine P, Keane MG, Mohler E, Ojo A, Rahman M, Ricardo AC, Soliman EZ, Steigerwalt S, Townsend R, He J, Chronic Renal Insufficiency Cohort (CRIC) Study Investigators. Sodium excretion and the risk of cardiovascular disease in patients with chronic kidney disease. JAMA. 2016;315:2200–10.

33. National Chronic Kidney Disease Fact Sheet 2017 –data from 2011–2014 National Health and Nutrition examination survey and CKD-EPI equation (listed at bottom of fact sheet). https://www.cdc.gov/kidneydisease/pdf/kidney_factsheet.pdf.

34. National Kidney Foundation. K/DOQI clinical practice guidelines for chronic kidney disease: evaluation, classification, and stratification. Am J Kidney Dis. 2002;39:S1–266.

35. Navaneethan SD, Kirwan JP, Arrigain S, Schreiber MJ, Sehgal AR, Schold JD. Overweight, obesity and intentional weight loss in chronic Kidney disease: NHANES 1999–2006. Int J Obes. 2012;36:1585–90.
36. Navaneethan SD, Schold JD, Arrigain S, Jolly SE, Nally JV Jr. Cause-specific deaths in non-dialysis-dependent CKD. J Am Soc Nephrol. 2015;26:2512–20.
37. Palmer S, Vecchio M, Craig JC, Tonelli M, Johnson DW, Nicolucci A, Pellegrini F, Saglimbene V, Logroscino G, Fishbane S, Strippoli GF. Prevalence of depression in chronic Kidney disease: systematic review and meta-analysis of observational studies. Kidney Int. 2013;84:179–91.
38. Palmer SC, Vecchio M, Craig JC, Tonelli M, Johnson DW, Nicolucci A, Pellegrini F, Saglimbene V, Logroscino G, Hedayati SS, Strippoli GF. Association between depression and death in people with CKD: a meta-analysis of cohort studies. Am J Kidney Dis. 2013;62:493–505.
39. Prescott M. The role of the nephrology social worker in team training for patient nonadherence. Nephrol News Issues. 2004;18(36–7):41.
40. Remer T. Influence of diet on acid-base balance. Semin Dial. 2000;13:221–6.
41. Roshanravan B, Robinson-Cohen C, Patel KV, Ayers E, Littman AJ, De Boer IH, Ikizler TA, Himmelfarb J, Katzel LI, Kestenbaum B, Seliger S. Association between physical performance and all-cause mortality in CKD. J Am Soc Nephrol. 2013;24:822–30.
42. Sallstrom J, Carlstrom M, Olerud J, Fredholm BB, Kouzmine M, Sandler S, Persson AE. High-protein-induced glomerular hyperfiltration is independent of the tubuloglomerular feedback mechanism and nitric oxide synthases. Am J Physiol Regul Integr Comp Physiol. 2010;299:R1263–8.
43. Saran R, Padilla RL, Gillespie BW, Heung M, Hummel SL, Derebail VK, Pitt B, Levin NW, Zhu F, Abbas SR, Liu L, Kotanko P, Klemmer P. A randomized crossover trial of dietary sodium restriction in stage 3–4 CKD. Clin J Am Soc Nephrol. 2017;12:399–407.
44. Sherman RA, Ravella S, Kapoian T. A dearth of data: the problem of phosphorus in prescription medications. Kidney Int. 2015;87:1097–9.
45. Stolarz-Skrzypek K, Kuznetsova T, Thijs L, Tikhonoff V, Seidlerova J, Richart T, Jin Y, Olszanecka A, Malyutina S, Casiglia E, Filipovsky J, Kawecka-Jaszcz K, Nikitin Y, Staessen JA, European Project on Genes in Hypertension. Fatal and nonfatal outcomes, incidence of hypertension, and blood pressure changes in relation to urinary sodium excretion. JAMA. 2011;305:1777–85.
46. Tucker SM, Mason RL, Beauchene RE. Influence of diet and feed restriction on kidney function of aging male rats. J Gerontol. 1976;31:264–70.
47. United States Renal Data System (USRDS) Annual Data Report [Online]. Available: https://www.usrds.org/2018/view/v1_07.aspx. Accessed 12/10/2018.
48. Walser M, Hill S. Can renal replacement be deferred by a supplemented very low protein diet? J Am Soc Nephrol. 1999;10:110–6.
49. Winkelmayer WC, Mehta J, Chandraker A, Owen WF Jr, Avorn J. Predialysis nephrologist care and access to kidney transplantation in the United States. Am J Transplant. 2007;7:872–9.
50. Winkelmayer WC, Owen WF Jr, Levin R, Avorn J. A propensity analysis of late versus early nephrologist referral and mortality on dialysis. J Am Soc Nephrol. 2003;14:486–92.
51. Zelle DM, Klaassen G, Van Adrichem E, Bakker SJ, Corpeleijn E, Navis G. Physical inactivity: a risk factor and target for intervention in renal care. Nat Rev Nephrol. 2017;13:318.

Chapter 19
Summary and Conclusion

Jaime Uribarri and Joseph A. Vassalotti

Keywords Lifestyle · Nutrition · Fitness · Mindfulness · Cardiovascular

> **Key Points**
> - Professional healthcare education typically does little to address nutrition and physical activity and mindfulness, which usually form a very small part of medical school curricula.
> - The evidence for these lifestyle interventions is reviewed in detail with practical tips for the busy clinician.
> - Four dietary approaches that are emphasized include the Mediterranean, DASH, and plant-based diets as well as the low-AGE diet.
> - Physical activity with practical interventions for walking and resistance training and its relationship to cardiovascular outcomes are reviewed.
> - Adequate sleep as part of a complete healthy lifestyle is emphasized.
> - The importance of mindfulness, spirituality, and yoga as effective therapies for the receptive patient is developed by several authors.
> - Particularly for people with established chronic medical conditions, lifestyle modification is an important adjunctive therapy for cardiovascular disease, chronic kidney disease, diabetes, and other chronic ailments.

Introduction

The editors' experience as nephrologists with several decades in clinical care has culminated in great respect for the importance of nutritional interventions as well as an appreciation for the frustration of our patients in navigating the forbidden approach to food choices. Perhaps this is best expressed by experts as the "is there anything left to eat" dilemma [8]. Although this experience mostly applies to individuals with chronic kidney disease, the approach to healthy nutrition concepts can also be applied

J. Uribarri
Division of Nephrology, Department of Medicine, Icahn School of Medicine at Mount Sinai, New York, NY, USA

J. A. Vassalotti (✉)
Division of Nephrology, Department of Medicine, Icahn School of Medicine at Mount Sinai, New York, NY, USA

The National Kidney Foundation, Inc., New York, NY, USA
e-mail: Joseph.vassalotti@mssm.edu

© Springer Nature Switzerland AG 2020
J. Uribarri, J. A. Vassalotti (eds.), *Nutrition, Fitness, and Mindfulness*, Nutrition and Health,
https://doi.org/10.1007/978-3-030-30892-6_19

to patients with other medical conditions and to the general population. This book incorporates the complete spectrum of healthy lifestyle, which also considers physical activity or fitness and mindfulness, based on the available evidence. The book supports healthcare professionals with a holistic approach to medicine recommending a lifestyle that should prevent the development of and/or slow chronic disease progression, independently of or synergistically with medications. Drug therapy is the emphasis of traditional medical education. Although medications are not specifically discussed, lifestyle therapies can be considered as adjunctive to drug therapy. For example, high sodium intake blunts the effectiveness of diuretics, angiotensin-converting enzyme inhibitors, and angiotensin receptor blockers in the treatment of hypertension, and therefore decreased sodium intake will improve the effectiveness of these medications [1]. The scope of the book is intended to apply to adults in the medical outpatient setting or even to healthy subjects who are motivated to remain this way throughout life.

Nutrition

Part I of the book describes several comprehensive nutritional interventions. Instead of focusing on a magical beneficial food or a deleterious unhealthy one as is often the case in the media or advertisements, an approach that incorporates the patient's lifestyle to consider healthy dietary patterns is more likely to be impactful. Unfortunately, processed products are the most widely available, inexpensive, and often most convenient food choices [3]. Moreover, surveys of primary care clinicians and cardiologists show that 90% or more believe their role includes providing patients with nutritional information in the context of the majority reporting minimal or absent nutritional education during training [4, 5]. The three major dietary patterns that share low-processed food content with demonstrated significant health benefits in trials are the dietary approaches to stop hypertension (DASH) diet, the Mediterranean diet, and the plant-based diet. These are not really "diets" in the sense of the lay perception of an extreme usually short-term approach to weight loss, but a long-term approach to health or even a way of living. The best way to individualize the use of one of these healthy eating patterns or modified patterns is with an interdisciplinary approach that may include a registered dietitian to incorporate the patient's personal preferences, financial constraints, and comorbidities and complications, such as hyperkalemia or heart failure.

Chapter 1 on the DASH diet reviews the literature that demonstrates this pattern of eating is efficacious in lowering blood pressure, improving lipid parameters, achieving weight control, and reducing risk of chronic diseases. The DASH diet composition is similar to the Mediterranean diet, except that lean dairy products are the major source of fat. Clinicians can play a critical role in promoting DASH use, since adherence to the DASH pattern remains low throughout the USA across demographics. The authors offer practical tools and useful tips for clinicians to implement the DASH eating pattern with their patients.

The comprehensive review of the Mediterranean diet in Chap. 2 includes the Mediterranean diet pyramid, which is particularly useful to understand with olive oil as the main source of fat using traditional foods from wide variety of fresh and local and season products prepared with traditional recipes. The medical literature is described supporting the Mediterranean diet's cardioprotective properties and beneficial effects on the incidence and control of the clinical features of metabolic syndrome, obesity, diabetes mellitus, neurodegenerative diseases, and aging. The Prevención con Dieta Mediterránea (PREDIMED), a multicenter interventional randomized controlled study involving 7447 subjects, clearly demonstrated that participants that followed the Mediterranean diet had lower incidence of major cardiovascular events versus those following the control diet [6]. Recently this study received a great deal of attention, requiring reanalysis and republication that confirmed the findings [7]. Personal preference is an important consideration to determine if implementation of this diet fits the lifestyle of an individual patient.

Chapter 3 on plant-based diet discusses the substantial evidence from multiple observational studies and clinical trials supporting the beneficial effects of plant-based dietary patterns for reduction of cardiovascular risk mediated at least in part by reducing hypertension and type 2 diabetes and improving overall health. The myth that plant-based diets are tantamount to inadequate protein intake is addressed with careful planning and nutritional education. Thus, plant-based nutrition, which is not necessarily purely vegetarian or vegan, should be recommended as part of an overall cardiovascular prevention or management care plan in the motivated patient.

Chapter 4 on low-AGE diet presents data on reduction of oxidative stress and inflammation biomarkers in several populations. Large-scale clinical trials must be performed to replicate these preliminary results using hard outcomes, in addition to biomarkers, to substantiate the benefit of this approach. An attractive aspect of the low-AGE diet is the emphasis on slow cooking of foods with indirect heat to minimize browning and avoid charring. Therefore, this diet can be easily incorporated to the other eating patterns, including the Mediterranean, DASH, and plant-based diets.

Intermittent fasting, defined as eating only for 8–10 hours daily, has received significant attention recently and can also be incorporated into other healthy patterns. The editors chose not to include intermittent fasting as a chapter, while the evidence for efficacy is still being investigated.

Chapter 5 on healthy drinks emphasizes the importance of incorporating beverage choices, which are hidden calories that account for approximately 20% of calorie intake and almost half of the added sugar according to the average contemporary American intake. The substitution of plain water, either tap or bottled, for sugar-sweetened beverages is a simple and inexpensive intervention. Artificially sweetened beverages are probably less healthy than water but generally preferable to sugar-sweetened beverages.

Chapter 6 on beneficial herbs and spices reviews the available evidence to support the use of these as condiments and beverage enhancers. The most robust evidence from trials of short duration is for the herb green tea and the turmeric spice. A plan for necessary additional investigation and engagement of regulatory agencies in the evaluation of the benefits and risks for herbs and spices is outlined.

The last chapter in this part, Chap. 7, on integrating healthy eating and drinking into daily life emphasizes the role of the registered dietitian and the use of resources and tools for healthy eating such as the *2015–2020 Dietary Guidelines for Americans*. Strategies for healthy eating are offered including volumetrics, mindful eating, and intuitive eating. Of interest, the chapter also describes how to use the Internet and social media to find reliable information and tools for implementing healthy dietary patterns.

Fitness

"Sitting is the new smoking." This aphorism attributed to public health professionals demonstrates the under-recognized hazards of a sedentary lifestyle are as concerning as tobacco use [2]. Accordingly, the Part II of the book deals with physical activity and yoga. A growing body of observational data and more recently randomized trials support the importance of physical activity for chronic disease prevention and management. The sedentary lifestyle is a risk factor for cardiometabolic morbidity and all-cause mortality, even when controlling for confounders [2].

Chapter 8 on aerobic physical activity focuses on walking and bicycling as the most practical among many forms of aerobic exercise. Evidence is reviewed that practicing regular moderate-intensity aerobic physical activities decreases the risk of many of common chronic diseases and systematic aerobic exercise training can be incorporated into the treatment and rehabilitation of those conditions. Walking, as the most basic form of aerobic activity, is acceptable and safe for the largest population of adults who can participate in many variations. Walking is particularly attractive for those who resist or are unable to participate in other forms of aerobic activity. Cycling is the second most useful form of aerobic exercise to recommend to patients, particularly as a mode of transport with health and fitness benefits similar to those of walking. Unfortunately, safe and convenient cycling requires skills, adequate function of many senses, knowledge of traffic rules, and suitable environmental infrastructure. Practical tools for the healthcare professional to promote walking and cycling participation during a brief clinical encounter are outlined.

Chapter 9 on resistance activities, which include weight machines, free weights, and resistance tubing or bands and body weight activities, provides a stimulus to the neuromuscular system that is essential for neuromuscular health, healthy aging, and independence. Resistance activities are an effective treatment for enhancing neuromuscular capacity and physical function with aging to prevent muscle wasting associated with aging. Evidence is reviewed supporting participation in resistance activities for individuals living with chronic conditions such as diabetes, cardiovascular diseases (CVD), and chronic kidney disease (CKD).

Chapter 10 on yoga integrates a wide range of strategies, categorized into lifestyle and values-related commitments, physical practices, breathing practices, and interior practices. Yoga is suitable for individuals of all body shapes, physical abilities, ages, emotional states, cognitive capacities, and demographics. Once a practice has been established with a qualified teacher, yoga can be engaged in by nearly all patients at relatively low cost. Yoga is a powerful wellness practice and an effective intervention or adjunctive treatment for physical challenges (e.g., musculoskeletal conditions, chronic illness, metabolic disease, and cancer) and mental or emotional symptoms (e.g., depression, anxiety, stress, anger, attention deficits, trauma histories). Suggestions to build a referral network of yoga teachers and therapists will allow clinicians to guide patients to yoga resources that can have a significant effect on their well-being, symptom tolerance, and course of treatment.

Mindfulness

Part III on mindfulness reviews concepts and techniques supported by a growing body of evidence for beneficial implementation for the receptive patient. Modern living fills minds with information from the constant chatter of cell phones and other electronic devices that may make mindfulness challenging to practice but perhaps even more important to consider. Mindfulness is not a practice for everyone. Mindfulness is not appropriate in certain circumstances and may carry risks for patients with psychosis or major depression. The practice also requires willingness to participate.

Chapter 11 on the health benefits of meditation reviews the evidence to support the intervention for promoting or maintaining physical and mental health, cognition, and wellness. Most of the evidence cited is based on systematic reviews and meta-analyses of randomized controlled trials with a few individual randomized trials included. Of importance, not all studies in this field are robust or well-designed, and most reviews still called for additional investigation. The author recommends that the clinicians have a personal mindfulness practice to help them understand the usefulness in offering implementation for their patients.

Chapter 12 on the health benefits of spirituality notes research on the physical and mental health benefits of religiousness and spirituality that have surged in the past few decades. Religion is described as having an affiliation with a denomination that has a structured set of beliefs with activities that are organized and reflect long-established traditions. Comparatively, spirituality is a broader concept, extending beyond religious experiences that are frequently associated with the search for connection with the sacred or transcendent. Most research published to date has focused primarily on assessing the impact of religiousness rather than spirituality, but considerable debate regarding the operationalization of these terms continues to persist. The chapter also addresses the challenges that arise from conflicts between the clinician's own beliefs and the beliefs of the patient. In addition, there is variable appreciation by clinicians of the importance of cultural competency. While most of the research highlights positive relationships between health and spirituality, some negative relationships have also been identified. A simple practical question that can be incorporated into a brief clinical encounter is offered. "Is there anything about your spiritual beliefs you want to share that might help us care for you?"

Chapter 13 is on resilience, a term widely used currently. Resilience is defined as the ability of a person to adapt or rebound quickly from change, illness, or bad fortune. There is evidence demonstrating higher levels of resilience are associated with improved health outcomes in chronic disease and increase one's ability to cope with certain medical diagnoses. Simple techniques to coach patients to enhance their levels of resilience include practicing gratitude, identifying one's core values, deepening relationships, and goal setting.

Chapter 14 on health benefits of sleep describes sleep as essential for survival and notes that adequate sleep duration is necessary for optimal daytime function. Unfortunately, societal demands and increasing rates of sleep disorders prevent individuals from obtaining enough sleep. Each of us has an optimal sleep duration that, if uninterrupted, can optimize daytime function. Living a healthy lifestyle, reducing stress, and adopting a bedtime routine are the best ways to achieve this goal. Despite attempts to manipulate sleep quality and quantity, either pharmacologically or behaviorally, sleep patterns are surprisingly challenging to modify. Even though people can become adept at concealing the effects of compromised sleep on daily function, there are simple steps the clinician can take to identify whether an individual is obtaining adequate sleep quality and quantity. Understanding the myriad ways in which sleep can be compromised and learning how to identify the signs of poor or inadequate sleep will help clinicians formulate a plan to correct these issues. Tools for the assessment of sleep that can play an important role in the detection of sleep apnea and other sleep disorders are suggested.

Chapter 15 entitled Integrating Mindfulness into a Routine Schedule: The Role of Mobile-Health Mindfulness Applications describes tools that are making mindfulness accessible to a wide audience. Mindfulness apps and face-to-face mindfulness courses by teachers with personal experience and expertise in mindfulness each have unique advantages and disadvantages. Randomized-controlled studies of mindfulness apps are scarce, but preliminary reports suggest positive effects in clinical and nonclinical populations and outcome domains.

Integrative Approach in Different Populations

Part IV integrates the prior sections into an approach for the general population and populations with CVD and CKD. Chapter 16 deals with electronic health (eHealth), an important tool to leverage in chronic disease prevention across the lifespan. eHealth technologies transcend geographic boundaries to efficiently deliver programs and information to the general population about physical activity, nutrition, and mindfulness, three critical and modifiable health behaviors to prevent chronic disease. Despite the generally low quality of commercial eHealth programs, patients continue to use them and report positive outcomes. Discouraging patients from using eHealth due to their inconsistent quality may negatively risk future disclosures and compromise the patient-practitioner dynamic. This chapter provides the current state of eHealth programs for physical activity, nutrition, and mindfulness. It highlights the need for clinicians to engage in proactive discussions with patients about eHealth. Clinicians must understand patients' motivations and desires for eHealth programs and the process used to achieve their goals. Patients with a high degree of eHealth literacy are more aware of their health-related wants and needs from an eHealth program, and they know how to overcome adversity and negotiate with the technology, program, and other users to achieve that goal. Being aware of the current state of eHealth literacy and the factors that enhance this skillset across diverse audiences at risk for chronic disease is critical for culturally adapting and tailoring conversations to promote its prevention.

Chapter 17 addresses CVD, the major cause of morbidity and mortality in the developed world. Due to the economic impact of CVD, low-cost interventions are of particular interest. Physical activity is an underutilized, but critical, component of primary and secondary prevention of CVD. Meditation and mindfulness may have a role in prevention of CVD, though there is inconclusive evidence at this time. Dietary patterns have been found to significantly influence cardiometabolic risk factors.

Chapter 18 on the integrative approach to CKD, a complex medical condition affecting millions of individuals across the globe with diabetes as the leading cause in the USA. CKD often impacts multiple organ systems of the affected individuals and various aspects of their personal and social life. Thus, only an integrated multidisciplinary approach can provide comprehensive and holistic care to address the complex needs of this patient population. The chapter emphasizes various nutritional requirements in patients with chronic kidney disease as well as recommendations for the intake of proteins and various electrolytes. The author describes the key roles played by the family, other social supports, dietitian, social worker, and nephrologist in selected cases. The importance of recognition and treatment of depression in this patient population along with addressing their exercise needs is also described in detail.

Conclusion

In summary, this book is a journey in ideal, integrated, all-encompassing way of practicing medicine. Although development of newer medications has made a tremendous impact on patients' survival, undoubtedly drugs are not enough to avoid or prevent the many chronic noninfectious diseases that have reached epidemic proportions in the Western world. The role of the right nutrition and physical exercise has become increasingly apparent in recent decades, and although we lack interventional trials, the associations between these two parameters and overall better outcomes are becoming undeniable. More difficult to integrate and study are the less quantifiable aspects of human behavior such as mindfulness and spirituality; nonetheless, experience shows a substantial association between these practices and good health maintenance. We are not against the pharmacological approach, but time has come to make sure we approach the patients comprehensively and include a serious practice of prescribing eating patterns, exercise, right sleep, and mindfulness. We believe the above approach can also be followed by anyone, not necessarily overtly ill people. This book will help engage and motivate clinicians incorporate practice lifestyle medicine into their hectic schedules as an adjunctive therapy to medications. In addition, healthcare professionals should consider modeling health living to serve as role models for their patients and society.

References

1. Agarwal R. Resistant hypertension and the neglected antihypertensive: sodium restriction. Nephrol Dial Transplant. 2012;27(11):4041–5.
2. Baddeley B, Sornalingam S, Cooper M. Sitting is the new smoking: where do we stand? Br J Gen Pract. 2016;66(646):258.
3. Cooksey-Stowers K, Schwartz MB, Brownell KD. Food swamps predict obesity rates better than food deserts in the United States. Int J Environ Res Public Health. 2017;14(11):1366.
4. Crowley J, O'Connell S, Kavka A, et al. Australian general practitioners' views regarding providing nutrition care: results of a national survey. Public Health. 2016;140:7–13.
5. Devries S, Agatston A, Aggarwal M, et al. A deficiency of nutrition education and practice in cardiology. Am J Med. 2017;130(11):1298–305.
6. Estruch R, Ros E, Salas-Salvado J, et al. Primary prevention of cardiovascular disease with a Mediterranean diet. N Engl J Med. 2013;368(14):1279–90.
7. Estruch R, Ros E, Salas-Salvado J, et al. Retraction and republication: primary prevention of cardiovascular disease with a Mediterranean diet. N Engl J Med. 2018;378(25):2441–2.
8. Kalantar-Zadeh K, Tortorici AR, Chen JL, et al. Dietary restrictions in dialysis patients: is there anything left to eat? Semin Dial. 2015;28(2):159–68.

Index